A Good Birth,
A Safe Birth

P9-DMU-822

A Good Birth, A Safe Birth

Third Revised Edition

Diana Korte
and Roberta M. Scaer

CONTRA COSTA COUNTY LIBRARY

The Harvard Common Press
Boston, Massachusetts

3 1901 03066 3712

With affection, to all the women we know in La Leche League who helped us toward the good births, breast-feeding, and mothering of our children.

And to all the other mothers who have shared their stories with us.

ﻉﻟ

The Harvard Common Press
535 Albany Street
Boston, Massachusetts 02118

Copyright © 1992 by The Harvard Common Press

All rights reserved. No part of this publication may be repro-
duced or transmitted in any form or by any means, electronic or mechanical, including photocopy, recording, or any
information storage or retrieval system, without permission
in writing from the publisher.

Third revised edition published in 1992 by The Harvard
Common Press.

Printed in the United States of America. Printed on recycled
paper.

Library of Congress Cataloging-in-Publication Data

Korte, Diana.
    A good birth, a safe birth :   choosing and having the
childbirth experience you want   /   by Diana Korte and
Roberta Scaer.   —   3rd rev. ed.
        p.   cm.
    ISBN   1-55832-042-3   (cloth)
    ISBN   1-55832-041-5   (paper)
    1. Childbirth. 2. Childbirth—Psychological aspects. 3.
Pregnant women—Family relationships. 4. Hospitals,
Gynecologic and obstetric. I. Scaer, Roberta. II. Title.
RG652.K67   1992
618.2—dc20   92-9757

Cover design by Joyce C. Weston
Cover photograph: E. P. Jones Company

10   9   8   7   6   5

Contents

Acknowledgments

We continue to be grateful to our husbands, Gene Korte and Bob Scaer, and all eight of our children—Kathy, Mike, Andy, and Amanda Scaer; Juliana, Aren, Drew, and Neil Korte—for their help and encouragement.

Special appreciation also goes to the women in Colorado, Maryland, and Washington who worked on the original three surveys that launched the first edition of this book. Thanks, too, to the thousands of women who participated in these surveys and to all the others who continue to tell us their stories.

We offer a round of applause to the hundreds of researchers around the world who make the information in a book like this possible. And special mention this time goes to matchmaker Lynn Moen of the Birth & Life Bookstore, and publisher Bruce Shaw and his outstanding staff at The Harvard Common Press, particularly editor Leslie Baker, for their enthusiasm, goodwill, and efficiency.

Finally, thanks to our major influences and forerunners in the world of pregnancy, birth, and breastfeeding. Here they are alphabetically: American Society for Psychoprophylaxis in Obstetrics (ASPO), Robert Bradley, Donna Ewy, Ina May Gaskin, Doris Haire, Rhondda Hartman, International Childbirth Education Association (ICEA), Marjorie Karmel, Sheila Kitzinger, John Kennell, Marshall Klaus, La Leche League International (LLL), Ashley Montagu, Niles Newton, Karen Pryor, Madeleine Shearer, David and Lee Stewart, and Suzanne Arms Wimberly.

The authors of this book are not physicians. All matters regarding your health require medical supervision. The suggestions contained in this book are not substitutes for professional medical advice. You should consult your physician before you follow suggestions in this book. The authors and publishers disclaim any liability arising, whether directly or indirectly, from the use of this book.

Introduction

Eight years ago, when the first edition of this book was published, we told you that the two trends in childbirth were moving in opposing directions. They still are. One trend is the growing number of hospitals providing homelike accommodations, including Jacuzzis and microwaves, plus the more than 140 out-of-hospital birth centers (with more than 40 in the works), which numbered in the dozens only a few years ago.

The other trend is high-tech childbirth. We've had routine IVs, labor induction, and cesareans for years. Now there's a growing emphasis on tests and procedures of all kinds. It starts early in many parts of the country, with pregnant women of all ages being encouraged to undergo prenatal testing. It continues with the use of the electronic fetal monitor (EFM) during labor for 75 percent of women (and before labor for some), as well as the ubiquitous ultrasound offered routinely in at least three ways (scans, Dopplers, and external EFMs).

And in the last eight years, the cesarean rate has increased from one in five births to nearly one in four. However, the good news about cesareans is that the rate has begun to drop, due primarily to the increase in the number of vaginal births after previous cesareans (VBAC).

What about homebirths, the defenders of all-natural, no-interference pregnancies? They have shrunk even more in the last eight years from 2 to 3 percent of all births to less than one percent today, according to a 1991 report from the National Center for Health Statistics. However, high tech is present in some homebirths, too, with the use of the Doppler instead of the traditional low-tech fetoscope. (Both are hand-held devices used to listen to the fetal heart tones, but the fetoscope doesn't use ultrasound.)

Which trend is growing the fastest? No doubt about it: Despite the leveling off of our cesarean rate and the upswing in the number of VBACs, high tech continues to dominate childbirth. If you're like most pregnant women, it's as much a part of your pregnancy and birth today as is your big belly. For most of you, your decision-making about high tech is likely to be when and for how long you will use which of these pregnancy and birth tools, not whether you'll use them at all. The issue now is to use birth technology wisely and not be seduced by it.

Though there are more choices in the United States for birth attendant and place of birth than probably anywhere else on this planet, women mostly give birth one way here—with a doctor in a hospital. And over the last eight years, despite the availability of these choices and with the exception of an increase in the use of midwives and VBACs, options in the birth process have become less—not more—flexible.

Birth plans, for instance, with their list of mothers' preferences during labor, birth, and hospital stay, were designed to help women get what they want. But today birth plans often carry little punch except for those women whose requests match their physicians' usual obstetrical routine. And the change in insurance coverage for those of you who have prepaid plans (with their limited choice of health-care providers and hospitals) can curtail your options even more—unless you're willing to pay additional cash out of pocket.

Each nation's culture is reflected in how women experience birth, and that's true here as well. Most American women expect labor to be painful and anticipate using a variety of drugs. And both expectations are met. However, women always vary widely—no matter where they live—about the "normal" amount of pain they experience, just as the "normal" length of labor and the "normal" number of days vary widely in pregnancies.

A 1988 study comparing labor pain experienced by women in teaching hospitals in the Netherlands and the United States found that the Dutch women did not expect to experience as much pain and used far fewer drugs for pain relief than American women. "There is in Dutch birth participants a deep-seated conviction that the woman's body knows best and that, given enough time, nature will take its course, whereas birth in America was characterized as much more of a 'medical event'," noted one of the study's authors. In the Netherlands most women are cared for by midwives, which suggests that women are helped and encouraged in a variety of non-drug pain relief methods; 35 percent of Dutch births still occur at home. As old-fashioned and unscientific as that sounds to many of you, nearly twice as many Dutch babies survive per capita (even after allowing for racial differences) than in the United States.

But we don't live in the Netherlands; we live in medically oriented North America, where birth conjures up much fear and anxiety. And too many laboring women have been threatened with comments such as, "If you don't get going on your labor, we're going to give you Pitocin (or a cesarean)," which can increase their discomfort and pain, sometimes leading to panic and a body's total shutdown of labor.

Due no doubt in part to stories like this, we found that many of the original 2,000 survey mothers weren't satisfied with their birth experiences. According to the questionnaire responses we've received from readers, most women giving birth in traditional hospitals with obstetricians today still aren't satisfied. (See Chapter 3 for an entirely different reaction from those women who gave birth elsewhere with midwives.)

Although most of you used a variety of tests and procedures during your pregnancy and birth, many also worry about the effects some of these interventions can have on your infant. And the older your child gets, the more critical some of you become. For those of you who had been looking forward to an unmedicated birth, some now feel guilty or defensive about erroneously believing that you "flunked" childbirth because you used drugs for pain relief.

Your comments came from forty-three states, seven Canadian provinces, and seven other countries; from as far as Malaysia and as near as the next block. One or both of us have replied to your letters (though some of you moved and our notes were returned). We thank all of you, and invite you once again to tell us what you think by sending us your questionnaire response. And though we've added more of your comments in this third edition, we apologize for not being able to add them all.

A few of you have bought many copies of this book to give to friends, and others have enjoyed passing around the same dog-eared copy. Many childbirth educators, La Leche League leaders, midwives, nurses, and doctors keep copies in their libraries. In addition, *A Good Birth, A Safe Birth* is offered in a number of mail-order catalogs and has been placed on many recommended reading lists.

Several dozen of you wrote early on to say that you were interested in organizing surveys or consumer groups. More often than not, those plans changed, and some of you decided to train as childbirth educators or midwives instead.

Perhaps the biggest trend we've seen in reader replies, particularly over the last few years, is the interest in and use of the doula, a woman who offers comfort and support during labor. And if you didn't have one of these compassionate women at your last birth, you plan to the next time.

Your stories have told us that for most of your births hospital routines are remarkably similar in the United States, from California to Maine. We noticed, however, that questionnaire responses show a big jump in the use of midwives in the last few years, and the births they attend are often more individualized. Your letters have also made it clear that your birth preferences can vary from pregnancy to pregnancy.

> I had two very different experiences with childbirth. My son (number-one child) was a twenty-seven-week preemie. I am still grateful that the interventions used were available. I feel all were necessary, and I have nothing but praise for the hospital, nurses, doctors, and technologists who contributed to saving our son. Three years later I gave birth to a healthy, full-term baby girl. Same doctors, hospital, nurses, etcetera. Also same interventions. It was a nightmare. I felt so helpless. I checked myself and my daughter out of the hospital against medical advice thirty-six hours after her birth because of all the interferences.
>
> —Manitoba, Canada

Just as one woman's Dr. Right is another woman's Dr. Wrong, one woman's good birth experience is another woman's misery.

> I was amazed how my body took control. With the first push or two, my water broke (I even got to do that myself!) while I squatted. A couple more pushes and I could see her head in the mirror. I reached down to touch my baby! Minutes later, she was nursing at my breast. The feelings of joy and awe at the experience of a natural delivery are hard to describe. But I can tell you that it was worth all the months of preparations, discussions with the doctors, and two days of contractions.
>
> —Ohio (third birth, following two previous cesareans)

> The information on anesthesia was extremely one-sided. You've pointed out only the negative aspects of it without giving examples of times when it is beneficial. I know from experience that an epidural can be a sanity saver, and turn what would otherwise be a nightmare of prolonged, unbearable, uncontrollable pain into a calm, happy, positive birth.
>
> —Connecticut

Most of you have attended childbirth education classes, and

though you were satisfied overall, nearly all of you had suggestions for more information you wish had been offered. Many of those suggestions had to do with information about pain relief ("realistic discussion of pain, not fairy tale") or discovering what options were really available ("not just what doctors want us to hear"). Many readers were especially critical of hospital-based classes, and thought that instructors "pushed drugs" and "didn't tell us about risks versus benefits of *anything*."

Reminiscent of our comments in previous editions, most of you found the best advice about breastfeeding came from friends, La Leche League, childbirth educators, midwives, and books. Now you also can get the help of more than 1,000 lactation consultants. (See "International Lactation Consultants Association" in Appendix D.) Family members still tend to give advice that falls either in the "really helpful" or the "really terrible" categories. Hospital nurses, obstetricians, and pediatricians fared the worst in the advice category overall, though there were some exceptions, and family practice doctors tended to be rated more helpful than not.

Nearly every chapter has new research confirming the conclusion we made in the first edition about a good birth being also a safe birth. We provide information about options that women want, including new data from reader questionnaires, and about the seldom discussed sexual pleasures of pregnancy, birth, and breastfeeding. Types of birth attendants (midwife and doctor) and of places of birth (hospital, birth center, and home) are compared. We present a demystified view of doctors and nurses so that you can understand why they do what they do. From cesareans to circumcision, from prolonged pregnancy to newborn jaundice phototherapy, the risks and benefits of modern American childbirth interventions are described.

We encourage you to appreciate your pregnant and new mother feelings. As your best guarantee of having a normal vaginal birth once you're in the hospital, we suggest that you plan in advance to have helpers—mate, doula, and perhaps a monitrice (your personal ob nurse)—with you. And as "husband" doesn't compute for the 27 percent of you who are single when you give birth, unless the research specifically mentions husbands, we've used the words *mate* or *partner*.

We've listed our names alphabetically again, with each of us revising our half of the book. And because many of you asked which of us wrote what, we provide the following: Roberta wrote chapters 1, 3, 6, 7, 8, 9, 12, the Epilogue, and appendices B, C, and E. Diana wrote the Introduction, chapters 2, 4, 5, 10, 11, 13, 14, and appendices A and D.

Most of you who read this book will be working outside the home throughout your entire pregnancy and returning to your job within three to six months. Some of our suggestions may seem to be too much bother for the amount of time that you have, especially when you're interested in making your pregnancy and birth as easy as possible, not more complicated. We think the issue remains choice, not what you pick. Do what works for you, take what you want from this book, and ignore the rest.

1

What Women Want

I believe the best environment in which to deliver a baby
would be within the ob wing, but in a more casual,
homelike setting. I think a new mother should be allowed
to have as much interaction with family members as she
feels up to—including other children, parents, spouse....
The new baby should be allowed in the patient's room
during these family gatherings if the parents so wish. I
would also encourage as much mother-infant interaction
as possible during the stay, interaction hopefully com-
mencing immediately after delivery. I also feel "standing
orders" for medication prior to and following delivery
should be replaced with individualized recommendations.... Congratulations for caring enough to conduct this
important survey.

—Survey*

As health-care users, we have the right to have a big say in those
services that affect our welfare so critically and cost us so dearly. But
instead of finding out what people want and need in their health
care, doctors and other health-care providers too often tell us what
we'll be getting. So far, that's worked because hospitals and doctors
have had a monopoly in their business. But in at least one area of
health care—childbirth—doctors and hospital administrators now
are trying to respond to what women want.

Today more and more women know what they want to have
happen in their childbirth experience. Really, they've known all
along, but for years no one ever asked them what they wanted.

In the late 1970s, three unique studies responded to this over-

---

*All quotes from women throughout the book are from the three maternity prefer-
ence surveys cited or from our readers, who are identified by state or province.

sight. More than 2,000 women were asked to rate hospital maternity options in three different cities. They represented the Northwest (Wenatchee, Washington), the Mountain States (M.O.M. Survey, Boulder, Colorado), and the East Coast (C.O.M.A. Survey, Baltimore, Maryland)—a cross-section of the nation.

Women of very diverse educational and economic backgrounds agreed on what's important in maternity care.

- They want their partner or the baby's father to be present for the labor, delivery, and recovery, and to have unrestricted visiting rights.
- They want a lot of contact with their babies, immediately after birth and throughout their entire hospital stay.
- Women who breastfeed want effective help from nurses and doctors.
- They want their other children to visit them and to see and hold the new baby.
- They want cooperation and assistance from the hospital staff—doctors and nurses—in using prepared childbirth techniques.

The hundreds of women who sent in the questionnaire in the back of the book or phoned or spoke to us in person strongly agree with the first four of the five most important needs from the survey results: the partner's presence, baby contact, breastfeeding help, and seeing their other children. Women continue to see childbirth as a social event in the broadest sense: It either unites the family unit or pulls it apart. They want the time around the baby's birth to be one that strengthens relationships and welcomes the new baby. Women have changed their view of the fifth need identified in the surveys. Our readers are turning to doulas to get the help they need in the hospital.

Partner's Presence

The battle to have the partner present at labor and a vaginal birth has been won at most American hospitals. But there are still places where a "significant other" is not allowed with the woman. In the case of cesareans (about one in four of all births), the partners often are made to wait in a separate room.

Women are in strong agreement on this issue: nearly all believe that the partner's presence at all times, during labor and delivery and after the birth of the baby, is the most important issue. Here's what two of them said:

> The doctor told my husband to go home and get some rest. He stayed. Four hours later, at midnight, the doctor came back and again told him to leave. He stayed, and we snuggled in bed. After the birth, he had planned on staying with me in our private room until I left the hospital, but the nurse told him this was against hospital policy even though the hospital pamphlet indicated otherwise. Later, the night nurse came in with a cot for him. Against policy, huh?
>
> —Ontario

> My husband was invaluable. He was there every minute and tirelessly pressed my back through every contraction of my very long labor. He helped me calm down at several points and after the birth did everything possible to care for me and our son. He was and is a wonderful father and husband.
>
> —Virginia

Research supports women who want to have their partners present during labor and delivery. Psychologist Deborah Tanzer, in 1968, was the first researcher to study husband participation in childbirth. She found that when the birth was unmedicated and the husband was present, the marriage was strengthened. One-third of these women described their births in such blissful terms that Tanzer concluded that they had what psychologists call a "peak experience," one of transcendent ecstasy. In contrast, none of the women who were alone in labor reported a peak experience. Apparently, the husband's presence was required for women to experience that kind of intense joy, and for women to view their husbands more positively after the birth than before.

Jane and James Pittenger, family counselors and childbirth educators, studied why some parents were more satisfied with their marriages after the birth of their babies and found great pleasure in their new roles, while others described severe strain in their marriages. The satisfied couples had taken the time to study together during the pregnancy about birthing and parenting, had chosen doctors who assisted and supported them, rather than ones who took control of the birth, and were together in labor and delivery.

Contact with Baby

A vital concern for women is the contact they have with their babies. They want their babies with them from birth, so that the mother's body, not an incubator, warms the baby; so that the mother can start breastfeeding as soon after delivery as possible; and so that the parents can become acquainted with their new baby as soon as it is born.

> When the baby came out the nurses tried to snatch her away, but my doctor told them the baby would be staying on my tummy. An hour later back in my room the nurses took her, saying my doctor ordered the baby out because I wasn't doing well. I later found out they lied—he *never* said that.
>
> —New York

> After delivery they brought him to me in a little plastic bassinet. I felt sorry for him in the bassinet doing startle after startle. I asked to nurse him (famous last words—he's four and still nursing). The nurse said he wouldn't nurse well yet. Timidly I asked to try. Anything to stop him from startling like that. She said, "Oh, all right—this is what you do.... My, he has a strong suck." Bless his heart.
>
> —New York

> I had a problem getting the nurses to bring me my baby on demand. They seemed so secure in the knowledge that they knew what was best for me and my baby. Imagine how they must treat a first-time mother!
>
> —Ohio

During their hospital stays, mothers want a great deal more contact with their babies than is now possible in many hospitals. Many want their babies with them night and day, with the choice to use the nursery for short intervals; hospitals call this "rooming in." Significant numbers of mothers want no separation at all from their babies.

The strong desire of mothers to stay close to their newborn babies is nothing new. Ashley Montagu was one of the first scientists to zero in on the critical importance of mother-baby contact immediately following birth. In his book *Touching*, he makes a link between labor contractions and touching after birth: "These uterine contractions of labor constitute the beginning of caressing of the baby in the right way—a caressing that should be continued in very special ways in the period immediately following birth and for a substantial period of time afterward."

A usual hospital routine is for the newborn baby to be removed to a heated bed or incubator to warm him. Mothers who have wondered why their own bodies cannot warm their newborns will be reassured by nurse Celeste Phillips's research on heated cribs versus mothers' arms. She found that newborn body temperature was as well maintained when babies were wrapped and held by their mothers as by the incubator. Because she noted cold delivery rooms during her research, Phillips further suggests keeping the babies warmer by raising the delivery-room temperature regardless of whether babies are in their mothers' arms or an incubator.

The current practice of routine, day and night drug prescriptions following normal childbirth interrupts maternal-infant attachment, mothers tell us. Women feel too drugged at night to care whether they see their infants. One woman reports she was told by a nurse that she was the only woman during her three-day hospital stay who refused the routine painkillers during the day and sleeping medication at night. Women may not know they can refuse such routine medications or that normal childbirth does not require them.

Mothers say they prefer having their babies with them so they can immediately offer the breast when their newborn awakens. This lessens the painful breast engorgement common with mothers who feed their babies on a schedule. "Another very, very exciting and interesting thing we have found regards weight gain by the newborn," says Mayer Eisenstein, a homebirth physician in Chicago, writing in *Safe Alternatives in Childbirth*. "I was trained that it takes seven to ten days for a newborn to regain its birth weight, and I believed it. But we found our homebirth babies gaining very well, usually exceeding their birth weight by one-half to one pound by one week of age. We interpret this to be the result of no maternal separation."

Many mothers who have experienced this kind of complete contact with their baby during their hospital stay report that they do not have the difficult adjustment from hospital to home described by other mothers whose babies spent long periods of time in the nursery. Research supports women in this also.

For years mothers accepted as inevitable the adjustment problems from hospital to home. Staying up all night with a crying baby the first night home seemed to start the awful, constant fatigue that wears down new mothers. "She's asleep when I'm awake, and I want to sleep when she's awake," became the common new mother's complaint. Every new mother and baby need time to adjust to each other. Sleep and nursing patterns that are mutually satisfying to mother and baby develop fastest when mother and baby are together from birth on, reports psychiatrist Muriel Sugarman. Multiple caretakers, different nurses on changing shifts who care for newborns left in nurseries, interrupt the progress of the mother and baby's adjustments to each other. In fact, from her comprehensive review of the literature on maternal-infant attachment, Sugarman suggests that multiple caretakers of the newborn prolong the period of time needed by mother and newborn to adjust. New mothers and babies need lots of uninterrupted time to be with each other.

Continuous rooming in contributes to healthier babies and more babies breastfeeding, reports Gene Cranston Anderson, a professor of nursing at the University of Florida. Babies using continuous rooming in cry less. Mothers are able to respond quickly to the early cues of mouthing and the hand-to-mouth movements the babies make when they need to nurse. Also, infants in their mothers' arms in the first hour of life do not startle; babies in the hospital nursery startle an average of twelve times that first hour.

Anderson thinks that in the first four to five days after birth infants are at health risk from crying and startling because these actions cause irregular breathing and a temporary switch back to fetal blood circulation. Her review of the literature also suggests that crying and startling are not good for the baby because they briefly raise the baby's blood pressure, which may lead to other health problems in vulnerable infants. Anderson found that continuous rooming in is the rule in Europe, where breastfeeding rates are high and infant mortality is low.

Mothers of premature infants can ask for a special kind of contact with their babies called "Kangaroo Care." Originated by Hector Martinez in Bogotá, Colombia, this practice is used widely in Europe for premature infants. Kangaroo Care involves placing the baby, dressed only in a diaper, between his mother's bare breasts under her clothes. The skin-to-skin contact promotes easy and frequent breastfeedings, and the mother's own body temperature moves up or down as needed to keep her baby's temperature within normal limits. Infants can go to Kangaroo Care as soon as they are stabilized—some within minutes of birth, some not for weeks. Time in Kangaroo Care varies from as little as one hour a day to most of the time. Fathers, too, can give the benefit of skin-to-skin care to their infants. Worldwide research reviewed by Anderson shows that premature infants given Kangaroo Care cried much less, slept better, breathed more regularly, and went home sooner. Mothers were more successful breastfeeding and felt more confident in caring for their babies.

What is this age-old experience of maternal-infant bonding that mothers have always been aware of and scientists are now studying? This attachment is a unique, intense, learned relationship between two people, a long-term commitment between mother and child. It begins when their eyes meet at birth, and just may be the strongest kind of link humans have with one another. Babies arrive with their attachment antennae well in tune. A newborn loves to look at a face. It seeks out the mother's eyes, and may mimic an act, such as sticking out the tongue. As its body is cradled by mother, the baby hears the heartbeat it has known for months. The child feels warmth and softness, detects mother's scent, and recognizes her voice. Brought to the breast often, the alert baby takes the warm sweetness of its mother's milk. The infant is secure and content. No more are babies looked upon as passive, unresponsive creatures who should be relegated to newborn nurseries.

Certainly the research on maternal-infant attachment most widely influencing doctors and hospital routines and supporting women's ideas is that of pediatricians Marshall Klaus and John Kennell. Their early-bonding studies were stimulated by knowledge of a high rate of child battering among children who spent their first weeks in preemie nurseries separated from their mothers. Welcoming mothers into the nurseries and encouraging as much contact as possible between mother and child seemed to prove to be a successful abuse preventive for many preemies.

Once again, mothers have been right all along. Doctors, nurses, and hospital administrators need to listen when women say it is vital to have their babies with them from birth, rooming in, with the choice to use the nursery for short intervals.

Effective Help with Breastfeeding

Most mothers want to breastfeed their newborns, but many are not receiving support and information from doctors and nurses that will help them nurse successfully.

I felt that I knew nothing about how to be a mother and relied very heavily on the nurses to tell me what to do and how to do it. A lot of the breastfeeding information they gave me was not entirely accurate.

—New Hampshire

The nurses were very helpful. They offered suggestions to make breastfeeding more comfortable for me and answered my many questions without making me feel dumb.

—Survey

Every single one of the nursery nurses had her own theory about initiating a breastfeeding, and most of their ideas were useless. Two nurses were exceptions; without their support and encouragement I would've given up.

—South Carolina

In 1961 only 18 percent of newborns in the United States were breastfed. The breastfeeding rate peaked between 1982 and 1984 at 62 percent. Now, according to La Leche League, less than half of newborns are exclusively breastfed at hospital discharge. Speaking at the 1991 LLL conference in Miami, lawyer Mary Ann Kerwin noted the U.S. Surgeon General's goal for the year 2000 of 75 percent of newborns nursing at hospital discharge and 35 percent nursing at six months. Calling the 1990s the "decade of decision," Kerwin identified four factors in the decline of breastfeeding: childbearing women working for employers lacking on-site day care and breast-milk storage facilities; the media showing bottlefeeding as the norm; the ready availability of synthetic milk, also known as formula; and health-care professionals not knowing how to help.

Our readers agree that they often do not get good help with breastfeeding, and large numbers identified obstetricians, pediatricians, family doctors, and hospital nurses as the least helpful. Hospital nurses, however, were noted as being helpful just about as often as other readers found them unhelpful—something we see as progress. Still, many breastfeeding newborns go home from the hospital with bottles of synthetic milk or water, or nursing through a breast shield placed over their mothers' nipples—problems that stem from poorly informed nurses and doctors.

As far back as 1967, Niles Newton and Michael Newton reported in the *New England Journal of Medicine* that failure in breastfeeding can often be traced to the doctor or the hospital experience. The surveys and our readers confirm this is still true. Drugs given to mothers during labor affect the ability of the infant to suck readily at the breast. Also, regulated, restricted, short breastfeedings advocated by many nurses in hospitals lead to reduced milk yield, poor weight gain, more nipple soreness, and greater likelihood of ending the breastfeeding altogether, according to the Newtons.

"The babies of our human ancestors were probably carried and nursed frequently for over 99 percent of our species' existence," says John Kennell. In those cultures where successful breastfeeding continues for an average of two years, the mother and infant are inseparable from birth, and breastfeeding is so frequent that it appears to our eyes to be almost continuous. Kennell compares the fat and protein content of human milk to other animals', and concludes that human milk was designed for babies to be almost continuous feeders.

If breastfeeding results in more contact with the baby, it also means a larger time commitment on the part of the mother. In this modern world of fast-paced living and lots of demands on our time, why do it? Because hundreds of studies attest to the biochemical superiority of breast milk. Pediatric researcher Jane Pitt says, "There is hardly an antiinfective mechanism I can think of that we know of in the body that does not show up in breast milk."

In *Nursing Your Baby*, Karen Pryor and Gale Pryor, mother and daughter, give complete information on the physical and emotional benefits of breastfeeding. They report a study showing that compared to breastfed babies, "artificially fed babies were four times as likely to be sick, and during the first two months, sixteen times as likely," and the illnesses were more serious in artificially fed babies. The Pryors offer data showing that breastfeeding for months, rather than weeks or not at all, has positive health effects "far into adult life," including fewer cases of allergies, obesity, and diabetes.

Synthetic milks simply cannot duplicate all the discovered and undiscovered elements that give such a health advantage to a breastfed baby. No synthetic milk can match the changing composition of human milk with the baby's needs and age. Even the mothers of premature infants naturally manufacture milk particularly suited to their babies' special needs.

However, simply breastfeeding because of a sense of duty to the baby isn't sufficient to keep most mothers breastfeeding very long. Niles Newton, La Leche League, and most successful nursing moms point out the physical and emotional pleasure that is a natural part of the mother's breastfeeding experience. This pleasure bond between mother and infant is what keeps the mother breastfeeding her baby in the face of difficulties.

The Pittengers describe the advantages of breastfeeding for the partner, too, noting that fathers or other partners do not need to express their love for their baby by putting a bottle in its mouth. "In exchange, fathers gain an active, more responsive, sweeter smelling, and healthier baby, and exposure to the breastfeeding style of parenting with its frequent parent-child interactions, touching, and play," say the Pittengers. Almost all the partners of mothers who have nursed successfully feel that the support and protection they gave them was crucial to the success of the nursing relationship.

For mothers to breastfeed, positive information and support are essential. With an outside network consisting of La Leche League, lactation consultants, and midwives, many mothers are able to overcome breastfeeding difficulties that begin in the hospital. But the issue remains: Moms want doctors and nurses to give the very best information available on breastfeeding.

Visits with Other Children

Women's desires for a strong family unit at the time of birth extend to their other children. Mothers want their other children to see the baby and mothers want to be able to see their other children—not waving through a window from a distance, but up close so they can talk to them, hug them, and reassure them.

> I enjoyed having our two older children (ages three and five) visit me and the baby in the hospital. There were no traumatic spells of crying because they got to see the new baby and they were with both my husband and me as a family unit.
>
> —Survey

> I would have liked to have my children visit me in my room (as opposed to the smoky visitors' waiting room) and have them touch and handle the baby. My parents were also disappointed to find that they could not hold the baby in my room or even visit while he was with me. They had held my first two children within hours of their births at a different hospital.
>
> —Connecticut

Of the three surveys, the one in Baltimore was the only one to ask mothers whether they wanted their other children present soon after birth. An overwhelming 88 percent want their other children there in the period following birth, during the recovery time.

I feel sisters and brothers should be able to hold the newborn as soon as possible after the birth, and that restrictions on family visitations be eliminated. After all, family means more to a baby than a nurse who works in a nursery.

—Survey

Again, mothers are way ahead of many professionals in recognizing the needs of their other children. In *Parent-Infant Bonding*, Klaus and Kennell refer to several studies showing that children who do not visit their mothers in the hospital are very distressed. These children showed "emotional distance" when their mothers tried to hug them after coming home: The children "either stiffened or turned away." Children who had visited their mothers were happy to see them at the end of the hospital stay: "Surprisingly, even one short visit seemed to allay some of the children's anxieties."

Very few research reports compare the reactions of siblings who have been present at birth with those who have not. Nurses Sandra Anderson and Leta Brown contributed a much-needed survey of the reactions of children present for a sibling's birth compared with children who were not present. The positive reactions of the children seeing their sister or brother born continued in the months following the birth. The children who were present showed less regressive behavior (for example, fewer accidents in recently toilet-trained children) and less abusive behavior toward the new baby. In their book *Children at Birth*, Marjie and Jay Hathaway, through photos and prose, show the intense interest of brothers and sisters in their newborn sibling.

"What we're seeing," says David Stewart, of NAPSAC, the National Association of Parents and Professionals for Safe Alternatives in Childbirth, "is that there is a biological prime time for attachment for all those who are present, regardless of age." Mothers whose other children are present at the birth or come in immediately after birth and see and hold their new sibling report that their older children have a deep concern for the baby's welfare.

Using a Doula for the Birth

Nearly 99 percent of American babies are born in hospitals. Mothers go to hospitals to get what they believe is the best care for themselves and their babies. We were not surprised, then, to find that the survey women and our readers believe strongly in getting informed, positive help from the hospital staff and doctors during labor and birth.

Voluntary comments from mothers about staff help (or lack of it) during labor and birth were abundant.

> The nurse needs to know when to help the husband help his wife or when to help directly—an art.
>
> —Survey

> I believe my labor would have been shorter if my husband and I had received support and encouragement from the nursing staff. I kept pushing incorrectly but nobody helped me improve my technique. Finally, another nurse was wonderful and encouraging.
>
> —Colorado

> One nurse especially was amazingly helpful during a particularly hard part of labor when I couldn't handle what was happening to me. She lay on the bed with me, held my hands and locked eyes with me, helping me to breathe in ways that got me through it, and talked me through the contractions. She showed my husband what to do for me that would be most helpful.
>
> —New Hampshire

> I asked for pain relief late in labor (having been told not to be a martyr by the doctor and in my childbirth class). The nurse said, bless her, "I can give it to you, but you're so far along it's really not going to help much." Even though I was in pain, I was relieved to hear that.
>
> —New York

In a typical hospital, women are often disappointed if they expect frequent help and encouragement from the nurses and their doctor.

A laboring woman's doctor no longer arrives at the hospital when she does, staying with her through the hours of labor. Now he comes to check her and shows up for the delivery, but mostly he keeps in touch by phone, leaving the routine labor care to the nurses. If anesthesia is needed, he can call in an order to the anesthesiologist on duty.

Nursing care, too, has changed from a hands-on comfort role "to one relying on technology, including pharmacologic [drug] methods of pain relief," report professors Ellen Hodnett and Richard Osborn. In their study of routine nursing care, the authors observed a "near absence of physical comfort measures provided by nurses." The availability of nurses to help a laboring woman varies enormously from one hospital to another, but their paucity generally reflects a nationwide shortage of registered nurses. Whether enough nurses are present in the hospital and whether they offer frequent hands-on comfort very much affects the care a laboring woman receives. Recognizing that if they are going to get the kind of one-to-one help from another woman they want in labor, our readers in large numbers are using doulas.

A doula is another woman who has had a normal birth and offers continuous comfort, support, and encouragement to the woman during labor, birth, and immediately after birth. Susan Carey, a childbirth educator, describes her role as doula: "My 'job' is a hand-holder. Backrubber. Brow wiper. Basin holder. Hall walker. Picture taker. Encourager. Actually this description sounds like a—you guessed it—*mother*."

Mothers sometimes act as doulas for their daughters, but most of our readers used other women as their doulas.

The doctor said she loved seeing me and my son-in-law in action, working together to help my daughter. She used the Jacuzzi for five hours of her labor until transition. She's a swimmer and during contractions she would roll over and move in the water. After the birth I lay down with her. The nurse took both our blood pressures, which were low and the same! That's unusual for me because I've had high blood pressure in the past.

—Mississippi

My doula was immensely helpful. Her calming influence kept us all working together and her backrubs saved me! I have found that I really need the support of a woman during my births.

—Connecticut

The positive effects of a doula on the health and welfare of mothers and babies are extraordinary. In 1982 John Kennell said, "If I had told you today about a new medication or a new electronic device that would reduce problems of fetal asphyxia and the progress of labor by two-thirds, cut labor length by one-half, and enhance mother-infant interaction after delivery, I expect that there would be a stampede to obtain this new medication or device in every obstetric unit in the United States, *no matter what the cost*.... There is a real hazard that the supportive companion will be considered unscientific and less important than medical interventions, because it does not fit the medical model of care." Kennell, speaking at the "Birth, Interaction, and Attachment" conference, was describing the first two doula studies in Guatemala carried out by a team of researchers (including him). At that time he also foretold the slow acceptance of the doula by hospital staffs and doctors.

In 1991 a third doula study was reported in the *Journal of the American Medical Association*. This time Kennell, Marshall Klaus, and their team of researchers studied a large group of women at a U.S. hospital where high-tech interventions in labor were common. (See Chapter 7 for an explanation of interventions.) One group received routine hospital care; in the other group, each woman had a doula. Doulas were highly significant in making childbirth safer, healthier, and less costly.

How common was an intervention or complication by group?

Intervention/complication	No Doula (%)	Doula (%)
Pitocin	43.6	17
Epidural*	55.3	7.8
Forceps	26.3	8.2
Cesarean section	18	8
Fever in mother	10.3	1.4
Sick newborn	24	10.4

*Does not include epidural use for forceps or cesarean section.

The intervention and complication rates for the women without doulas are fairly typical of most other U.S. hospitals. However, the rates are shockingly higher than when a doula is used. For women without doulas, Pitocin is used over two and a half times more often; epidurals are used over seven times more often, even when not needed for forceps or cesarean sections; forceps are used over three times more often; cesarean sections are more than twice as common; more than seven times as many mothers have fever; and more than twice as many newborns become sick in the forty eight hours after birth

The study's authors question whether women's male partners can have the same kind of effect in reducing interventions and complications They referred to the research of Bertsch *et al.*, showing that while male partners touched laboring women 20 percent of the time, doulas touched the women 95 percent of the time. When questioned whether a woman's partner would accept the presence of a doula, Kennell said that in an ongoing study of doula care with couples, the men are very enthusiastic about the emotional support they feel they get from the doula.

Because using doulas would prevent the use of expensive interventions and decrease hospital stays of mothers and infants by preventing illness, Kennell estimates an annual savings of $2 billion to the U.S. health care system. The authors finish their report by writing: "While there may be financial savings, the physical and emotional benefits of doula support for the welfare of mothers and infants make a compelling case for the review of current obstetric practices.... For those who provide care for mothers during labor, the challenge is to turn to obstetric technology only when necessary, relying instead on the practice of continuous labor support to help the birth process follow its natural normal course."

Research Backs Women's Wants

It is abundantly clear that research strongly supports women's preferences. As health-care users demand change, they can have great confidence in their feelings about what is right for them and their families. Says Shannon Pope, who spearheaded the Wenatchee, Washington, survey, "Never for a moment allow yourself to feel that, because you are a layperson, your viewpoint in childbirth is any less accurate or less valid than that of the person you are trying to influence. If you are a woman, you will be discounted on the basis of your 'obvious inability to separate the emotional aspects of childbirth from the factual.' But you have the advantage of recent scientific studies and *common sense* on your side! If you are a woman who has already experienced childbirth, you have the advantage of firsthand knowledge, and unless the person you are dealing with is also a person who has experienced childbirth, you are unique in possessing this area of knowledge."

At this point many of you may be thinking: If research supports what women want, why in the world don't hospitals and doctors just give it to them? Why do I have to make an effort to get what I want? We've thought about that question a lot.

The only satisfactory answer seems both simple and complicated, and it took writing this book for us to answer it for ourselves. *Hospitals and doctors think that what they are doing is best, is right, is safe for the majority of women and babies.* Doctors' beliefs about what the best care is determine hospital policies.

Women's preferences in childbirth include a very broad view of birth; the *social*, the *psychological*, and *spiritual* aspects are as important to women as the *physical* act of giving birth. The doctor's viewpoint is different. He focuses on the *physical* act of giving birth. In other chapters we will examine the belief-system of the doctor and how the way he views birth determines how it must be treated. A key issue in understanding doctors and in getting what you want is how the word *safe* is used. How is "safe" measured? How do you define "safe"? Doctors feel free to act as they do because of the way they use maternal mortality and infant mortality figures to measure safety.

Because of what doctors believe about childbirth and how they view safety, they intervene in most births. To intervene means to get in there and get that baby out by applying technology. The doctor takes decisive action to speed or to end the labor and get the baby delivered. Intervention procedures are being carried out on a massive scale. Women are beginning to understand that one intervention leads to another, and the doctor may find himself on a treadmill he cannot stop, ending with a cesarean delivery.

Satisfaction with Childbirth

Today's high-tech, drug-based care assumes that pain management and pain relief are women's most important needs. According to this view, control or absence of pain will lead to satisfaction. Although no research supports this idea, some reports say women accept and seek out a high-tech birth. *Mothering* magazine editor Peggy O'Mara reported the findings of perinatal psychology speaker Robbie Davis-Floyd. She found that some professional women do not value the childbirth experience because they objectify birth. Because these women do not see birth as a personal experience, they welcome drugs and medical intervention for childbirth.

Satisfaction in childbirth is much more complex than the simple matter of pain relief. Reported in *Psychology Today*, the pain/pleasure findings of some British researchers counter the belief among doctors and nurses that pain relief is the first priority of most women. Questioned a year after birth, most women who gave birth without anesthesia rated their childbirth satisfying and pleasurable, although they had more pain than anesthetized women. Significantly more women who had anesthesia were dissatisfied, and fewer remembered the birth as pleasurable.

> I was completely satisfied. The only awful thing about it was he was posterior and I had terrible back labor. I went from two to five centimeters dilation in an hour when I relaxed in a tub of hot water. Then after walking a short time, I got the overwhelming urge to push. Because I wasn't fully dilated, the birth assistant helped me lie on my side. I screamed in pain trying not to push. Then the birth assistant helped me walk for a while to see if that would help dilation. I literally clung to the walls, the pain was so awful. Soon I was ten centimeters dilated and ready to push. I even got to catch him and while doing so announce he was a boy. All I can say is that it couldn't have been better. I was quite happy.
>
> —Maryland

Other British researchers (Josephine Green *et al.*) found that interventions in labor and delivery made women less satisfied and feel less in control. "This was true for minor interventions such as shaves, enemas, and episiotomies as much as for major ones like forceps deliveries and cesarean sections," say the authors. In this study of 825 women, those with interventions felt they "could not get comfortable precisely because the staff, the drugs or the equipment were depriving them of that fundamental degree of control over their own bodies."

From her research on childbirth satisfaction with psychologist Larry Bugen, Sharron Humenick, University of Wyoming nursing professor and childbirth educator, says that pain relief is not the key to satisfaction. The woman's feelings of mastery, of control and coping well, and of having an active part in decisions about her labor are the most important reasons a woman feels satisfied with the birth, says Humenick. She adds that health-care providers and many women themselves "remain unaware of how much women may personally benefit from active participation in birth. As a result, for many women, epidurals rather than supportive coaching have become the first line of defense in coping with the rigors of labor. In the process, active participation, self-actualization and the balance between technology and touch may be lost."

Internationally known childbirth educator Sheila Kitzinger believes that the woman's feeling of power or powerlessness in childbirth is the most important key to satisfaction. In her booklet "Some Women's Experiences of Epidurals," she wrote, "A central issue in women's birth experiences is that of control: whether they are able to maintain control over what happens to them and their bodies, or whether control is taken from them and they are deprived of autonomy."

> Over the next few months after birth, I grew more and more angry. Here I was, a woman who understood pregnancy and birth intimately, who was conversant with the lingo that is used in obstetrics, who knew what she wanted. If I was intimidated and assaulted (I feel like I've been raped!) by medicine (whether intentionally of not) then what happens to other women? How did things get this way?
>
> —Ontario

Another report that relates childbirth satisfaction to feelings of mastery comes from Penny Simkin, childbirth educator and author of *The Birth Partner*. Simkin found that "the women with high satisfaction described feelings of accomplishment, control, increased self-esteem and/or confirmation of worth. Most of those with low satisfaction expressed disappointment or anger that they were not in control. Those with high satisfaction remembered their doctors in positive or humorous terms, and their nurses as being supportive. All of those with low satisfaction had negative memories of both their doctors' and nurses' words and actions."

> I was mostly unsatisfied. Only happy to have the baby! I was given an epidural (for my c/sec) by an anesthesiologist who hated my nurse. I was so tense and uncomfortable with him snapping and acting condescending toward her. I didn't care for her—but *him!* He was gruff, rude, uncaring, and unprofessional.
>
> —Texas

Beyond the joy of giving birth, I found another satisfying experience while in the hospital. The staff was consistently gracious, involved in my care and my excitement over childbirth. The best way I can describe it is that I felt loved and "mothered" by the nursing staff.

—Survey

Simkin concludes, "There is more to a healthy outcome than the survival of the mother and baby. A sense of maternal fulfillment and personal self-worth are other hallmarks of a healthy outcome, and these can be effected by the people who are with the women."

Women are right to take a broad view of the birth experience, to consider the social, psychological, and spiritual aspects as important as the physical act of giving birth. Meeting women's preferences makes the birth more safe. When a woman's preferences are met, she needs less intervention and has fewer complications for herself and for her baby. Chapter 3 demonstrates over and over that a good birth is a safe birth.

"The challenge for all of us—childbirth educators and advocates, parents and concerned providers—is to give birth back to mothers," wrote Beth Shearer, codirector of C/Sec. "Words I wrote for ICEA's 25th Anniversary seem even more relevant today: 'Perhaps it is time to change the emphasis from "family-centered" birth to "woman-centered" birth. When women feel in touch with their own needs, free and strong enough to ask for them, and confident they will be met, the needs of their babies and their families will be met at the same time, regardless of the method of delivery.' The choice between mothers' and babies' 'rights' is a false choice. If mothers are taken care of well, they will take care of their own babies better than the 'experts.'" The needs of the mother, father, and other siblings can all be met in a safe birth. Where you have your baby, who your birth attendant is, what options you have, and what interventions the doctor uses are all negotiable. You can have your baby the way you want to.

2

The Pleasure Principle

It's a glorious experience. I know there are a lot of people who say, "Oh, I hated being pregnant." I felt exhilarated and really wonderful.... It (second birth) was two days of labor, but not bad, not hard—it was easy.

—Actress Demi Moore, on *Oprah* (1991)

If you're like most women, you think of childbirth as a necessary experience of pain and exertion in order to get the end product: the longed-for baby. But while birth *is* these things, a seldom-discussed fact is that it can also be a time of great pleasure.

If childbirth can produce pleasure, then why are so many women dissatisfied with their birth experiences? For one, standard hospital birth practices, from the shaving of your pubic hair to routine episiotomies, destroy much of this pleasure potential. Another reason is that we've not been taught that our reproductive functions—all of them—are designed to give us pleasure.

Sexually, women are not carbon copies of men. Our sexuality involves far more than just making love, important as that is. Aspects of sexuality that women experience but men don't include the increased sexual energy a woman can feel before menstruation, the relaxing spurt of milk from her breasts when her milk lets down, and the tug of her baby's rhythmic sucking on her nipple.

Most sexual research concentrates on intercourse. But while women's other sexual functions have been overlooked in comparison, enough research exists to help us describe some of the similarities between sexual arousal and women's reproductive functions.

Sexual Arousal and Pregnancy

In both sexual arousal and pregnancy, breasts enlarge and nipples become sensitive. There's also extra blood flow and lubrication in the vagina, and hormone production soars. And, according to sex researchers Masters and Johnson, among others, masturbation is common during pregnancy, even if never experienced before. However, not all pregnant women are hovering in a permanent state of sexual arousal. Many other influences—fatigue, nausea, or worry—can affect a pregnant woman's sexual desires.

Your sexual interest during pregnancy probably fits one of the following four descriptions:

- It doesn't change at all during pregnancy.
- You feel tired and nauseated from day one. After the first few months, you don't feel as sick, but you're not much better. Though you need your partner to hold and comfort you, sexual intercourse is not a priority. In fact, you might prefer doing without it.
- You may be sleepy and sometimes nauseated in the first trimester, but in the second trimester you marvel at your energy and you feel wonderful. Your desire to make love is greater than ever before.
- You vibrate with good health throughout the pregnancy. Your senses are more acute than ever. Food is appetizing, and you've never had a moment's queasiness. Your desire to make love with your mate continues to increase right up to the time of birth.

Whichever description matches your experience, you're in good company—other women have felt the same. An unchanged sexual response is the least likely, while increased desire in the middle trimester is the most common. But whether you're turned on or turned off, want an orgasm or not, your feelings are normal, and may vary from pregnancy to pregnancy.

Oxytocin: The Caregiving Hormone

Researchers have found another parallel in sexual arousal during intercourse, birth, and breastfeeding. A seldom-studied hormone, oxytocin—which we label "the caregiving hormone"—flows in a woman's body during all three stages. In intercourse, this hormone's release is triggered by orgasm; in labor, by the onset of contractions; and in breastfeeding, by each letdown of milk.

Unlike many other hormones, oxytocin is generated in sporadic bursts rather than in a steady stream. With orgasm or milk letdown, an oxytocin burst can produce a euphoric sensation. Its release, however, is easily inhibited. Just as orgasm in lovemaking can be stopped by sudden noises, many a labor's progress has been halted by an inhibiting hospital environment. Nursing mothers sometimes report their milk letdown slowing or stopping when they're criticized, fatigued, or unhappy.

Parallels: Birth and Intercourse

During sex, women do not want their concentration disturbed, and in undrugged and uninhibited labor their reaction is the same. Social inhibitions decrease as orgasm nears or as unmedicated labor progresses. The uterus rhythmically contracts, and a tense, almost tortured, look appears on the face. In both intercourse and labor, women find themselves deep-breathing, feeling sensations of pressure and stretching, or emitting sighs, groans, even screams.

> I bellowed gloriously as I pushed her out. It felt great to yell, but it freaked out the nurses and doctors. Lamaze teachers aren't supposed to "lose control." I didn't. It just felt right to yell, sort of a war cry.
>
> —Colorado

Masters and Johnson data demonstrate that the uterine contractions during orgasm follow the same recorded pattern as those of the first stage of labor—differing only in intensity. Caressing the breasts, in fact, can get a slowed labor going again by stimulating uterine contractions.

When women are not fearful or anxious and have a supportive environment, passionate emotions are released and sensory perceptions are heightened—just as they are during intercourse. Regardless of how much pain they have endured, once into the second stage of labor, the pushing stage, many women report pleasure. In the early 1980s, British researchers confirmed that women who give birth without anesthesia suffer more pain than anesthetized women do, but they also experience greater pleasure. As Northwestern University psychologist Niles Newton points out, pain and pleasure are not opposites. It's quite possible to experience both simultaneously. Clearly, however, every woman's reactions to every labor will vary, and one woman's pleasure will be another's unrelenting pain.

In my first birth I was literally screaming for something, but my doctor told me it was too late—the baby would be born in five to fifteen minutes. Bless his heart! The euphoria and high after that was something else. Better than after the best sex!

—Washington

I think you have too much emphasis on how pleasurable child-birth is without a proper balance of the reality of pain. I didn't find it so wonderful physically. Emotionally, yes, but physically sometimes it can be really hard and hurt.

—Texas

Just as more sexual experience will enhance your physical capacity for sexual pleasure, pregnancy all by itself—regardless of what kind of labor and birth you had—will do the same. Researcher M. J. Sherfey reports that in many women (as long as obstetric damage doesn't intervene), pregnancy brings an increase in the volume of blood flow in the pelvis, enhances the capacity for sexual tension, and improves orgasmic intensity, frequency, and pleasure.

The Natural Eroticism of Breastfeeding

The similarities between lovemaking and breastfeeding are also strong: The uterus contracts, the nipples become erect, the breasts receive extensive stimulation, and the skin flushes. Soon after a baby is put to the breast, a letdown brings the milk to the infant. Although the hormone oxytocin is responsible for this milk-ejection reflex, nursing mothers don't usually have orgasms when their milk lets down. Many nursing moms do describe a feeling of well-being. However, first-time mothers may need a month or two before they can recognize the letdown sensation.

It is common for a mother to leak breast milk during lovemaking. Some mothers then worry needlessly that there won't be enough milk for the baby's next feeding, but there always is. While some couples find milk-filled breasts an added sexual pleasure, others don't. Either reaction is normal, of course.

By the time your baby is three months old, he typically will have been put to the breast more than 700 times. For many women, this frequent contact enhances the response of their erogenous zones, especially if they occasionally nurse the baby skin to skin, unclothed. Breastfeeding's enhancement of your sexuality, however, may not be noticeable until after you have weaned the baby.

Other Links to Birth Pleasure

- *Heightened Emotional Awareness.* This increases during pregnancy and birth, just as it does during sex, in a mixture of risk and trust.

  In pregnancy, you'll probably experience highs and lows. Though you may be criticized for being "too emotional," these feelings are a necessary preparation for caregiving: They make you feel more responsive to your baby and help you experience more pleasure in this role. As your pregnancy progresses, you look for calm reassurance and support from those who care for you as well. Many women, accustomed to managing their lives, are amazed by this need for support.

- *Desire to Be Touched.* Researchers stress that the sexual pleasure derived from childbirth requires a calm, nurturing environment. An optimal birth is made up of more than careful and caring hospital procedures and loving supporters, however. It's understanding many women's desires to be touched in a loving way during labor (though some women prefer little or no touching because of the intense sensitivity of their labors).

  Studies confirm that many laboring women cope better with pain when there is constant support that includes touching. If you're like these women you might recover your equilibrium through a sympathetic hand on your arm, or a caress may blunt the stress of a contraction and give you new strength. Ensure that your desire for touching will be met by loving supporters. Have not only your mate with you in labor, but a helping woman as well. (See Chapter 11.)

- *Rewarding Brain Chemicals*. As in marathon races, birth requires enormous physical, mental, and emotional energy. Like a long race almost over, labor can cause excruciating pain, but our bodies offer a reward—brain chemicals—for this exertion. Known as endorphins or beta-endorphins, these chemicals are narcoticlike painkillers that circulate in the bloodstream. These natural opiates are released by hard exercise—vigorous walking, running, and cycling, for example. Some researchers speculate that this chemical release explains the euphoria that joggers call "runner's high." The cramping pains of childbirth release endorphins, too, as do the grimacing and grunting of many women in labor.

Sexual feelings will vary in any woman, whether during pregnancy, childbirth, or breastfeeding. In any case, it is important to broaden your knowledge about your sexual self and expand your appreciation of your body. Always remember that whatever you feel, and whatever you want, is right for you.

3

If You Don't Know Your Options, You Don't Have Any

No one can tell a woman how to make the choice that is best for her. There is no one *right* choice. Today there are more choices and more support for trying than ever before in American history, which also leaves women with the burden of choice.

—Gail Sheehy, *Passages*

For every one of you reading this chapter there is the strong possibility that within a fifty-mile radius of where you live you can find both a place for giving birth and a birth attendant that you will like. You may have to change your idea of place of birth, you may have to change your idea of a birth attendant, or you may have to pay for the care you want rather than take the care your insurance dictates. But different kinds of options are coming so fast, it is difficult to keep up with the new possibilities. Find out what's available in your area.

The movement to humanize hospital maternity care started in the 1950s. The two main thrusts of this movement—called "family-centered maternity care"—were to keep mothers and babies together while in the hospital and to ensure the partner's presence before, during, and after birth. In the late 1960s, childbirth education had reached enough birthing women so that they began to "vote with their feet"— that is, they started going to those doctors and hospitals where the partners were not only allowed but *encouraged* to be present. This was the crack in the door to change in hospital maternity policies.

Today acceptance of the partner's presence at a vaginal delivery is universal in American and Canadian hospitals. Many cesarean mothers are still denied the father's presence at delivery, however, and while it is easier in many hospitals for mothers to get their babies on demand, interference in family togetherness is still widespread. So, women continue to "vote with their feet" and go to those hospitals where they *can* get what they want.

Some women with their babies due *now* see changes in hospitals as turtle slow. They see their only choice as voting the hospital out altogether and opting for an out-of-hospital birth—at home or in a birth center. While the actual percentage of out-of-hospital births is small, the threat of women opting for out-of-hospital births is another reason hospitals have made changes demanded by consumers.

NAPSAC, the National Association of Parents and Professionals for Safe Alternatives in Childbirth, was founded in late 1975 by Lee and David Stewart at a time when there were very few alternatives to the traditional hospital delivery. Interviewed in November 1991, the Stewarts said the national NAPSAC office receives 500 requests a month from all over the United States for literature and information. "The most frequent question we get—in the hundreds every month—is 'Where can I get a competent midwife or doctor for a home birth?'" said David Stewart.

He estimates one percent of all births are planned home births. "The difficulty in getting accurate figures comes from the lack of registration of some home births," he said. "Parents don't want to call attention to themselves by registering a home birth. They fear harassment of themselves or the direct entry midwives they tend to use." Nurse-midwife Kittie Ernst is director of the National Association of Childbearing Centers. Interviewed in November 1991, she reported 140 out-of-hospital birth centers, each with an estimated 150 to 170 births a year. "Some have many more than that," she told us, "and two birth centers, one in San Diego and one in Fort Lauderdale, are planning for 2,000 births a year." A rough estimate for out-of-hospital birth centers is 30,000 births a year.

Although the actual percentage of out-of-hospital births is small, the threat of women opting out of the hospital is an important reason why hospitals have made changes. Annually, childbirth represents more than a $20 billion business in the United States. Hospitals and doctors have a strong economic motivation to get you—and keep you—as a customer. Hospital administrators know that women make most of the health-care choices for a family, and that a woman's choice of hospital for her baby's birth almost always becomes her choice for other hospital needs.

Nearly all women still choose to deliver in a hospital. So although the out-of-hospital birth numbers encourage homebirth and birth-center advocates, and frighten most obstetricians, the numbers barely twitch birth statistics. The numbers are tiny compared to the millions of babies born each year in U.S. hospitals.

Where to Have Your Baby

There are four different places where you may choose to give birth:

- In a traditional hospital with labor, delivery, and recovery rooms
- In a hospital with single room maternity care
- In a birthing center outside the hospital
- At home

The most important means of evaluating a place of birth is safety. We will do that for each option. Another way to evaluate is by cost. The cost of care paid by insurance, by a government agency, or directly by the woman is very different by place of birth. Any hospital birth is expensive, averaging $4,300 for a one-day stay and including the doctor's charge. A cesarean delivery averages $7,600. These figures include no newborn complications, which can escalate the costs to $12,000 or more. The average birth center charge is $2,800. The average homebirth charge is $600 to $2,000, depending on whether a midwife or doctor is used. (These are 1992 figures and are likely to be higher in large cities.) The average hospital birth cost is for a normal delivery without complications. As you will see, normal birth remains normal much less of the time in a hospital setting.

The third way of evaluating where to have your baby is to look at how satisfied women have been with each option. Sixty percent of our readers who delivered in a traditional hospital were *not* satisfied. Those who delivered in military hospitals were unanimous in their dissatisfaction, asking us to *do something* about the bad care they feel they received. About three-quarters of those readers using single room maternity care were quite happy with their birth experience. Nearly one in three readers using single room maternity care also had a midwife as a birth attendant and interventions at a fraction of those reported in traditional hospitals. That high a proportion of midwives and that low rate of intervention in single room maternity care is not typical nationally. We believe it is part but not all of the reason for the high satisfaction of our readers. Twenty percent of readers using single room maternity care were not satisfied.

Nearly 100 percent of our readers using a birth center outside the hospital or homebirth were very satisfied. Interventions were nearly absent outside the hospital. There is a clear connection between a woman's dissatisfaction with childbirth and intervention in labor and delivery.

A fourth way of evaluating where to have your baby is to look at the likelihood of intervention for each place of birth. The fewer interventions there are, the less risk there is to mother and baby. With fewer interventions there will be fewer problems as a result of intervention, fewer cesareans, and, we believe, a safer, more satisfying birth for mother and baby.

With less intervention, mother, baby, and father (or partner) are more likely to have a strong attachment to each other, and this fragile new family will have the mutually loving start they need. The pleasure principle, the full expression of a woman's sensuality in birth, operates best with the least intervention. And, finally, with less intervention a woman feels more that she has "given birth" rather than that she has been "delivered." Her enhanced self-esteem from this achievement helps the woman in her new role as a mother. "The sense of achievement from a good birth experience is the strongest stimulus I know to greater self-esteem and effective functioning," said nurse-midwife Ruth T. Wilf. In contrast to this, the greater the amount of intervention the more likely the mother will feel that others took control of her body and her childbirth experience. She is more likely to feel she was passively rather than actively involved in giving birth. Regrets about the birth and lowered self-esteem are the frequent results.

What was done to me at the military hospital shouldn't have been done to a dog. I was not allowed to eat or drink. After multiple tries by the nurse, the anesthesiologist had to be called to put in the IV. I wasn't allowed to move my arm. After nine hours I was only at four to five centimeters with an epidural that never took on my left side. The doctor said he'd have to do a c-section. I felt everything on my left side even though they gave me more epidural. Finally they pulled my son out and gassed me. When I woke three hours later, my husband told me we had a beautiful son. I neither cared nor wanted to see him. My husband could have sold him that very minute and I wouldn't have cared. How ashamed I am of those feelings now. I can never fully describe the agony or the scars that I will carry for the rest of my life.

—New Jersey

Traditional Hospital

Birth in a traditional hospital will often resemble the birth described by Jenny in Chapter 7: It will be organized according to the obstetrician's belief that birth is a physical procedure with significant risks.

The laboring woman is first put to bed in the labor room, then moved to the delivery room. Delivery is often a surgical procedure (vaginal delivery with episiotomy and use of forceps, or a cesarean delivery) following an actively managed labor. She is then moved to a recovery room before being transferred to the postpartum room, where she will stay for the remainder of her time in the hospital. Her baby is removed from her at birth and placed in a central nursery.

The choices a mother may make in her labor and delivery vary greatly among hospitals. Some hospitals offer a great deal of flexibility; in other hospitals, almost all mothers experience the same routine. You can get what you want if you act ahead of time by choosing the hospital where policies are very flexible.

According to the American Hospital Association, most women choose the hospital for delivery before they choose their doctor. We suggest you may need to choose "Dr. Right" (see Chapter 5) first, find out where he works—he may deliver at more than one hospital—and then decide on the hospital. Or if you choose a hospital first, find the doctor there whose practice style matches your preferences. Another key to getting what you want in a traditional hospital is to have labor support from a woman friend (your doula) as well as your partner.

The rate of interventions at most traditional hospitals is very high. In November 1991 a nurse told us that women in her hospital want "a quick fix" and "don't want to hurt." The doctors tell women what they will be having (an epidural) and tell them to come to the hospital early. Women often arrive at the hospital only one centimeter dilated—"too soon," she said. Several doctors give epidurals at two centimeters dilation and "the women are happy with this," we heard. The women are put to bed when they arrive, hooked up to an external monitor and soon given an epidural. Because they are "bed-bound" so long in labor, they often need Pitocin to help their labor along.

That hospital's intervention rates are about as high as is possible and birth is a completely managed event there. Ten to fifteen percent of women are induced. With exceptions too few to count, all women receive a partial prep, enema, IV fluids, fetal monitor, and epidural during labor. Vaginal deliveries all are in the lithotomy position (on the back with legs in stirrups) and need episiotomies. We weren't surprised to hear that with this kind of management, one in three deliveries is by cesarean section.

Certainly, that hospital is unusual in the complete management of normal birth and the wholesale use of interventions. High rates of intervention are typical in traditional hospital settings, however. And the interventions carry great risk of complications for mother and baby. Very little has been done to document this risk.

Family practice doctor Lewis Mehl, director of the Institute for Childbirth and Family Research in Berkeley, California, completed one study of safety in home versus hospital birth. Mehl found the incidence of complications to mother and baby in a hospital birth was far greater than in a homebirth. Because the rate of intervention is likely to be extremely low where the choice is for an unmedicated birth at home, we agree with Mehl that it is the high rate of intervention that results in the greater risk of complications to mother and baby.

Mehl compared matched populations of 1,046 women planning homebirths to 1,046 women planning hospital births, with all the women defined as "low risk."* (The homebirth mothers included those who needed a hospital even though a homebirth was planned.) The hospital-birth women were more likely than the planned homebirth mothers to have had the following: high blood pressure during labor (five times more likely), severe perineal tear (nine times more likely), postpartum hemorrhage (three times more likely), and a cesarean (three times more likely).

The babies born to the planned hospital-birth women also had a higher complication rate than the babies born to planned homebirth women. In the hospital group, the infants were six times more likely to have had fetal distress before birth, four times more likely to have needed assistance to start breathing, and four times more likely to have developed an infection. There were no incidents of birth injuries in the homebirth group, yet there were thirty infants in the hospital group with birth injuries.

Another study compared complications and safety in a birth center versus a hospital. Robert C. Goodlin reported in the medical journal Lancet on 1,000 births of low-risk women delivering in the traditional

---

* A "low risk" designation means that these mothers had no complicating factors of age, medical history, or socioeconomic problems that might lead to difficulty with childbirth. For a more complete discussion of the somewhat controversial "low risk" designation, see Chapters 5 and 6.

labor and delivery area versus in a hospital birth center separate from the traditional area. No IVs, monitors, or anesthesia were used for the 500 women in the birth center. Only 6 percent of them had minimal doses of drugs for pain during labor, and the women ate, drank, and moved about as they wished.

In comparison, interventions were high among the 500 low-risk women who delivered in the traditional labor and delivery areas of the same hospital. All had IVs; 81 percent had the electronic fetal monitor; 70 percent had moderate-to-high doses of drugs for pain; and 30 percent had epidurals.

The following chart shows the difference in complications between the two groups.

Complications	Regular Birth (%)	Birth Center (%)
Mother		
Failure to progress in labor	18.3	5.2
Labor augmentation	21.2	3.1
Cesarean section	9.2	2.8
Infant		
Fetal distress	5.3	.3
Meconium-stained fluid	11.9	2.3
Meconium aspiration	.2	1.2
Scalp infection	1.2	0
Jaundice	12.6	2.4
Neurological abnormalities	.6	.2

Mothers delivering in the traditional area were three times more likely than mothers delivering in the birth center to have their labor diagnosed as "failure to progress," and seven times more likely to have their labors speeded with Pitocin. In the traditional area mothers were over three times more likely to have a cesarean section. Before they were born, the babies delivered in the traditional area were seventeen times as likely to experience fetal distress and six times more likely to have meconium-stained fluid, another indication of possible distress. After birth, the infants born in the traditional area were three times more likely to have neurological abnormalities. They were six times more likely to have jaundice, a growing problem in pediatrics, possibly related to the much higher rate of Pitocin and other drug use in the traditional area. (See Chapter 14.)

Just over one percent of the traditionally delivered babies got scalp infections from the use of electronic fetal monitors. Because the monitor was not used in the birth center, there were no scalp infections. Follow-up for an average fifteen months after birth showed that 2.4 percent of the infants born in the traditional area were victims of child abuse, while none of the infants born in the birth center were abused. The babies born in the birth center were more likely to breathe in meconium, a potential problem. Goodlin believes this reflects the absence of drugs in the babies, who were more vigorous. Out of the six significant categories of labor or birth complications for infants, the birth center babies did much better than the traditional hospital babies in five categories.

Many professionals who use birth centers believe that a better outcome for mother and baby is the result of two important factors. The first is the greatly reduced use of intervention. The second is the homelike setting itself, which results in a less anxious and more effective labor. Goodlin suggests that low-risk women benefit from a "service which seeks to reduce apprehension and insure tranquillity."

To sum up the traditional hospital:

- Insurance coverage available.
- Birth takes place in several different rooms: labor room, delivery room, usually a recovery room, and a postpartum room (for the hospital stay after birth).
- Baby is taken to a central nursery.
- Immediate availability of emergency equipment.
- No one-to-one nursing care because nurses are responsible for several patients.
- High possibility of medical intervention.
- High risk of complications for mother and baby, regardless of a predetermination of "low risk."

Hospital Single Room Maternity Care

Whenever hospitals are being rebuilt, administrators are switching to single room maternity care. Using this option, a woman labors, delivers, recovers, and sometimes stays for postpartum care all in the same room. This choice pleases hospital personnel, doctors, and many childbearing women.

Costs to the hospital are greatly reduced by more efficient use of space, equipment, and staff. Multiple-use rooms are full more often than rooms that can be used only for labor, delivery, or recovery. Fewer rooms are required. Expensive equipment is moved from room to room as needed. Depending on her shift, the same nurse can be available for a woman through labor, delivery, and recovery, something both nurses and patients appreciate.

Although rooms are homelike, emergency equipment is immediately available. The bed is convertible and can be broken away to place the women in the lithotomy position. Doctors find the rooms adapt easily to the use of interventions and technology. Because doctors feel comfortable that the setting allows them to use any intervention except for a cesarean, women with all levels of risk can use single room maternity care.

Single-room care is also a response to women's demands. Family-centered care and individual choice is much more easily met in this setting than in a traditional hospital. Women get the feeling that they have more control over what happens to them because their care can be individualized.

> My husband was *not* with me. He was with our two-year-old, who needed him more. The midwife, doula, and I got to the birthing room about 6:30 in the evening. I had to push immediately. No one even turned on the lights—the sun was setting and the room was bathed in a nice pink light. I sat there and ate orange slices between pushes. The pushing was hard work and I tired of it quickly. I asked my doula, "Why did I have another baby?" She said, "Eat another orange slice." The midwife said, "Here—feel your baby's head" and with her help I pulled Alejandro out. He was nice and plump and annoyed. I nursed him in the bed I delivered him in.

> —New York

As of 1991 just over half the women who gave birth within the previous twelve months used single room maternity care, according to Inforum, Inc., a marketing information company—a dramatic increase from 1988 when nearly two-thirds of births took place in separate labor and delivery rooms. Inforum's annual telephone survey conducted by the Gallup Organization also showed that most of the women surveyed would have used single room maternity care if it had been available to them.

Women can be confused when they look for this option. Joan Nathan, spokesperson for the American Hospital Association, told us that 75 percent of hospitals giving maternity care offer "a combination labor/delivery unit with a homelike setting." But only one-third of those hospitals have single room maternity care. Most hospitals with this option have traditional areas and one or more rooms labeled "birth rooms."

Some hospitals have strict screening for birth rooms that acts as a barrier to women who want to and could use them. For example, we know that there are some hospitals that do not permit laboring women into their birth rooms until they're at least three centimeters dilated (one good reason for staying home as long as possible). The women are not sent home, but admitted to the regular floor.

Usually this strict screening is instituted because the doctors are not committed to providing a real alternative to a traditional birth. Ross Planning Associates reports that "birthing rooms were good public relations tools, but they had low rates of use because they were not, in general, supported by the medical staff." The widespread use of single room maternity care shows that most doctors do accept birth rooms, but some doctors still resist them. If you like this option, you'll need to know your doctor's preference. Also the fact that a hospital may offer both traditional and birth rooms can be confusing to the woman trying to choose a place of birth. When you are investigating your own hospital options, go beyond the words, for example, "birthing rooms," you are given. Ask for a detailed description of that hospital's services, using our description as a starting point.

Research is needed to see if single room maternity care reduces complications, including cesareans. One large study comparing hospital policies with the use of interventions was reported in 1987. Researchers Judith Lumley and Brian Davey surveyed thirty-six Australian hospitals in which 44,000 babies are born every year. The survey compared intervention rates with hospital policies regarding family-centered maternity care and flexibility of options. The study showed no relationship between a hospital's flexibility and the rates of intervention. The researchers stated "that it is clearly possible for a hospital to have implemented family-centered maternity care and still have very high intervention rates. There is no guarantee that changing hospital policies toward flexibility or sensitivity to parents' wishes will do anything at all about the use of oxytocin, forceps or cesarean delivery. A commitment to minimal intervention is necessary."

That kind of commitment was made in 1976 when obstetrician Richard Stewart and the certified nurse-midwives with him in a group practice changed the whole maternity unit of Douglas General Hospital in Decatur, Georgia, and made single room maternity care and low intervention the standards of care. Women are admitted regardless of risk factors except for excessive prematurity. Women in labor before the thirty-second week of pregnancy are transported to a regional neonatal intensive care hospital. All others—women with diabetes, hypertension, twins, the need for induction, or previous cesareans (many are delivered vaginally)—receive the same low-intervention care. In 80 percent of all the births the midwife is the birth attendant (and is with the laboring woman from admission). If the birth turns out to be complicated and needs the obstetrician's presence and expertise, as in twin or breech births, he comes in, but the midwife often completes the birth.

The expectant couple comes to the hospital when labor is well established. Women are encouraged to walk and assume any position that gives the most comfort. Solid food in early labor and drinks as labor progresses are encouraged. Preps are not done. Enemas are given only if the laboring woman asks for one. Amniotomy (breaking the bag of waters around the baby) is not done. The cesarean rate is 13 percent (including repeat cesareans); forceps use is 2 percent. Of the vaginally delivered women, 25 percent had drugs for pain, 10 percent had anesthesia, and 27 percent had episiotomies. Maternal and infant outcomes are excellent.

"Babies do not need to be delivered by obstetricians," Stewart told us. "Babies *need* to be delivered by midwives who give absolutely superior care." So sold on midwifery care are Stewart and his wife that when their daughter was born, the Stewarts had the midwife on call as their birth attendant. "The obstetrician has been the star of the show too long," Stewart emphasized. "That's why childbirth is handled the way it is. The star of the delivery is the mother. Although many women want alternatives, they are uncomfortable questioning their doctors. Women are going to have to work to get what they want," he concluded.

To sum up:

- Insurance coverage available.
- Labor, delivery, and recovery in the same place.
- Central nursery available and may be overused.
- Immediate availability of all emergency equipment.
- No one-to-one nursing care because nurses are responsible for several patients.
- An alternative accepted by doctors.
- Almost all women can use single-room care.
- Satisfaction of women can be high; the family unit can be kept together. Twenty percent are dissatisfied.
- High possibility of medical intervention.
- Little research available measuring complications rates.

- Some hospitals offer birth rooms but prevent most women from using them.

Out-of-Hospital Birth Center

In 1975 there were five freestanding birth centers in the United States. By 1991 there were one hundred and forty centers with more than forty in the planning or building stages, according to Kittie Ernst, director of the National Association of Childbearing Centers (NACC). Freestanding birth centers are unique in many ways. The setting is homelike. Routines are absent. Birth is viewed as a normal process to be respected but not feared. The woman has the constant attendance of the midwife or doctor. Intervention and drug use are minimal or absent. Instead, the setting is an encouragement to all to wait out a difficult or prolonged labor and, instead of intervention, to offer the women comfort measures and other help by word and touch. The midwives' or doctors' attitudes of flexibility and support for whatever the woman wishes contribute most to her feeling of control.

Because a woman feels free to respond to her needs, she walks, stands, kneels, or sits as she wishes during her labor, and assumes any delivery position with which she is comfortable. Her partner can hold and comfort her, as can any other support person present. The mother's children can be present for whatever part of the labor and delivery she or they want. Birth becomes a family affair and often includes several close friends as well.

Most freestanding birth centers are several minutes away from the hospital that serves as backup for complicated deliveries. To ensure safety for women who wish to use their services, birth centers are strict in screening for health problems or complications during pregnancy that may require a hospital birth. Birth centers have emergency equipment available for the birth attendants to resuscitate a baby at birth or to stop a maternal hemorrhage, the two most frequent serious complications at birth.

About one in five women who apply to an out-of-hospital birth center will be declared ineligible, either at the first prenatal visit or sometime during the pregnancy. "Horrendous emergencies can always be linked to risk factors predictable before labor and delivery," said nurse-midwife Linda Ross. This strict screening pays off for the pregnant women and for the birth center. During labor only one woman in eight requires transfer to a hospital—usually for delayed progress in her labor. When transfer is needed, the midwife or doctor usually accompanies her to the hospital to deliver the baby, thus maintaining continuity of care. Check your chosen birth center to confirm whether this is done.

Continuity of care throughout the childbearing cycle is part of the birth-center philosophy. All care, from early pregnancy through labor and delivery, postpartum, and baby care, is given by the midwife in the same place where the woman will deliver.

Educating the parents is another crucial element of birth-center philosophy. "Maternity care is viewed as a process of education to promote a healthy, safe, and satisfying birth outcome in which there is a high value on the feelings and wishes of the family during childbirth," said Ruth Watson Lubic, director of the Childbearing Center, Maternity Center Association, New York City.

Because birth is viewed as a normal process and as an important beginning to a healthy family, the mother-to-be is encouraged to take responsibility for her health care during her pregnancy and delivery as a first step in taking care of her baby. Educating the parents to be responsible for their baby's birth is viewed as the best preparation for their assuming the responsibility of raising their baby. "Knowledge is power," said Kittie Ernst, speaking at a *Birth* journal conference. "The more parents understand the more powerful, in control, and confident they are going to be."

All freestanding birth centers are characterized by "parent power," says Ruth Wilf, of With Woman Nurse Midwifery Services, Philadelphia. Families are not only encouraged but expected to design their own highly personalized birth plans. Parents are encouraged to make all the decisions about who will be present at the birth, what the labor and delivery positions will be, and when they will be discharged. They are told to bring to the birth center anything they want to eat (many birth centers have kitchen facilities), and to do just about anything they want to do during the birth experience.

Unmedicated childbirth is advocated by freestanding birth centers. "We guarantee you won't have an epidural unless it's absolutely needed," Ernst told us. "We practice midwifery, not obstetrics. An epidural allows the woman to escape from the birth experience. For many women we see, a midwife-assisted, natural delivery may be the first success a woman has had."

"You are designed to give birth without drugs," nurse-midwife Loretta Ivory tells her clients. She also encourages women to remain at home as long as they want to. "Women at term pregnancy, including women having their first babies, know when to come to the birth center if they have been encouraged by their birth attendant to listen to their own feelings." She describes how she handles the question of when a woman should come to the birth center. "When a woman calls me and says, 'Should I come in?' I say, 'Do you want to?' and if she says, 'Well, I don't know, I thought you'd tell me,' then I say 'Stay home.' However, when she calls and says, 'I want to come in,' then it's time to come in."

Although intervention is very low in all freestanding birth centers, most provide analgesia for those women who request it. All women who choose The Natural Childbirth Institute in Culver City, California, have unmedicated births, nurse-midwife Robin Ozerkis told us. (A numbing injection is given after birth for suturing an episiotomy, if needed.) Intervention and complication rates are very low. Fewer than 3 percent of births are augmented with Pitocin. (Pitocin is given only after transfer to the hospital.) Fewer than 3 percent of the deliveries need forceps or vacuum extraction; less than 50 percent of the women have episiotomies; and the primary cesarean rate is under 7 percent.

Many of the babies born at The Natural Childbirth Institute have their sisters and brothers present at their birth. Founders of the institute Vic Berman and Salee Berman encouraged the presence of siblings from the time the institute opened in 1975. (The Bermans have since left the birth center.) The institute was one of the chief sources of photos for the Hathaways' book, *Children at Birth*.

The American College of Obstetricians and Gynecologists (ACOG) and the American Academy of Pediatrics have issued statements opposing all out-of-hospital births "because of a lack of information to support out-of-hospital births," according to the organizations. The American Public Health Association took a stand in 1979 that birth could be safe outside the hospital and endorsed freestanding birth centers on the basis of research then available. After a literature review the Institute of Medicine of the National Academy of Sciences reported in 1982 that much more good information was needed and that "reliable information about the safety of all birth settings is lacking." We had no proof, at that time, to say that the hospital was safer or as safe as an out-of-hospital birth. In the next decade the evidence supporting out-of-hospital birth came in.

In 1982, the same year the institute report came out, researchers Anita Bennetts and Ruth Watson Lubic reported an evaluation of 2,000 births from 1972 to 1979 in eleven freestanding birth centers. The authors were denied information on low-risk women delivering in hospitals as a source of comparison "primarily for political reasons," the authors report. They settled for evaluating the centers.

Outcomes were excellent. The neonatal death rate for birth-center infants *including transfers* was 4.6 per 1,000 births. Pediatrician Paul Branca of Thomas Jefferson Medical College, Philadelphia, said, "The outcomes for the birth centers studied were at least as good (maybe even slightly better) as outcomes for hospitals for a comparable group of mothers during the same time period."

One criticism of the birth-center studies that were being published was that women who chose birth centers were a "self-selected group" and could not be compared to any group of low-risk women delivering in hospitals. A self-selected group, the argument went, would need fewer interventions and have better outcomes because the women took better care of themselves. In 1986, Anne Scupholme, *et al.* compared a self-selected group with an assigned group in a birth center. Each group had 148 women. Because of overcrowding in a hospital, lower-risk women were assigned to the nearby freestanding birth center. The assigned group differed from the self-selected group in that the women were younger, poorer, and less educated, and a higher percentage were nonwhite, qualities that are often considered to make women at higher risk of potential problems.

The researchers found no differences between the groups in outcomes. Interventions were few, complications were low, cesareans were few (five percent), and satisfaction was high in each group. The authors concluded that self-selection is not what determines the excellent outcomes in freestanding birth centers and that "women assigned to a birth center for care can be as successful in using the care as women who are motivated to select the birth center."

"Safety, satisfaction, and savings characterize freestanding birth centers," reports Kittie Ernst. At the 1989 *Birth* journal conference and later that year in the *New England Journal of Medicine* she presented the results of a national, descriptive study of 11,814 women giving birth in eighty-four centers, the largest study ever done of freestanding birth centers. The data from the study showed low intervention rates and good outcomes for mothers and babies.

Midwives managed three-quarters of the births, doctors the rest. Monitoring was almost always done by portable Doppler or fetoscope rather than by electronic fetal monitoring. Nipple stimulation (7.7 percent) was used over Pitocin (1.4 percent) to enhance labor. Twelve percent of the women were transferred to hospitals in labor, primarily due to delayed progress. Pain-relieving medication was not withheld if the mother asked for it (57 percent of the women had it at some point in labor), but other comfort measures were used more often. During labor 95 percent of the women ate or drank, 43 percent took showers or baths, and 35 percent had body massages.

Women were encouraged to assume the positions of their choice during labor and delivery. Eighty percent delivered in positions other than lying down on the back (the lithotomy position was not used). Sitting and side-lying were the most common choices. Twenty-two percent had episiotomies.

The cesarean rate was 4.4 percent (one-third of those transferred to hospitals had cesareans). The neonatal death rate, *including trans- fers*, was 1.27 per 2,000 births, comparable to the best results for de- liveries of low-risk women in hospitals, according to Ernst.

Satisfaction with the birth centers was so high among the women in the study that virtually all of them (99 percent) said they would recommend the birth center to friends. Although costs varied from center to center, Ernst reported that they are often half that of a tra- ditional hospital delivery and 30 percent below hospital single room maternity care. In response to the cost effectiveness of freestanding birth centers, insurance coverage is now widespread.

The Department of Defense includes freestanding birth centers in Champus, a program that allows dependents of armed-services per- sonnel to get civilian medical care. Champus requires that the birth center be accredited by the Commission for Accreditation of Free- Standing Birth Centers. A nonavailability statement is not needed; that is, the dependent can still use the birth center even if military childbirth care is available.

Some readers of this book are members of an HMO, a health main- tenance organization, in which members prepay a fixed amount for all medical care and must use the health-care providers employed by the HMO. Depending on the local HMO, birth centers may be in- cluded on the approved list of childbirth providers. In some areas, doctors on the boards of the HMOs have kept birth centers run by midwives off the list.

To sum up:

- Insurance coverage available.
- Labor, birth, and recovery in the same place.
- No separation of mother, infant, and mate.
- Equipment available for most common obstetrical emergen- cies; hospital backup provided.
- Very strict screening for admission.
- Complete pregnancy, birth, postpartum care, and pediatric care given at the birth center.
- Highly individualized and personal care, usually by midwives

- Interventions nearly always few; birth viewed as normal.
- Twelve percent transfer during labor to regular hospital for delivery.
- Risk of complications very low.
- Parents educated and guided to take responsibility for their own health care.
- Satisfaction very high.

Home

> Should babies be born at home? What a question! Where else should they be born, if not in the home? The hospital? But I had thought that a hospital was a place where one went for relief from sickness or injury. I would not have thought, had I not known it to be a fact, that the most important event in the life of a family, the birth of a child, was celebrated away from home, away from the family, in a hospital.
>
> —Ashley Montagu,
> *The Home Birth Book*

Homebirth isn't seriously considered by most North American and European women today, with the exception of Dutch women. This is not true in the rest of the world, where the vast majority of babies are born at home. However, a small but growing percentage of women believe, as Montagu does, that the home is the best place to give birth, a place of celebration in the midst of one's family, and that the hospital is a place of medical refuge.

The number of babies born at home in the United States is small in relation to the millions born in hospitals. In many states, the percentage of babies born at home is one percent or less. In a few states, the percentages are much higher. In Washington, for example, more than 4 percent of all births take place at home.

The cost of homebirth is minimal compared to a hospital birth. Almost all of the cost, in fact, is the birth attendant's fee, up to $1,000 or more. Very few state insurance regulations cover the cost of homebirth.

People who choose a homebirth vary widely in their lifestyles and economic status. Their reasons for having a homebirth almost always have to do with a strong desire to have a self-directed rather than doctor-directed experience, to enhance family unity, and an inability to get what they want at a hospital. These parents see childbirth as a normal process. They believe that the addition of a new family member should take place in a way that is most helpful to welcoming the new baby. The parents embrace full responsibility for decisions they make. The child is theirs forever, wherever it is born; the responsibility for the best outcome is theirs.

Most families who choose homebirth do so in an atmosphere of widespread disapproval, meaning they are often forced to carefully examine the reasons for their decision. In the area of safety, they see two key hospital hazards: the risk of infection and high rates of intervention in normal births. They are willing to accept the risk of not having surgical delivery immediately available because they believe screening for risk can be done. They believe that homebirth is safer for a normal mother and baby than a hospital birth.

The report of the Institute of Medicine of the National Academy of Sciences described in detail the research needed to evaluate birth settings and safety for mother and baby. Researchers need cooperation of doctors and hospitals so that comparisons can be made between out-of-hospital and in-hospital births. So far, that cooperation is sadly absent. Many obs are so convinced that any kind of out-of-hospital birth is unsafe that they will not sanction any research.

What research there is, however, suggests that homebirth is as safe or safer than hospital birth when women are attended by skilled birth attendants. Lewis Mehl carried out the first study comparing a group of women who gave birth at home to a similar group of women who gave birth in a hospital. (The results appear earlier in this chapter, on page 37.) This study suggests a much better outcome for the homebirth group.

During a decade of work that extended into the 1980s, English research statistician Marjorie Tew compiled the strongest evidence supporting the safety of homebirth. Tew used British birth data covering hospitals, planned homebirths, and "general practitioner units" (GP units) similar to freestanding birth centers. Data from 1970 was available to classify 16,200 births into risk categories of very low; low; moderate; high; and very high. The perinatal mortality rate (PNMR) is the number of deaths of babies during and around the time of birth per 1,000 births. The PNMR was used to compare outcomes for hospital births and planned out-of-hospital births, including home and GP units.

At each level of risk, perinatal mortality was lower out of hospital. Except for very high-risk births, the differences in PNMR were what statisticians call statistically significant, meaning the differences are great enough that we may assume with confidence they reflect real differences. At the very low and low levels of risk, hospital births had a two-to-three times higher rate of perinatal mortality. At a moderate level of risk, the hospital PNMR was more than eight times greater than out-of-hospital PNMR. Even at a high level of assigned risk to the birth, the hospital PNMR was over three times higher.

In 1990, reporting in the *NAPSAC News* and in her book *Safer Childbirth?*, Tew extended her analysis and research. For the 1970 data she described a "gentle" increase in PNMR over the levels of risk in out-of-hospital birth. Tew suggested that "low interventive methods effectively protect against death across a range of predicted risk. Conversely, the steeply rising mortality rate over the range of predicted risk in hospitals seems to confirm Michel Odent's [former head of Pithiviers Maternity Unit in France] dictum that the fetus, already at increased risk, is less able to withstand the stresses of obstetric interventions."

Tew reported 1985 British data that confirmed the older data. At a lower level of risk, PNMR was seven times higher in hospital. At a higher level of risk the perinatal death rate was four and a half times higher in hospital. Out of the hospital, "birth was very much safer to mothers in both the lower and higher risk groups." She examined 1986 birth data from the Netherlands, where one-third of births are at home. The country as a whole has excellent maternity care and outcomes. However, PNMR for hospital births was six times higher than for homebirths. The Dutch data also allowed birth attendant comparisons. Looking at pregnancies of normal length, PNMR was ten times higher for obstetricians than for midwives. For obstetricians "the average risk status [of women] at delivery was not much higher than that of midwives' deliveries. It could not possibly account for a PNMR ten times as high for obstetricians as for midwives," decided Tew.

"The British and American experience, now powerfully supported by the Dutch results, tells us convincingly that homebirth and midwives are indeed 'safer than we thought,'" concluded Tew. "Together they offer the safest option. The danger of home as a place of birth does not lie in its threat to the healthy survival of mothers and babies, but in its threat to the healthy survival of obstetricians and obstetric practice."

Rona Campbell reported on her survey of British homebirth research (including Tew's earlier research) at the International Homebirth Conference in London in 1987. Campbell was meticulously careful to phrase her conclusions with scientific accuracy. She said that an experiment called a randomized control trial (see description of RCT in Chapter 6) was needed to determine with certainty that one or the other place of birth was the safest. She summarized the evidence to date:

> There is no evidence to support the claim that the safest policy is for all women to deliver in hospital. For women having a planned homebirth, the risk of perinatal death appears to be low, particularly for women who have already had one child. Morbidity (illness, infection or other complications) is higher among mothers and babies cared for in hospital. Most women with experience of home and hospital delivery prefer home delivery.

Marsden Wagner, an official with the World Health Organization (WHO), spoke at the same conference.

> The World Health Organization supports the more traditional forms of health practices such as homebirth. Just for the record, let me read to you out of the WHO publication *Having a Baby in Europe:* "It is important to remember that it has never been scientifically proven that the hospital is a safer place than the home for a woman who has had an uncomplicated pregnancy. Studies of planned home birth in developed countries with women who have had uncomplicated pregnancies have shown morbidity and mortality rates for mothers and babies equal to or better than hospital birth statistics. These studies have also found significantly fewer interventions used in home births."

A unique experiment in homebirth continues to take place in rural Tennessee in a spiritual community of families called The Farm. On The Farm or in the surrounding area over 1,700 babies have been born at home. All were attended by Farm midwives who learned their skills through practical experience and apprenticeship (called empirical midwifery). Statistics for these births (including the 4.7 percent of all births transferred to the hospital during labor) contradict most hospital obstetrical statistics. Intervention is almost nonexistent. Ninety-eight percent of the women gave birth with no drugs or anesthesia; 28 percent had episiotomies; less than 1 percent were given Pitocin to stimulate labor; less than half of one percent of deliveries required forceps; and the cesarean rate was 1.8 percent. Complications are usually managed at home. Nine out of eleven sets of twins and two-thirds of the breech babies (thirty-three of forty-nine) were born at home.

Ina May Gaskin, The Farm's head midwife, wrote, "unless home birth is considered by a society to be a valid option worthy of social support, it is easy to lose the knowledge that birth is a normal process. When all maternity care is in the hospital, it becomes fragmented, and caregivers lose their skills and the knowledge of how women's bodies function in pregnancy and labor. The cost in human lives and suffering is uncounted but catastrophic."

To sum up:

- Insurance coverage unlikely, but costs low.
- Parent responsibility is high for finding a skilled birth attendant and for ensuring hospital backup.
- Regular prenatal care essential to reduce risks.
- Approximately 15 percent transfer to the hospital during labor; one out of four first-time mothers.
- Interventions minimal.
- Complication rates extremely low.
- Risk of infection is low because the mother is not in an alien environment.
- Birth experience is directed by the parents.
- Mothers may feel more relaxed in their own territory.
- Siblings can easily participate in the birth at their own pace.
- The baby is part of the family from the beginning.
- Satisfaction very high.

Choosing Your Birth Attendant

You have four choices for a birth attendant: an obstetrician, a family practitioner, a certified nurse-midwife, or a direct-entry midwife. For a few parents who are unable to find a birth attendant they are satisfied with, a fifth choice is possible: themselves.

Obstetrician

Whether a woman expects to have a healthy, normal pregnancy, or whether she has been labeled "high risk," most American women choose obstetricians as their birth attendants. Obstetricians—surgeons trained to handle any gynecological or obstetrical problem—deliver three out of four U.S. babies. Many women like the idea of having a specialist for their baby's birth, believing that, because the obstetrician can handle any complication that may develop, they have the best care available at all times.

In Chapter 4, we describe the obstetrician's training and practice. In a four-year residency the ob/gyn-to-be spends less time on obstetrics than gynecology, with some months in anesthesia, pathology, and endocrinology. He becomes a surgical specialist in diseases of the female reproductive system.

Most obstetricians believe birth to be a time of highest risk to the baby and feel obliged to get the baby out as quickly as possible. They view a woman's birth canal as dangerous to the baby and believe that intervention is necessary in almost all births.

Family Practitioner

Family practitioners, who deliver about 15 percent of U.S. babies, are medical doctors who have taken an additional three years of residency after medical school.

A family practitioner chooses his specialty because he wants to treat the whole family. This is often the main reason some women prefer to go to a family practitioner for obstetrical care: They like the fact that he already knows the whole family, and they prefer the continuity of care. Because the family practitioner's philosophy is to give primary care to the whole family, many family practitioners have a policy of delivering their obstetrical patients whether it is their night on call or not.

Family practitioners view birth as a normal process. Because they take care of newborns just as pediatricians do, they often see the complications from interventions. They view intervention in labor and delivery as risky and see themselves as skillfully using interventions only when necessary.

Certified Nurse-Midwife

Certified nurse-midwives, who deliver roughly 7 percent of U.S. babies, according to Inforum, Inc.'s Gallup survey for 1991, are registered nurses with an additional two years of midwifery training. During these two years, the student midwife participates in over 100 normal deliveries. "The new nurse-midwife has more experience in normal childbirth than the average family practitioner," says Silvia Feldman, author of *Choices in Childbirth*. "She rapidly accumulates so much experience thereafter, working full time with normal births, that she soon knows more about managing normal pregnancies and childbirths than the average obstetrician." Certified nurse-midwives always have the support of a backup obstetrician, and many work in joint practice with obstetricians.

The nurse-midwife's practice is limited to managing the maternity care of mothers whose progress through pregnancy, labor and delivery, and postpartum is normal. During training a certified nurse-midwife is taught to recognize an abnormal situation in pregnancy or birth, and to refer mothers to, or seek consultation with, a specialist. Education of the pregnant woman is a basic part of the philosophy of certified nurse-midwives. They view this education as helping the woman to participate in her own health care.

"Historically, midwives have viewed themselves as experts in the normal birth, skilled assistants to the birthing woman's efforts, trusting her body's own powerful ability to give birth naturally and safely," says nurse-midwife Rebecca Barber. Because they share this viewpoint, certified nurse-midwives believe intervention to be risky, and prefer a more "hands-on" approach, with the skillful avoidance of drugs. What some see as a disadvantage of the midwife—that she is not trained to do the surgery necessary in complicated deliveries—others see as the main advantage. Her primary effort is to assist the childbearing family in having a normal delivery. "She is better equipped to give complete care to the normal [woman] than is her obstetrician physician colleague," said Ruth Lubic.

Certified nurse-midwives are now the birth attendants for a growing number of U.S. births, both in hospitals and in freestanding birth centers (and some at home). To meet the expanding need, all schools of midwifery are increasing their enrollments, according to Kittie Ernst. A shortage of certified nurse-midwives has held back growth in the number of birth centers, Ernst told us.

Ernst described another solution to training more midwives. A community-based educational program gives registered nurses the chance to study midwifery wherever they live. Registered nurses who are not near one of the university midwifery programs can get a master's or doctorate degree in nurse-midwifery from Case Western Reserve University in the off-campus, self-paced program. Ernst designed the curriculum for the program, which is administered by the Frontier School of Midwifery and Family Nursing in Kentucky (phone: 606-672-2312). "It won't be long before insurance companies and government agencies catch on to the lower cost of midwifery care and realize that certified nurse-midwives should be giving obstetrical and gynecological care to all healthy women—that's 75 to 80 percent of all women," Ernst said. "For every obstetrician/gynecologist there should be four nurse-midwives."

Direct-Entry Midwife

Direct-entry midwives enter training "directly," without having first qualified as a nurse. Commonly known as lay midwives, they deliver one percent of babies in the United States each year, reports David Stewart of NAPSAC. Their training varies. Some have completed midwifery and licensure programs in England, others have trained at a birth center run by direct-entry midwives, such as the Casa De Nacimiento (House of Birth) in El Paso, Texas, and still others have learned by training and apprenticing with experienced midwives.

Licensure and legality of practice vary also. As of this writing no Canadian province has legalized the practice of direct-entry midwifery. "The practice is definitely illegal in nine states in the U.S. and in 15 states it is legal," Terra Palmarini, midwife and coauthor of *Pregnant Feelings*, told us. "In the rest no legislation deals with direct-entry midwifery, putting its practice in a grey area of legality." Palmarini suggested that women contact the Midwives Alliance of North America (MANA) or their local health department for their state or province's status and referral. NAPSAC offers a *Consumer Guide* which includes a directory for alternative birth services.

Direct-entry midwives have the same commitment to normal birth as certified nurse-midwives. The word *midwife* means "with woman." Most midwives give continuous one-to-one care through all stages of labor and birth, and some work with an assistant for the early stages of labor. Direct-entry midwives almost always deliver at home, though many hospitals permit the midwife to accompany a woman to the hospital when a complication arises and to remain with her through the delivery, which is sometimes completed by the midwife under a doctor's supervision and at other times is handled by a doctor. Direct-entry midwives are also being used as labor assistants for women choosing hospital births.

Yourselves

Very few American women choose to deliver their own babies without a birth attendant. When they do, it's usually because they are unable to find a birth attendant who will give them the kind of birth they want either at home or in the hospital. Gregory White, a homebirth family practitioner in Chicago, reports hearing from a registered nurse whom he had attended for her first three home deliveries. After she moved to Florida, she went to thirty different doctors, by actual count, to try to find a homebirth attendant. None would do it. Finally, she gave up and decided to have a do-it-yourself birth.

A number of do-it-yourself births are done by preference. Marilyn Moran of Leewood, Kansas, and Kathy Lanzolotta of Harborside, Maine, are the spokeswomen for this choice, believing that birth is a spiritual and sexual experience between mates that should not be intruded upon if the pregnancy and labor are going normally. Believing it inappropriate for a woman to give birth into a stranger's hands, Moran suggests that a woman give birth into the waiting hands of the baby's father or her partner. For those who choose a do-it-yourself birth, Moran says it is crucial to have prenatal care to give the parents continuing information on the woman's risk status, and for the parents to study as much material about birth as they can, so they know the signs indicating a possible complication requiring hospital assistance.

Measuring the Safety of a Birth Attendant

The best way to look at safety is to compare mother and baby death and complication rates for the different kinds of birth attendants. Obstetricians point to dropping maternal and perinatal mortality rates as proof of how well they are attending births. In Chapter 6 we point out that overall death rates don't prove that what one is doing is safe; only evaluations of each intervention used could prove or disprove that. But death and complication rates can be useful in *comparing* birth attendants by specialty.

Maternal mortality is based on the number of deaths of women per 100,000 live births. Maternal mortality rates in the United States are so good that it is difficult to distinguish any significant differences by specialty. The maternal mortality rate is less than one maternal death for every 10,000 live births. For comparison, you have a far greater chance (more than twenty times greater) of becoming pregnant after your husband has had a vasectomy than you have of dying in childbirth.

There are reported differences in *infant* outcome by specialty that can be useful in comparing birth attendants. The best outcomes for mothers and babies in the industrialized countries of the world are in those countries where many or most of the babies are delivered by midwives. As an example, highly ranked Sweden has almost universal midwifery. Drug-free childbirth and 100 percent hospital births are also basic to Swedish maternity care.

One of the very few direct comparisons of neonatal mortality rates for babies delivered by either midwives or doctors was presented in the *American Journal of Obstetrics and Gynecology* in 1971. The neonatal mortality rate is the number of infant deaths per 1,000 live births during the first twenty-eight days of life. For about three years state funds were used for a nurse-midwifery demonstration project at Madera County Hospital in California. During the program midwives managed "the vast majority of pregnancies and 78 percent of the hospital deliveries," according to the report. Birth became safer for the babies with midwifery care: Neonatal mortalities were more than halved and the prematurity rates went down by 40 percent. The program was terminated, despite good results, because of opposition from the California Medical Association. After doctors again assumed the care of women, neonatal mortality and prematurity skyrocketed. Over the next two and a half years, the neonatal death rate tripled and prematurity increased by 50 percent.

Published reports of homebirth and direct-entry midwifery care in Kentucky, North Carolina, Missouri, and Arizona in the U.S., and in Ontario in Canada, are available, showing excellent outcomes. For example, in the North Carolina study by the Centers for Disease Control, planned homebirths attended by direct-entry midwives had a neonatal mortality rate of four per 1,000 live births. In the same time period, the neonatal mortality in low-risk hospital births in North Carolina was seven per 1,000, not a statistically significant difference.

Marjorie Tew, whose work we referred to earlier in this chapter, has analyzed the most complete data on place of birth and birth attendant. Her first report of British data showed birth safer at home or in a general practitioner unit than in a hospital. Almost all births in hospital at the time of the study were attended by obstetricians. Yet the perinatal mortality rates were higher at every level of labor risk for the obstetrical units than for homebirth with midwives or birth centers with general practitioners. Tew's analysis of Dutch data gave more evidence for her conclusion that midwives are safer than obstetricians for most women.

Again in their careful, scientific way, Rona Campbell and Alison MacFarlane, social policy analysts, looked at Tew's data and analysis and reported that there was no proof that the obstetricians were responsible for the higher mortality rates. They did agree that there is some evidence that complications are higher among mothers and babies delivered in hospitals and cared for by obstetricians.

A comprehensive review of the literature on midwifery is given by David Stewart, author of *The Five Standards for Safe Childbearing*. His historical review shows that midwife-attended deliveries have neonatal death rates well below national averages. In many, if not most, of the studies the midwives were attending the poor and high-risk client, where one could expect *higher* neonatal death rates.

A current outstanding example of midwifery care is in North Central Bronx Hospital in New York City, reported by Doris Haire and Charlotte Elsberry, director of midwifery services at the hospital. Although 70 percent of the mothers are considered at medical or socioeconomic risk (i.e., poor and nonwhite), midwives care for most of them. One in ten women arrive in labor with no previous care and 10 to 12 percent of the women are addicted to drugs. With all these problems, the philosophy of care remains one of low intervention. Complications are usually low, and the cesarean rate is just over 11 percent. "Despite the odds, the maternal and infant outcomes are much better than one might expect," the authors report. The neonatal mortality rate *regardless of birthweight* is 9.2 per 1,000 live births. For infants weighing 2.2 pounds or more, the neonatal mortality rate is an unusual 3.7 per 1,000 live births. Sixty percent of the infants are being breastfed at discharge—"a remarkable percentage for such a disadvantaged population," said Haire.

Maternity systems based on midwifery have better mother and baby outcomes, according to the literature. "The data base for these figures is in the millions, is global in scope, and spans almost a century, up to and including the present," said Stewart. He estimates that if all the women delivering in the forty-year period between 1940 and 1980 had had a birth attendant with a midwife philosophy, mother and baby mortalities would have been halved and the rates of brain-damaged children and other birth injuries and complications in newborns would have been reduced by at least three-fourths. Over the forty-year period, according to his estimates, 1.5 million children were severely brain damaged because of medical procedures; and 45 million children suffered minimal brain damage who would have been normal, had unnecessary intervention in normal deliveries been avoided.

In 1985 the World Health Organization held a conference on the "Appropriate Technology for Birth." The WHO adopted a new series of recommendations that follow a "careful review of the knowledge of birth technology." The WHO reaffirmed that "the training of professional midwives or birth attendants should be encouraged. Care during normal pregnancy, birth, and afterwards should be the duty of this profession." Normal pregnancy care includes 80 percent or more of all births. The WHO recommends that professional midwives, either certified nurse-midwives or direct-entry midwives, care for all those women.

The WHO's policy on midwifery care has been in place for more than thirty years. Testifying before the California state legislature, the WHO's Marsden Wagner explained the balance needed between midwives and obstetricians to provide the best care. "Care during normal pregnancy and birth should be the duty of the midwifery profession. Midwives are trained to focus on the normalcy of pregnancy and birth, placing the needs and wishes of the mother first, and avoiding interventions unless absolutely necessary. Obstetricians, on the other hand, are physicians trained to focus on pathology and to intervene. When the balance does not exist, the surgical interventions in birth rise to levels that most experts worldwide believe to be far beyond what is necessary."

The philosophy of care, not the title of the birth attendant, is decisive in safe care for mother and baby. The safest philosophy of care involves:

- Prenatal education and screening
- Continuous one-to-one labor support by a skilled labor attendant, who may also be the birth attendant
- The view that a woman's body is designed to give birth safely to her baby in her own unique way
- The belief that intervention should be used only when the need is greater than the risk

This philosophy is common among midwives, but can be found among some family practitioners and obstetricians, too.

Women at low complication risk have much greater rates of intervention and complication for themselves and their babies in hospitals than in alternative settings, either in a freestanding birth center or at home. Your chance of a normal birth is related to your choice of a birthplace and a birth attendant.

If you are willing to look, you have a great chance of finding a place of birth fairly near you that will satisfy your needs in childbirth. Many hospitals have eased their policies to allow flexibility in their routines. With your partner, a woman friend, and an agreeable birth attendant, you can have a good and safe birth in many hospitals today.

4

Understanding Doctors

I'm proud of what I do. I'm proud that I've gone to school and become an educated person. I don't think I'm better than anyone else. We doctors are not pillars of society. We are part of society. Who's a pillar? The guy who sweeps out a gas station, pays taxes, doesn't commit any crimes, goes to church, loves his wife. Isn't he a pillar of society?

—Obstetrician*

Most of you will have a doctor, probably an obstetrician, as your birth attendant. To get a good and safe birth, you need to understand your doctor. She's a unique person, with her own background, training that has shaped her thinking and beliefs, and her own pressures and successes.

Residency

After four years of college and another four years of medical school, new doctors choose graduate medical education specialties, or residencies, as they're more commonly known. (Year-long internships, in which new graduates sampled all the medical specialties, are no longer used, according to the American Medical Association.) The number of required residency years varies, and ranges from four for ob/gyns and three to four for pediatricians to three years for family practitioners.

Residents often put in up to 100-hour work weeks and seldom go home, despite objections voiced in medical journals and the media in the last decade about the health effects of such a schedule. This

---

* This anonymous doctor's comments follow throughout this chapter.

concern is not only for the doctors themselves, but for the people they treat, who, due to physicians' possible reduced mental and physical functioning, might be misdiagnosed and treated inappropriately.

> I was in surgery seven hours from seven A.M. until two in the afternoon. Usually there were a half dozen or more operations, and I'd make rounds in between or after. The afternoons and evenings were for admitting new patients, performing physical exams, writing up charts, and prescribing tests or medications.

Typically, most of an ob/gyn's training is in surgery. Surgeons at their best are finely trained technicians. Learning to use technology is crucial for them, so that they can intervene automatically and quickly in lifesaving situations.

> Obstetrics is the least scientific of all specialties. Traditionally, the bottom half of the medical class went into obstetrics. When I was in training, we still listened with a headscope. That was the state of the art. We were afraid to do a c-section and we knew nothing about the fetus. Now in fifteen years there has been an explosion of technology in obstetrics.

In the 1970s technology was added to the ob/gyn training program, making it a more challenging residency to new doctors. But it's more than the appeal of science. "A lot of medicine is drudgery and trivia," one doctor told us, giving his opinion why doctors so readily accept new technology in their practice. "Medicine is often like an assembly line [a common complaint of the patient also]. New techniques and technology are exciting. They are like new toys, and you think you are doing things better. You become part of relentless progress."

> Unless residents are trained to keep technology in perspective, I can see where they would get on a treadmill and rely upon machinery too much. Nurses are the same way. I was trained in the in-between era, where I saw both worlds. There is a place for technology, but people tend to rely on it too much. Doctors and nurses who are trained at high-tech centers have to make a conscious effort to not allow high-technology procedures to be their only tools. That's not easy. If that's the way you were trained, you'll be uncomfortable changing.

The most important skill for many ob/gyns, from their point of view, is not delivering babies; it's surgery. This is an emphasis that is often not in women's best interests.

Residents are eager to do surgery. There is pressure on residents to find surgery because there is never enough to go around. I don't think I'm overtrained for surgery. I don't think you can ever be surgically overtrained. But you can very easily be under-trained. You can quickly get in the habit of doing surgeries that don't need to be done when there are alternatives, too.

Ob/gyn residents, like other specialists, treat low-income women almost exclusively. These women are the most likely in our culture to be high risk, and the least likely to ask questions. This treatment, plus the normal vulnerability of pregnancy, labor, and birth, guarantees that many of these women will not object to any procedure done to them, and an ob/gyn resident is not encouraged to discuss with a patient what she wants.

I tell residents that they are going to find a different world when they go into private practice. Nobody ever told me that when I was a resident. If I said to a patient during my training, "You need a hysterectomy," she never said, "Why?" She said, "Yes, doctor, thank you, doctor." In my practice, there is a lot of consumer interest, and questions and more questions.

Doctors who specialize in family practice treat the whole family—not just the pregnant woman. Like pediatricians, family practitioners in their three-year residencies often will see the same child and that child's family for many visits. A family-practice doctor contrasted his own residency training for us with the training he saw in ob/gyn: "I had fifteen patients of my own that I took care of from the very beginning of their pregnancy to their labor and delivery, and then I took care of their babies until I finished my three-year residency. That kind of follow-through in patient care is something you don't get at all in the standard ob/gyn training." Patients at major medical centers usually see a different ob/gyn resident for each visit and yet another stranger at the birth.

As a resident, I used to see forty to forty-five people in a three-hour clinic. I might have seven patients in labor at one time. All I could do was make a snap judgment, a quick decision. I couldn't really sit down and talk to people. There just wasn't enough time. I have a real easygoing practice now. I see about half the patients that the average obstetrician does. I've made it a point not to treat my patients in my private practice the same way we treated

women during my training. A doctor can change just like everybody else. It just depends on how human he is.

The resident obstetrician typically believes that she will learn all
she needs to know about childbirth in her residency. That may leave
her suspicious of any ideas that are different from what she learned.

> I delivered 2,000 babies in my residency. If the patients didn't
> get medication, it was a rare exception. In fact, I was told that
> I failed in my duty if I did not provide the patient with med-
> ication. I trained in a big-city ghetto hospital. There the women
> wanted and needed medication. There was no prenatal edu-
> cation, no Bradley or Lamaze classes. Most of the women were
> not married and didn't want to be pregnant. They didn't want
> pain. There was no reward for them to have that child, and so
> in that situation, if I didn't provide them with anesthesia, I
> wasn't doing my job. That's what I was there for.

Many an obstetrician feels that if understanding women's birth
pleasure were significant, she would have been taught that in her
training as well. "Sure, I saw women experiencing pleasure in their
births," the late obstetrician Jane Patterson told us, "but I was choosing to ignore it. Childbirth was a painful, uncomfortable experience,
and maybe the next day after it was all over, then they were happy.
But with the actual experience itself? No. That was the way I was
taught."

> I am way overtrained to deliver a perfectly healthy woman
> who is having her third child, who is going to go into spon-
> taneous labor. She doesn't need a board-certified and
> surgically trained obstetrician for that delivery nine out of
> ten times. One out of ten she might. My training makes it
> hard for me to sit on my hands and just wait and watch.

One obstetrician described the transition from training to private
practice to us by saying, "Physicians are trained in a high-pace setting and have to unlearn rigidity, haste, and intensity." Asking an ob
to "sit on her hands" and wait for nature to take its course goes
against training and experience.

Along with the attitudes and knowledge gained through medical
training, physicians have six other influences that more or less—
depending on the individual doctor—affect your care.

Special Influences on Doctors

1. Fear of Malpractice Suits

Malpractice is more than a specter for many obstetricians; it's a reality. Your physician knows colleagues who are being sued and may have been sued herself, since 77.6 percent of ob/gyns have been sued at least once, according to a 1990 report of the American College of Obstetricians and Gynecologists. That strongly influences what your doctor may or may not do during your pregnancy and birth.

> I talk to other doctors, and they are worried. This is especially true when I'm doing an ob consultation. I've read in the newspapers about doctors who deny that the fear of malpractice influences their decisions. Well, that's not true. Privately, we know a very large portion of an ob's decisions are based on the legal implications. It gets worse every day. The agencies that handle our malpractice policies come and give risk-management seminars for doctors.

The anxiety level about malpractice suits among most obstetricians is high, and for many of those who've been sued, it's the most stressful experience of their lives. "The shadow of malpractice falls over our every act," states Ralph S. Emerson in the *Bulletin of the American College of Surgeons*. And often legal advice encourages "defensive medicine." Lawyer James J. Pagliuso, in his article "Situations to Avoid If You Don't Want to Be Sued," stated: "I believe obstetricians and hospitals are taking substantial medicolegal risks if they don't undertake at least external monitoring from the outset of active labor." And when doctors are sued, judges usually hold physicians liable when they don't use technology.

> I have people who come into my office and they say, "Why haven't you done the ultrasound yet?" and I say that I don't think it is indicated, and they say, "Well, my girlfriend had an ultrasound, and I want an ultrasound; I want to see the baby." "You'll see your baby in six months," I say. "Well, I don't want to wait," she tells me. She'll get her ultrasound. And strictly because if ever there was an anomaly or the slightest thing wrong, she is going to say to me, "Why didn't you do the ultrasound when I asked you to?" So I am pressured to do it. I don't do everything that a patient demands, but those kinds of pressures I cooperate with because I don't want to lose my practice.

I have to earn a living, and I like what I do. I'm basically just like everybody else. If you work in a factory, and the guy down the line does something wrong and gets fired for it, you are not going to repeat his mistake. It's the same with obstetricians.

Who's the least likely to get sued? The doctors who listen and talk to their patients. The fear of a malpractice suit in your doctor's mind might cause you to receive unnecessary interventions, from extra office tests to a cesarean. (The cost of so-called defensive medicine is estimated to be $15.1 billion each year, according to the American Medical Association.) Prevent defensive medicine from interfering with your pregnancy and birth by doing your part in developing a partnership with your doctor.

2. Insurance Companies

About 85 percent of Americans have health coverage. For them nearly all hospital bills and two-thirds or more of doctors' fees are paid by insurance. This coverage allows most patients to buy services from both doctors and hospitals without concerning themselves about price, though this is starting to change. In a turnaround from the early 1980s, now many of you who have insurance belong to a prepaid health plan that offers comprehensive medical care for a fixed fee. And these plans do not always cover all the expenses once paid for by the free-choice insurance plans.

When a hospital buys ultrasound machines and electronic fetal monitors, the administration is counting on insurance companies to pay the tab—and that means using the machines. Insurance (ultimately the patient) pays for all those other extras in the hospital, too—from IV bottles and Pitocin to epidurals and anesthesiologists, nursery fees and baby bottles, sleeping pills and other medications. Although your doctor doesn't get a cut of the insurance company's payment to the hospital, insurance companies reinforce the inclination of the ob/gyn to *do* something by virtue of what procedures they choose to pay for. (A few physicians, however, get a finder's fee from certain hospitals for bringing in new ob clients.) Costs for cesareans, for instance—a surgical procedure—are usually reimbursed 100 percent. This is not always so with vaginal births.

Obstetricians have incentives to use technology during pregnancy, too. Insurance companies routinely pay for prenatal tests. Critics of the American medical industry point out that physicians with diagnostic equipment, such as ultrasound machines, in their offices use that equipment more than physicians who use independent labs to do the work. Generally, you'll get more tests of all kinds if they can be done in your doctor's office. This is not to say that your doctor doesn't believe these procedures are necessary, but their use is sometimes a habit, rather than thought out specifically with you in mind.

Knowing your physician's incentives to use technology during both your pregnancy and birth, perhaps, when the question of tests, ultrasound, or hospital procedures comes up, you can discuss the pros and cons *for you*, with a clear explanation of the risks/benefits before automatically agreeing with your doctor's suggestions.

3. Drug Education

There continues to be controversy over the drug education that physicians receive. Some say that doctors receive more information from drug companies than is appropriate. Most of these companies offer endless free samples to doctors, starting when they are medical students and continuing through their private practice years.

Others point out that pharmacology takes up one-seventh of a physician's national board exam, and many doctors work hard to keep up with drug information.

Regardless of who's right about where doctors get their information, or whether they're influenced by pharmaceutical company largess, many physicians continue to prescribe drugs widely known to be ineffective or dangerous.

4. Personal Income

The typical ob/gyn in 1990 netted (after expenses, including the payment of a malpractice insurance premium, and before taxes) $202,430. This is more than twice the average 1980 ob/gyn income, based on reports from *Medical Economics,* and a fact that is contrary to typical media coverage that assumes doctors' incomes have dropped because of malpractice insurance and lawsuits. Because ob/gyns are surgeons, they continue to be among the highest-paid specialists. A pediatrician earns about half as much ($104,937), a typical nurse earns $28,000 to $38,000, certified nurse-midwives earn $33,000 to $38,000 (in 1988), and full-time, homebirth lay midwives who charge for births earn an estimated $20,000 to $30,000 annually.

I know a lot of doctors who drive Chevrolets and Toyotas, have modest homes, and don't play golf every day. And they have a hard time paying their bills. I am under the same pressures as everyone else, so I want to make more money, too. Until I was into my thirties, my top yearly income was $18,000. That's not a lot of money. I was married early and had two children. I had $25,000 in loans to pay back, and it cost well over $50,000 to start my practice. Right there is a lot of incentive to make some money and make it fast. Many physicians think they deserve it. I don't know how to argue with that, because this is a money-oriented society, and that's status and that's America.

5. *The Doctor Surplus*

Predicted in 1980, the doctor surplus has come to pass, with the number of doctors having grown proportionately faster than the population. Although some ob/gyns left obstetrics because of higher malpractice premiums, others dropped obstetrics and its intense competitiveness to concentrate on gynecology, because it is more lucrative and has better hours.

More doctors, however, doesn't mean lower prices. Over the last decade, ob/gyns, along with most other doctors, have increased the fees for and the number of medical tests and procedures that they perform. Many pregnant women have several ultrasound scans, routine Doppler use at prenatal visits, a prenatal test (amniocentesis, chorionic villus sampling, or alpha-fetoprotein sampling), and several uses of the electronic fetal monitor (stress and nonstress tests) before they go into labor—plus additional tests and procedures during labor.

Not only has the number of these tests and procedures increased enormously over the last decade, but sometimes—not to exaggerate the doctors' role in this increase—women themselves request some of these procedures as well. "Ten years ago," a family practitioner said, "my patients wanted no drugs, no interference during childbirth. Today they all want proof through technology that everything's fine. They all want amnio and wouldn't think of not using a fetal monitor."

To cope with the doctor surplus, ob/gyns not only raise prices, as much as possible they try to eliminate the competition as well.

I believe the demand for obstetricians in society will rapidly decrease. I think it should. We have too many specialists. There are women who do want an obstetrician, and they would no

more go to a midwife or a family practitioner than they would
live in an underground sod shack. I mean, they want an epidural; they want me; and they want to tell their friends that I'm
a specialist and I'll deliver the baby. There will always be that
demand. But that is going to be decreasing in the future, and
what are all those extra twenty thousand obstetricians going to
do? I've already lost some referring doctors because I have a
nurse-practitioner in my office and I work with nurse-midwives.

Obstetricians on occasion have made it difficult for some family
practitioners and many certified nurse-midwives to get hospital privileges. But the best example of the obs' efforts to eliminate competition is their battle against homebirths. Midwives who assist at
homebirths have been accused of crimes, and doctors who participate in homebirths—or who give prenatal or backup care to these
women—are often hounded by their peers. These doctors are threatened with loss of hospital staff privileges; their malpractice insurance
policies are often dropped; and they are frequently treated like out-
casts among other physicians.

Clearly many doctors believe it is not safe for any women, even
those who are healthy and have had prenatal care, to give birth at
home, although available statistics contradict that belief. However,
there's apparently an economic incentive at work as well. If birth can
take place safely with a family practitioner or midwife in attendance,
then fewer obstetricians are needed. With more obstetricians being
trained, there is bound to be increasing conflict of interest.

6. Pressures of Medical Practice

The reality of medical practice is not as simple as diagnosing a problem and providing a cure. Sometimes patients demand the impossible.

People expect more of doctors now. They don't expect mistakes. They are more aware of the shortcomings and faults that
take place in medicine. And there's been another attitude
change, too. If a woman delivers a baby that has a defect,
people are much more surprised. In the past, people understood that there wasn't much we could do about it.

Patients have high expectations of physicians, and so do other
physicians. Doctors expect all their peers to practice medicine much
the same way.

There are fads—new, unproven techniques—in medicine, and they come and go. It's easier to go with these fads, no matter how unscientific they might be. You can buck the trend better if you are an established authority in a large medical center. It's a lot harder to do that when you are just an ordinary workaday obstetrician. You have no credentials and no research to support your viewpoints. Therefore, you are compelled to practice what is called the "standard of care"; that is, what is reasonable in the community, what other obstetricians do. That's the threat, that's the problem. If you are outside the "standard of care," you are potentially leaving yourself open for liability, criticism, and loss of license.

The medical profession has always regulated itself. Now it's just beginning to be held accountable to different segments of society. And more and more, a physician is regarded as just another person doing business.

We don't police ourselves nearly as well as we could. We've got a long way to go, but I think attitudes are changing. The older doctors resent any policing of hospital procedures, because they've been God so long. Nobody ever questioned them before. "Medicine is not fun anymore," they say. "Everyone is telling us what to do and what not to do." I think the younger physicians coming up are going to practice in an era of peer review. People are going to know what doctors are doing. Due to liability concerns and consumer demands, hospitals and doctors are going to have to protect themselves through self-regulation.

Although many other professionals put in as many years of schooling and work as many hours in a week as physicians do, there remains a difference. Only physicians make life-and-death decisions, though nurses often feel that responsibility, too. And this is perhaps the greatest pressure of all. To add to the stress of making these decisions, many patients willingly give that power to doctors. Often we want the doctor to decide, thereby adding to her pressure to perform without error.

Physicians do want the best medical care for you. However, the typical doctor believes that, of the two of you, she's the best judge of what that is. Why else would you be asking her opinion? She not only believes she's right, she also has peer pressure from colleagues to not rock that boat called "the status quo."

But there is a right birth attendant for you. Our next chapter describes how to find "Dr. Right," a person who will be your health-care partner—not your boss. The search is yours, because ultimately you, and only you, are responsible for your health and well-being.

5

Finding Dr. Right

Women must realize first that they do have a right to say
how they want their babies delivered, with whom and
where.... Like everything else—one must care to have
things a certain way. If there is no strong desire, then the
doctor, as most people do, will follow whatever practices
that are convenient for him. We need to educate
women who will then demand proper services from
doctors and hospitals.

—Survey

Knowing your birth options is no guarantee that you'll get them,
but it's a start. Understanding your doctor's point of view based on
her training and background is also a necessary step. Next in getting
the birth you want is not only choosing the right birth attendant, but
establishing a relationship, based on thorough communication, that
works in the best interests of you, your baby, *and your doctor.*

Because more than 90 percent of you will choose a physician, we
call your birth attendant Dr. Right. For most of you, she is an obstetrician; for others, a family practitioner; for a few, an osteopath. This
chapter tells you one step at a time how to find Dr. Right, what to do
once you're in her office, what to say/do/ask when you're face-to-
face with her, and what questions you need answered.

If you're like most women in your search for an ob, you'll either
keep going to your current doctor or you'll ask friends for recommendations. Some women, research shows, add two more steps to
the search process. They look for a doctor who communicates well
and is affiliated with a hospital they want to use.

Here are some some suggestions for finding Dr. Right:

Make a List

I am again shopping for a doctor, a doctor who delivers at a hospital with practices I agree with. I would like to have a doctor who has a midwife working with him or her. I definitely know what I want and don't want next time and I will try not to get myself into an undesirable situation again. I plan to find out what I can about the doctor even before I see him or her, and then, during the first visit, make sure our ideas are in accord.

—Survey

Start with the recommendations of others and make a list. When getting names, ask why this person is being recommended. You'll soon discover that many of the reasons aren't sufficient. Would you choose your partner in your health care for *these* reasons?

- She goes to your church and lives in the neighborhood. (She may even vote the same ticket, but that doesn't mean she's enthusiastic about vaginal birth after cesarean [VBAC] or that she will help you avoid drugs in labor.)
- Your Aunt Sally says she has a wonderful bedside manner. (Your doctor probably won't get to the side of your bed until you're ready to deliver the baby.)
- She's the only woman doctor in town. If your number-one priority is a woman, and your town doesn't have midwives, then this is obviously a valuable piece of information to add to your list. But if one of your reasons for having a woman doctor is that she's more likely to give you what you want because she's a woman, don't count on it. Women doctors go through the same medical training that men do. Chances are, though, according to some research, a woman physician will pay more attention to your personal relationship with her than her male colleagues might. As most ob residents are now women, your chances of finding a woman practitioner increase all the time.

Some people also look in the yellow pages or their town's medical directory (available at the public library). That can help you get a geographical fix on the doctors in town. But mere names and locations don't tell you enough.

Physicians often suggest to consumers that a hallmark to look for when doctor-shopping is board certification. This term means that a doctor has completed the required years of medical training and, in addition, has passed a series of professional competency exams in her specialty. Board certification, in the case of obstetricians, however, may work against your having your baby your way, unless you're planning a cesarean or have a serious chronic illness. Board certification is no guarantee that your doctor will listen to your preferences, or that she has experience or interest in assisting you with your birth, free of unnecessary interference.

Check It Twice

There are three groups of people who can help you double-check your list: nurses who work on hospital ob floors, childbirth educators, and La Leche League leaders.

Before you call any of these, though, make up a list of key issues for your birthing experience, in order of priority. (If having a woman with you along with your mate is crucial, ask that question first—not last.) If you've never had a baby before, read a few books to help you think about what you want. Just because you've never had a baby doesn't necessarily mean you won't have strong preferences when the time for your labor and birth arrives.

Hospital nurses are proud of their ob units and are generally happy to help pregnant women who call for information, though some refuse to comment. The nurse can tell you which doctors are most likely to help mothers with unmedicated births; what the hospital's cesarean rate is and which doctors do the fewest cesareans; which doctors don't routinely have laboring women hooked up to IVs and fetal monitors throughout labor; and more. These hospital ob nurses can also give you the phone numbers of local childbirth educators and La Leche League leaders.

Most women giving birth in the United States attend childbirth-education classes. If you are in a class now, talk to your teacher. If you are not, you can still call a childbirth teacher. She'll likely be glad to help you. Also, consider contacting La Leche League, particularly if you plan to breastfeed.

Both of these groups of women are knowledgeable about birth and infants. They offer monthly meetings that attract large groups of women—pregnant or, in the case of La Leche League, new mothers, too. Though they may not give you direct physician or midwife referrals, they'll answer your questions about the reputations of the doctors on your list and about the care that individual hospitals in your area give to new mothers. As with all the people you are questioning, be specific with them about your preferences.

Along with these three information sources, there are two others that might be helpful—particularly when you're looking for the right hospital. In many cities local ads show a nurse ready to give you a physician referral, or hospitals are shown that advertise "birth planners." It's true that the women who answer the phones can give you a referral, but it will be to someone on their staff; it's their staff that is paying for the service. If you've chosen your hospital first, however, and are still looking for Dr. Right, this service might be helpful in narrowing your list of names. And if you have chosen Dr. Right and speak with a designated birth planner about your preferences at the hospitals with which your doctor is affiliated, then you might find out which hospital's menu of services has what you want.

Don't Forget the Birth Center and the Hospital

> Next time I will shop for a hospital as well as a doctor. Next time I definitely want rooming in; I definitely want my first child to be able to visit me in the hospital, and to see her new brother or sister; I want to be able to feed my baby after its birth and have a period of closeness with it. To me the issue of bonding is much more important than whether I have an enema, prep, or an episiotomy.
>
> —Survey

You need to find the right place to give birth as surely as you need to find the right birth attendant. However, if you have a medical plan that confines you to specific physicians and hospitals, you will not have the luxury of shopping around unless you're willing to pay even more out of pocket. (Most insurance plans do not pay 100 percent of maternity expenses.) (See Appendix A. Then convert those suggestions for changing hospital practices for all women into getting those changes for yourself if you're limited to a hospital that does not offer what you want.)

Ten Questions for Birth Centers

If you're considering a birth center, you won't need to find Dr. Right, as the person and the place are a package with the fee reimbursed by some insurance companies. Read over the questions for hospitals that follow, too, as some will apply to these centers as well. Most do not, because birth centers typically have low intervention rates and little opportunity for or interest in separating you from your baby, mate, or friends.

1. *Is your birth center accredited by the Commission for the Accreditation of Freestanding Birth Centers?* (Contact the National Association of Childbearing Centers listed in Appendix D for more information.)

2. *Are you staffed by certified nurse-midwives and nurse practitioners or by physicians?* Most birth centers have certified nurse-midwives on the staff even if there are doctors as well. If you're considering a center that doesn't have any certified nurse-midwives, be sure to ask about their hospital-transfer rate and use of drugs. (See Chapter 3 to find out how this birth center compares with others on all the issues in this list of questions.)

3. *How many of your clients transfer to the hospital?* Transfer rates vary among birth centers, and if your birth center has a higher rate than average, ask why.

4. *Are childbirth education classes, as well as prenatal, childbirth, and postpartum care, included in your fee?* They usually are, and the overall cost generally is far cheaper than hospital rates.

5. *How long are prenatal visits?* Midwives often spend up to an hour with you during each monthly visit.

6. *Who will be with me during labor and birth?* If there are several certified nurse-midwives, will more than one be with me? What chance is there that a midwife or doctor who I don't know will be there during labor?

7. *Is a home visit part of my postpartum care?*

8. *If my baby needs the care of a pediatrician at birth, how is that handled?*

9. *What's your cesarean rate?* Cesareans, of course, are not performed at birth centers, but women who need them are transferred to a hospital. At the same time you're asking this question, ask what are the reasons for the cesareans.

10. *What is your opinion of prenatal testing, and in particular, the use of ultrasound?* Do you use a Doppler (see "Ultrasound") or do you

use a fetoscope for prenatal visits and labor? In 1989 the American College of Obstetricians and Gynecologists (ACOG) said that fetoscopes are as good as electronic fetal monitors for monitoring normal births. However, many doctors and nurses are unfamiliar with their use, while midwives are quite comfortable using them.

Ten Questions for Hospitals

Some of these questions can be answered by nurses in the maternity unit. For the others, call the hospital or nursing administrator's office and ask who can help you.

1. *Do you have a one-room option in which I can labor, give birth, and recover? Is this room always staffed?* If this hospital mostly offers multiple-use rooms, they will always be staffed.

2. *What is the nurse-patient ratio?* Ideally, according to ACOG, there should be one nurse for every two women in early labor, and one nurse to one woman who is in the pushing stage. No one knows what the national average is, but reports suggest the typical ratio is not ideal. The nursing shortage makes it likely that many hospitals will be understaffed, particularly if several women are in labor at one time. If the hospital you're considering has a shortage of ob nurses, but in every other respect is the right hospital for you, you might want to consider hiring a private-duty nurse (a monitrice) for your labor. (More on that later.)

3. *What is your cesarean rate?* Nationally nearly one in four women have cesareans, but the rate at which they're performed at different hospitals varies enormously. Government research shows laboring women will usually get whatever is typical care at an individual hospital, so that's why it's important to match up your preferences with their routine.

Massachusetts and New York, among other states, require that hospitals provide you with the cesarean rate so that consumers have a basis for comparison. For information about other states, see the Public Citizen's Health Research Group listing in Appendix D.

4. *If a cesarean becomes necessary, can my partner stay with me in the operating room?* If the hospital says yes, ask which doctors, including anesthesiologists, arrange for partners or other helpers in the cesarean operating room. Though the presence of the mate is more common than it once was, that arrangement is not automatic, especially if you

are not legally married.

5. *How many other people can I have with me?* Can my doula (see Chapter 11) stay with me during my labor and come with me to the operating room as well if a cesarean is necessary? Some hospitals are willing for you to have two people, your mate and a doula, with you during labor. They are usually less enthusiastic about two people with you in the operating room, but it is possible to arrange this.

6. *What is your epidural rate?* In some hospitals the rate is 90 percent or more. If you want to avoid this drug, it's best to avoid hospitals where its use is standard, because that's what the staff is used to offering you for pain relief.

7. *Do you have a lactation consultant on staff?* This is a popular option with many women, and more and more hospitals have a person like this on staff. If they do, ask if she is accredited, and whether she's full time or part time. (It's possible that a part-time lactation consultant wouldn't even be in the hospital the days you're there.)

8. *Can my baby remain with me at all times from the moment of birth? When can my mate and other children visit?* Let them explain when your baby can't stay, rather than when he can, for a clearer understanding of hospital rules. (See a detailed discussion of rooming in in Chapters 13 and 14.) In some hospitals mates can remain with you twenty-four hours a day, and others have special visiting times for your other children.

9. *What is the average cost?* Costs vary, though Arnold Relman, former editor of the *New England Journal of Medicine*, suggests investor-owned or for-profit hospitals charge 15 to 20 percent more than other hospitals. Be sure and check your insurance coverage, as it's common now for individuals to pay a higher percentage of maternity costs than they once did.

10. *Does your hospital have a policy regarding required use of the electronic fetal monitor during labor?* Most hospitals do, for malpractice reasons. If yours does, ask what is the required length of time. It's usually between twenty and thirty minutes, although if you're using Pitocin, have an epidural, or are labeled high risk, EFM use is usually required for your whole labor.

Every hospital maternity floor has two sets of rules, only one of which is written. The written rule is the ob policy, which mirrors the local medical standard of care—or what most doctors believe to be good medicine. It's determined by the ob committee of the hospital, and includes issues such as EFM use or whether your mate can be with you during a cesarean. (See question 8 in "Ten Questions for Dr. Right," page 83, to find out about the unwritten rule.)

Begin Investigating Doctors

After you've done your homework and now have some names, the next step in finding Dr. Right is to ask all the questions you can on the phone, just like you did with birth centers and hospitals.

- *How much does maternity care cost?* In many cities, all obs charge the same fee. Family practitioners often charge somewhat less.
- *Does a nurse-midwife work in the office or does Dr. X work with homebirth midwives?* Many women prefer to work with midwives, and many more obs have these women working in their offices than was true only a few years ago.

  A smaller number of doctors also bravely work with direct-entry midwives in any one of several ways: They provide backup if a woman needs to go to a hospital, or they will provide access to the use of an ultrasound scan machine if she has a condition that might benefit from its use, such as a suspected multiple pregnancy.

  Occasionally, these midwives and physicians offer a partnership in which some women get what they perceive to be the best of both worlds. That is, the woman sees both the midwife and the physician separately for prenatal visits, and the midwife accompanies the laboring woman to the hospital and stays with her throughout labor. And although the physician will be present at the birth, often the midwife will either catch the baby herself or will guide the mate to do so. (For midwives who provide this service, see "Midwifery" in Appendix D for information about referrals.)
- *What is the scheduled length of the appointments?* The closer appointments are (ten to fifteen minutes apart, rather than twenty to thirty, for instance), the more likely it is you'll do a lot of waiting, as well as be rushed through your appointment when you do see her. Ask how long patients wait. (If it turns out that, for other reasons, she's Dr. Right, find out when you should schedule an appointment to reduce waiting—perhaps first thing in the morning, or just after lunch.)
- *Does she deliver babies at more than one hospital? If so, which ones?* Doctors in metropolitan areas usually work at more than one hospital, each with its own set of maternity options. Some arrange twenty-four-hour rooming in, for example;

many don't. (In your search for the best birth attendant and best hospital, you may have to resolve the dilemma of Dr. Right not being on staff at the best hospital.)

- *How many babies does she deliver in a month?* If it's fewer than ten, she's likely to give you more time and interest. If her number is closer to thirty, beware. Babies aren't born an average of one a day, and she may assist as many as five or six mothers in one day. If you are one of the five or six, you might rightfully be concerned whether you'll get adequate attention from her.

When you've gathered what information you can by phone and are interested enough to meet this person, then make an appointment. Traditionally, initial visits for pregnancy include an internal exam to confirm pregnancy. Just because it's still office routine in many places, however, doesn't mean you have to do it that way. You do not need to have a particular doctor examine your body to find out if she is the right one for you.

Schedule a Consultation Only

When you call, tell the receptionist that you want a get-acquainted appointment, because you are pregnant and are looking for a doctor. Some physicians charge for this ten- to fifteen-minute appointment, and some do not. If the receptionist tells you that all initial visits must include an exam, and she won't budge from that rule, we suggest you scratch that doctor off your list. Pelvic exams often make women feel uncomfortable, if not humiliated. Why have more than you need?

Here's why you should remove a doctor from your list who requires an exam during an initial visit. If you go ahead with the exam first, one of two outcomes is likely: You will find changing doctors extremely difficult even if the one who examined you is *not* Dr. Right; or, after she's examined you, the doctor is more likely to become aggravated at your questions, your taking your time to make up your mind, or your decision to change doctors. Remember, you are negotiating first whether this person is Dr. Right.

Some doctors (or more likely, office nurses) may argue that your pregnancy must be confirmed first by an exam before you do any talking. Let's say you have your consultation first, and then you decide she *is* Dr. Right. Now you have your physical exam, only to find out you're not pregnant, for heaven's sake. You may be embarrassed, but it's an honest mistake. It does happen. Know that you are that much farther along in your search for the right medical care when you do get pregnant.

Take Someone with You

When the time arrives for your consultation, take your mate with you if you can. An increasing number of partners go to prenatal visits, and many often have more questions than you do.

If your mate is unavailable, take another adult with you. More attention is paid to patients (whether in the doctor's office or in a hospital) if they are accompanied by another adult. The other person is effective whether he or she says one word, especially if she or he takes notes. Doctors, like the rest of us, are more careful when others are writing down their words. Besides, if you have someone with you, it's easier for you to keep to your agenda.

So, you and your companion arrive at the doctor's office. Now it may all go according to plan, and the two of you may be ushered into the doctor's office for your consultation.

Or what might happen is that the receptionist will invite you into an examining room and ask you to disrobe. Remind her that you're there for a consultation, and repeat your phone conversation.

Perhaps at this point, you'll think to yourself, it's not worth making a big deal about this. Sooner or later, I'll need to be examined anyway, you say. Go over in your mind why it's important to consult first, examine last.

- It's difficult to change doctors after that initial exam.
- You give the impression to the doctor that you will be her patient when what you need is information and time to decide.
- Many women find it difficult to meet a new doctor while flat on their backs, with their legs in stirrups, counting the dots on the ceiling tiles to pass the examination time.

These are some possible reasons. You may have others. So stick by your goal. This is a consultation appointment.

Resolve the Problem of Names

Many women tell us that it's important that they establish a tie with their doctor in which she's an equal, not a boss. It's well established that similarity in how we address each other encourages equality, particularly in an ongoing relationship. The use of names in this instance is not a matter of etiquette—it is an indication of power. So, now for that special problem: What do you call each other?

Nearly all midwives and many younger doctors prefer to be called by their first name, and they will tell you that. But what do you do if this doesn't happen, if you decide not to bring up the issue of names in advance, and if you call her "Doctor" and she calls you by your first name. (Women report this is more likely to happen with male doctors.)

There are three scenarios. (1) You can call her by her first name. (2) If first names are not your preference, ask that you be addressed by your last name, and continue to call her "Doctor." (3) Make no comment (but we suspect this is not an effective option for most of you, because if you're going to see this person fifteen or twenty times, the issue is not going to disappear).

Following are our ten questions to ask Dr. Right. Use what's appropriate from this list and add your questions as well. Keep interviewing doctors until you've found the right person.

Ten Questions for Dr. Right

Ask the questions that are most important to you first. Always pursue specific answers. A doctor's replies are based on her beliefs and training, and her personal experience colors every answer she gives you. Do not expect a doctor to be enthusiastic about something she has never tried before. Like the rest of us, doctors do best what they do most.

1. *Can my mate be with me at all times, including in the cesarean operating room?* This is first an issue of hospital policy, and then secondly a decision for each doctor.

2. *How many other people can I have with me at all times?* The role of the helping woman, the doula, is becoming more popular in American hospital births. Some laboring women prefer that they have two women there with them.

3. *What percentage of your patients do you deliver yourself?* You naturally assume she'll be there, but many a laboring woman has a rude awakening when an unknown doctor shows up at a time when she has enough strangers to cope with as it is. Now your doctor may say

(and many have), "Of course, I'll deliver your baby, except if I'm not on call or if I'm out of town." At first hearing, it sounds as though she'll be there. Check further. Ask, "About what percentage of your patients do you personally deliver—75 percent, 50 percent, 30 percent?" She'll have some idea.

We know from what mothers tell us, which is reinforced in recent studies, how important it is for most of them to have their own doctor there, especially if they have done a lot of research before choosing her. But as most of you will not have a guarantee that Dr. Right will be on call, ask to meet all the other doctors who cover for her and review your birth preferences with them.

4. *How much time will you spend with me when I'm in labor?* Women who have never had a baby before often anticipate that their doctor will be with them throughout labor—and a few actually are there for the duration. Most doctors, however, arrive closer to the time of the birth. If you ask this question outright, you will at least know in advance the realistic amount of time she (or whoever is on call) will be there, so that you can plan accordingly to rely on supporters.

5. *What is your cesarean rate?* ACOG suggests that a reasonable rate is something less than 16 percent; other observers believe a reasonable rate is even lower. Ask what her usual reasons are for performing cesareans. (Are they valid reasons?)

6. *What is your definition of "high risk"?* The following conditions, according to ACOG in 1991, are considered high risk: maternal diabetes, high blood pressure, heart or kidney disease, sexually transmitted diseases (such as AIDS and herpes), other viruses (including rubella and viral hepatitis), previous or current birth defects, multiple pregnancies, vaginal bleeding during pregnancy, breech position, postdate pregnancy (beyond forty-two weeks), alcohol and drug use, smoking, environmental hazards, radiation, prematurity, maternal age under sixteen or over thirty-five, convulsive disorders, chronic urinary tract infections, and severe anemia.

Your physician's list might include more or fewer conditions. Just as with the terms *bonding* and *rooming in*, the term *high risk* does not have a uniform accepted definition. If you are labeled high risk, don't assume that you will automatically have problems with your pregnancy. If the consequences of your doctor's high-risk label for you are upsetting, in that it requires you to do things you don't want to do (such as frequent use of ultrasound or stress and nonstress tests), get a second opinion.

7. *What is your usual recommendation if a pregnancy goes beyond forty-two weeks?* Some doctors automatically schedule a cesarean,

others induce labor, and still others just wait and see. No research supports intervention for this.

8. *What percentage of your patients have epidurals? Other drugs? Pitocin? Routine IVs? Confinement to bed?* (See Chapter 7 for other common birth interventions that you can add to this list.) You are likely to get what your doctor usually prescribes. Recall our discussion of the hospital's written rules (number 10, page 77, in "Ten Questions for Hospitals"). The unwritten rule is the doctor's protocol—her usual, routine recommendations for all patients. That's why hospital nurses could answer your questions about specific doctors.

9. *What is your recommendation for the use of the electronic fetal monitor (EFM)?* While the hospital itself is likely to have a policy in use when you first arrive, whether to continue using EFM is up to your doctor. She may say that she wants you to use the EFM during all of the labor because either there aren't enough nurses or none of them will use the fetoscope to monitor your labor. If you like everything else about her, and she is willing to waive the EFM if you have your own nurse, then hire a monitrice. You don't have to take potluck with the staffing.

10. *What is your recommendation for the use of ultrasound?* According to the Food and Drug Administration, 80 percent of women use ultrasound at least once during pregnancy. Ultrasounds are obtained most commonly with the following three instruments: (1) Doptone or Doppler—the hand-held fetal stethoscope with transducer that is placed against your abdomen and "broadcasts" your baby's heartbeat; (2) scan—a video screen with attached transducer that can determine your baby's gender and due date; (3) external EFM—one or two belts with transducer (to monitor baby's heartbeat) placed around your abdomen, or newer telemetry models that allow you to carry the transducer in your pocket.

Ultrasounds have no apparent immediate side effects, and not enough time has passed to know if they will engender long-term side effects. The FDA and the American Medical Association, however, recommend that ultrasounds be used with caution.

When you're offered ultrasound, ask yourself if its use this time will make a difference, and ask your doctor if there's an alternative. Could she use a fetoscope, for instance, to listen to the heartbeat during your prenatal visits? If you're positive of your menstrual dates (just as accurate as the scan), are not interested in discovering your baby's gender, and do not have any unusual occurrences, such as a larger than expected uterus, why not forgo the unknown risk and cost of the scan? And though EFMs are frequently used as nurse substitutes in the United States, ask to have a nurse who can use the fetoscope, or hire your own monitrice.

Get It in Writing*

> I have a very progressive doctor, and he asked me for a list when I was pregnant of what I wanted in my childbirth experience, in terms of anesthesia, enemas, preps, stirrups—the whole bit. I wrote it all out—including the labor, the delivery, the postpartum experience. He took my list; we went over each item. He said okay to everything that was on my list. It became part of my chart, and I never had any problems with anybody.
>
> —Survey

Somewhere about the fifth or sixth month of pregnancy, after you and your doctor have had several chances to talk over your desired options, it's time to get it in writing. Asking your doctor for her signature may seem to show a lack of trust on your part, but your doctor will not be with you all the time you're in the hospital. This signed paper takes your doctor's place. It also helps your health-care provider focus on you in particular.

Summarize your options clearly on paper. Get your doctor's signature on it, in case she's not there at the labor and birth or, more likely, doesn't get there until some hours after you do. Give a copy to each of the possible substitute doctors when you meet with them. Have Dr. Right's partners sign the agreement, and leave a copy with each possible substitute. When there's a question about this or that being different from the routine, just wave your paper and say, "My doctor has agreed to this. If you have any questions, ask her." If she refuses to sign the paper, write down her oral agreement and use the paper anyway.

Does that mean that your labor and birth will follow your birth plan to the letter? Not necessarily. On the one hand, your experience might mirror that of the Canadian woman who said, "During pregnancy number two I spoke to my obstetrician many times about my preferences. He assured me that 'if' all went well I could 'probably' have a delivery with no interventions. Too many ifs and probablys."

---

*...but understand that's no guarantee.

On the other hand, your experience might be like the woman from Kansas who recently wrote, "I had gone to my ob with my birth plan, ready for a fight. Instead I got smiles, reassurances, and a doctor who did nothing I did not authorize." We don't want to mislead you: There are no guarantees for your birth plan, though you'll increase your chances of its effectiveness enormously by having a doula. (See Chapter 11.) That's because once you're in labor, you're not likely to argue about birth-plan items if you're told that your child is "in danger." And forget about discussing an unplanned cesarean in a calm manner. You'll be in the throes of labor, likely feeling much pain, and worried about your baby.

We've learned from mothers that even if birth plans can't predict the final blueprint of your experience, these lists usually seem to help women focus on what's important to them and what's not. And remember: Your job is not done after you've passed out the list. You have to continually reinforce it. Repeat at every visit: "Remember, I'm the one who wants...."

Change Doctors Midpregnancy

During my first visits, my ob was thorough, very nice, and talked about her kids. She had been my gynecologist for years. When I was seven months pregnant, my husband and I took in our birth plan. The interview was a complete disaster. We wanted no routine Pitocin; she threatened us with possible infant brain damage if we didn't use it. When I said I didn't want medication, she said, "You can hurt as much as you please and you will." It went from bad to worse. When I said I didn't want a routine IV, she said she'd be "sloshing in my blood which would be all over the floor." Brain damage, agony, and death? Hardly the image of joyous childbirth I had imagined. I knew I had to change doctors and discovered it wasn't as difficult as I thought it would be. I was welcomed by the birth center I transferred to and was thrilled with my birth there.

—Colorado

What if you get this far—or even farther—in your pregnancy, and you discover this is not Dr. Right? You realize you can't compromise as much as she wants you to. Should you change doctors? The natural vulnerability and dependency of pregnancy work to keep women from switching, but some women do it. And their experiences, including that of a woman who changed doctors at eight and a half months, indicate that switching is not only satisfying for these women, but the new Dr. Right welcomes them.

Sometimes when pregnant women decide they must change doctors, they worry unnecessarily over how and what to tell the first doctor. You don't owe her a lengthy explanation, certainly not an apology. Your new doctor will handle the request for a transfer of your records, or she will ask you to call your former doctor's office and request that your records be transferred. You can let your former doctor know why you're transferring, but a brief letter is adequate. Most of the time, this will be the end of it. Don't expect her to agree with your decision or even to be civil about it. That's okay. It's your decision, not hers.

Know Your Negotiating Position

When a doctor answers a woman's questions, explains pertinent facts, and offers choices, the doctor gets an informed patient, one less likely to call anxiously at all hours with fearful questions. That means fewer time and energy demands on the doctor.

And, as pointed out previously, doctors who have trusting relationships with their patients have far fewer malpractice suits. Besides, consumers have a right to good communication, some doctors say. They believe it's the birth attendant's role to educate patients about their bodies so they can be informed partners in health care. It's like getting a warranty. Education goes with the product.

Also, doctors who are partners, not bosses, have less pressure on them to be godlike. Doctors know in their hearts that medicine is an inexact science. All of us can, and do, make mistakes—physicians included. Inviting a doctor to be your partner ultimately allows her to function at her best.

But let's also be frank. The doctor makes her living from helping women give birth. The more women she helps, the more money she makes. The doctor wins economically if you buy her services. And the word will get around very quickly (probably from you) that this doctor is one who supports women's preferences.

Be Clear About Rights and Responsibilities

You have a right to an explanation of, and the reasons for, any procedure that might be done to you by your doctor or the hospital. You also have the right to refuse any procedure. (The exception to this is the much debated issue of the twenty-one women who have been forced to have court-ordered cesareans in the United States since 1980.) You have the right to be informed of the probable consequences to you and your baby and of any alternative to that procedure. You must have a chance to weigh the benefits against the risks—or your physician risks malpractice liability.

You have to do your part, too. It's your responsibility, not the doctor's, to ask for plain English when you don't understand medical terminology. It's also your responsibility to keep notes of your conversations with your doctor regarding explanations of procedures and descriptions of drug side effects. Don't rely on memory alone, no matter how good a memory you have.

Communicate your preferences clearly, frequently, and repeatedly. If you don't, no one will read your mind; doctors are as poor at mind reading as the rest of us. Doctors have repeatedly told us that their patients don't tell them what they like and don't like. How can you blame your health-care provider for not giving you what you want if you haven't asked?

Not all of the steps we suggest may apply to your situation, or you may be reluctant to try every one. However, even doing one thing differently in your contact with your doctor is a sure sign of success. One step leads to another, and each time you try something new, it gets easier. A woman in labor is in no condition to fight with her doctor or the hospital staff. She must negotiate her options ahead of time. We also believe that a true partnership with your health provider—accomplished carefully visit by visit, question by question—is an important step toward personal satisfaction with the whole birth process.

6

Obstetricians' Beliefs About a "Safe Birth"

No doubt about it, if ten women went into the jungle to
have a baby, nine would walk out with healthy babies.

—An Obstetrician in Practice for Twenty Years

I think I should practice the best medicine. All of my
patients are hooked up to fetal monitors and IVs during
labor.

—The Same Obstetrician

You may wonder as you read these two quotes by the same obstetrician how he could say two things that seem so contradictory. Easy! Most obstetricians believe that a birth can be labeled "normal" only *after* the birth is over. As an eminent pediatrician wrote to the *Denver Post*, "There is no such thing as normal childbirth except after the fact." A prominent obstetrician said, "Normal pregnancy is really a retrospective diagnosis." Obstetricians believe that at the time they are handling your birth, they are handling a very dangerous situation, with most births at high risk.

A "High Risk" Label

Women who are "high risk" are simply more likely to have problems in their pregnancy or with their childbirth or baby than those who are low risk. The words *high risk* applied to a pregnant woman mean that she should be watched carefully for complications that may affect her or her baby. The factors that make a pregnant woman high risk are medical and social. The social factors known to make her high risk include being unmarried or poor, for example, and the medical factors include high blood pressure, toxemia, or other serious maternal diseases.

A high-risk labor includes women who have been labeled medically at high risk during pregnancy, and all premature and induced labors. (Some doctors see augmented labors as high risk also.) These labors can result in a normal birth, but they are more likely to need the birth attendant's intervention for the best outcome for mother or baby. High-risk deliveries include cesarean and breech births.

A high-risk designation does *not* mean a woman or her baby will have problems; one of the drawbacks with such labels is that the doctor or the pregnant woman may forget that. Once a woman is labeled high risk, the doctor and woman may act as if she or her baby *will* have problems, and unnecessary interventions might occur to end the pregnancy. For example, a doctor may tell a woman he wants to deliver her breech baby by cesarean section a week before her due date. That presumes that the woman or her baby will have problems if she is allowed to go into spontaneous labor and deliver vaginally. The doctor and woman have forgotten that the high-risk label is a decision made in the minds of those who use the words, and it may or may not really exist for that particular woman.

The words *high risk* are so widely applied today that most obs see them as applying to most of their patients. "We'll take [high-risk or difficult birth] patients the community hospitals can't, and we should," said an obstetrician at University Hospital of Denver. "But the term 'high risk' gets kind of muddy. What some are calling high risk is not what we're calling high risk."

Most obs believe they are handling a dangerous situation with all births, including the low-risk woman—the healthy, married woman who has carried her baby to term, has no serious medical problems, and has started labor spontaneously. Doctors point out that one-quarter of the admissions to neonatal intensive care units come from babies born to low-risk women, and more than half of the complications in childbirth occur in low-risk women.

"This seems to be a *damning defense* of the present system of obstetric care," said Doris Haire, president of the American Foundation of Maternal and Child Health. "It compels one to ask what proportion of these complications, which had their onset *during* labor and birth, are the direct result of aggressive obstetric procedures." She quotes G. T. Kloosterman, chairman of the department of obstetrics at the University of Amsterdam: "The spontaneous labor in a healthy woman is an event marked by a number of processes which are so complex and so perfectly attuned to each other that any interference will *only* detract from their optimal character. The doctor, always on the lookout for pathology and eager to interfere, will too often change true physiologic aspects of human reproduction into pathology."

Other observers also believe that obstetricians' interventions can lead to complications. In *Birth Trap*, Yvonne Brackbill, June Rice, and Diony Young give us a picture of the connection between high risk and interventions by calling it a "technological daisy chain.... Obstetrical interventions are not independent of each other."

In the *New England Journal of Medicine*, James Mold and Howard Stein used a term they borrowed from biology, a "cascade," which refers "to a process that, once started, proceeds stepwise to its full, seeming inevitable conclusion. This chain of events tends to proceed with increasing momentum, so that the further it progresses, the more difficult it is to stop. The participants in the process are often unaware that it is a cascade effect, and they frequently fail to recognize its cause."

"The cascade effect is frequently seen during labor and delivery... in uncomplicated pregnancies admitted to the hospital," say the authors. The interventions start, one leading to the other, with the electronic fetal monitor. "Labor may be slowed by the combination of inactivity and anxiety," leading to efforts to speed labor, and the cascade is underway. "The cascade of benign interventions to which physicians subject many women can lead to complications that lead to further interventions and more complications, and end in some final intervention—usually a cesarean section—that would not have occurred had not the cascade been set in motion." The cascade effect is fueled by the "anxiety" of the laboring woman and the birth attendant who cannot accept "the small risk of a potentially life-threatening condition," and "may be tempted to do something—anything—decisive to diminish their own anxiety."

The authors conclude: "Certain risks may be unavoidable. There are always going to be some bad outcomes, and we cannot subject every patient to aggressive testing and monitoring simply to avoid some very uncommon bad consequences in a few. This involves a difficult ethical problem, but it can often be solved simply by involving the patient in the decision-making process."

Doctors certainly do not believe that what they are doing causes complications in births and problems in the babies. "It is threatening to be told that what you are doing is not good, that you may have been hurting people," obstetrician Vic Berman told us. "Doctors simply can't say what they have been doing for twenty years is wrong. If it were wrong, *they* were hurting babies. That's a totally unacceptable idea."

The obstetrician's training and his peers (other doctors) tell him that what he is doing is right. And his everyday experience with complications in birth shows him he needs to get in there and do more, not less. Besides, interventions and technology make an obstetrician's practice more interesting. "Every doctor enjoys his intervention," obstetrician John Franklin told writer Alice Lake. "That's what his skill and training are for. Some think that nature is in constant need of improvement and others that nature can't be trusted."

A Safe Birth

If all childbirth is seen to be dangerous, the overriding concern of the obstetrician, naturally, becomes a "safe birth." Those are buzzwords we find obstetricians using frequently: "I can't do that because it's not *safe*." " I find an epidural is a *safe* way to deliver a baby." "The hospital is the only *safe* place for your baby to be born."

Women are very vulnerable when the doctor uses the words *safe* or *unsafe*. *Of course* you are going to do what you are told will ensure your baby's safety. But you will come far in the art of negotiating to have your baby your way if you understand what a "safe birth" means to many obstetricians. There are six key elements; a "safe birth":

- Is actively managed
- Is predictable
- Is controlled by the obstetrician
- Takes place in the hospital
- Is attended by an obstetrician
- Is solely measured by a live baby and a live mother

A "safe birth" is actively managed. Obstetricians believe childbirth is fraught with danger. They see complications every day. Their surgeon's training has prepared them to take charge of events and they do. They get in there and "manage" the labor and delivery, administering interventions that they have used many times before. But why use these procedures with all labors and births? An obstetrician explained to us, "You have to understand that we look at things virtually 180 degrees differently from you [childbearing women]. You are all saying this would be very pleasant and nice. Unfortunately, in medicine we have to do things for the minority situation when things go wrong. We'll never have a meeting of minds on this issue because you look at things from the opposite standpoint. We are doing things and setting up rules and regulations for the small number of cases that are going to be bad, not for the large number that are going to be good."

Obstetricians honestly believe that all women, and babies about to be born, deserve the very best in technology. A West Coast family practitioner described to us what it was like to work with obstetricians: "The impression I got was that if you didn't do all these fancy things for the mother and the baby, somehow you were not providing optimal care. Optimal obstetrical care was that which used all the new technology." Technology is essential to the active management of labor and delivery.

A "safe birth" is predictable. An actively managed birth is quite predictable. The obstetrician knows the risks of his procedures, and he has faith that he can handle them with another procedure, if necessary. For instance, if the epidural he's given slows a mother's labor, he can speed it up with Pitocin. If that same epidural prevents her from pushing, he can use forceps or a vacuum extractor.

His basis for measuring whether your labor is going "normally" comes from a generally accepted medical standard called the "parameters of normal labor." For instance, if a woman's bag of waters breaks, it is expected that she will soon start to labor and will deliver within twenty-four hours. And whenever labor begins, the woman is expected to deliver within twelve hours. When a woman is in what is called "active labor," after three or four centimeters' dilation, obstetricians expect her cervix to dilate at least a centimeter an hour. In the second stage of labor, the delivery, the belief is that a woman shouldn't have to push for more than one or perhaps two hours— less if she has given birth before. For the third stage, the delivery of the placenta, it's generally agreed that the woman should be given about a half hour before the birth attendant begins to extract the placenta. However, as one doctor told us, "Nobody waits that long. Everybody starts pulling on the cord sooner."

If your labor and delivery do not follow this timetable, the obstetrician's "creed" requires that he do something to bring your labor within the "normal" range. Using his tools of intervention carries some risk to the mother and the baby, but the obstetrician believes he can handle any complications that result from his own procedures. Two of the most common complications of "intensive obstetrical care," reported by Madeleine Shearer in the journal *Birth*, are newborn scalp infections (from fetal monitors) and maternal intrauterine infections. Both of these complications the obstetrician believes can be handled easily with antibiotics.

A "safe birth" is controlled by the obstetrician. Your doctor believes that he is giving you a safe birth and protecting your baby's interests when he denies you a part in the medical decision-making process. At a Northwest Regional International Childbirth Education Association convention, author Suzanne Arms spoke to this issue when she said, "Society now has experts who believe we must leave important life decisions to them, that they know best."

Doctors still hold to the view that they really do know what is best for you. As one doctor told us, "You do have to give us some credit for knowing technically what is best for the situation." Believing that he really does know what is best for you, he also supposes that you then have total trust in him.

Doctors' demand for absolute authority is the subject of *The Silent World of Doctor and Patient* by Jay Katz. Katz argues that anxiety and uncertainty are a part of the practice of medicine, but that doctors cannot live comfortably with these fears, thus hiding these fears behind their demand for authority and control over patients' lives. To give patients part of the decision-making process is a frightening prospect, so doctors present themselves to patients as all knowing. Seeing doctors as all powerful may comfort some women. But, because medicine is "an imperfect art," says Katz, doctors can't possibly live up to patients' expectations.

We become disappointed and criticize doctors for acting like gods. At one childbirth conference, the discussion turned to this issue, and a doctor responded with, "We'll stop being gods when you get off your knees." However, Katz suggests that mutual trust is a better basis for a doctor-patient relationship than blind faith. Sharing doubts, needs, and ideas results in better communication. He notes that this won't be easy until medical training begins to take seriously a doctor's communication skills.

Because obstetricians do not believe that women should make important decisions about their own deliveries, doctors sometimes become angry with inquiring pregnant women.

The obstetrician would say things like "I know you better than you know yourself," "I think your blood pressure is terrible and you'll probably have a seizure on the way out of the office," "I think you are too informed and are trying to diagnose yourself."

—Virginia

You may already have experienced your obstetrician's irritation; certainly a lot of women have. No one is necessarily immune. Suzanne Poppema, a family practitioner herself, was pregnant with her first child when she had this experience. She was seeing an obstetrician who was substituting for her regular doctor. He spoke of using the fetal monitor on all his patients. When she questioned him, suggesting that she didn't want to be attached to a machine, he became irritated. She later said, "I got the distinct impression that somehow I cared less about my baby than a woman who would have agreed that monitoring was the best way to go. When I shared with him the information that a very good study showed no evidence of benefit to monitoring low-risk labors, he said he didn't believe in the study. The impression I came away with was that, somehow, I wasn't quite as concerned about my baby as I should have been."

The experience of childbirth for the woman is too often unimportant to the doctor. As one pediatrician told us, "It's okay for the doctor to follow the wishes of the patient when it doesn't make any difference one way or the other. But we need to communicate to the patient those things she wants to do that are dangerous."

When we discussed the results of our survey with a surgeon, he unknowingly summarized the belief system of obstetricians in terms of control when he said, "You may know what women want, but it may not be what they need." Doctors believe that they alone know what women need. During the course of our negotiations with our local hospital, we came up against this belief system many times. In one session, a local obstetrician told us, "You need to understand our point of view. We are interested in medical safety, not TLC."

If the experience of childbirth for the woman is too often unimportant, the doctor's comfort is not. Since he controls the situation, he becomes the key person in the whole experience. The kind of bed or delivery table used, the labor and delivery position of the woman, and the temperature of the delivery room are all designed to contribute to his convenience and comfort, not that of the mother-to-be or the newborn infant. A nurse who has worked in newborn intensive care units was discussing with an obstetrician whether the cool delivery room could be contributing to breathing distress in the newborn. She asked him who he felt was the most important in terms of comfort in the delivery room, the infant or him. He replied, "I am."

Because of obstetricians' unwillingness to give up some control, women have lost an option in maternity care. Until about the mid-1980s, some hospitals offered separate birth centers within the hospital in response to women's demands. These birth centers operated the same way freestanding birth centers do today. The doctor was a life-guard with a flexible philosophy of care that used little intervention. Safety and good outcomes were unmatched by the care on the regular obstetrical floor. While these alternative birth centers—or ABCs, as they were called—enhanced the woman's control of her birth, they reduced the doctor's control. Careful record keeping from the ABCs showed that obstetricians did not like this alternative, according to Madeleine Shearer, reporting in *Birth* journal. One by one, the ABCs closed down.

Michel Odent, former head of the Pithiviers Maternity Unit in France, writes in *Water and Sexuality*: "How can childbirth be controlled? This is the foremost question for doctors." Most obstetricians firmly believe that their control over decision-making is an important key to a safe birth. We have shared with you research showing that a woman's satisfaction in childbirth depends on her feelings of control, of mastery, of being part of the decisions about her care. These needs are in conflict with a doctor who wants no part of sharing in decisions regarding the birth. Control by the obstetrician is the toughest issue you will face in negotiations. He believes he knows what is best. You need to know how he defines "best." You need to find out how your doctor handles normal childbirth.

A *"safe birth" takes place in the hospital*. If you believe that the active management of labor is best for all mothers and babies, then the associated risks of intervention are much too great to take place anywhere other than in a hospital. In this and other countries, midwives and doctors who deliver women at home or in birth centers are doing sophisticated prenatal screening of pregnant women to identify those who are likely to develop complications that require regular hospital care. However, because of their own personal experience with sudden emergencies in the hospital, most obstetricians do not believe that successful screening is possible. Therefore they reject any kind of out-of-hospital delivery, whether in a freestanding birth center or at home. One of the "Standards for Safe Childbearing" of the American College of Obstetricians and Gynecologists is that all births occur in hospitals. The obstetrician's training affects him in this belief also. "From the first day of medical training, a modern obstetrician is programmed to believe that attempting a home birth is a dangerous and irresponsible act," says Bruce Flamm, author of *Birth After Cesarean: The Medical Facts*. So strong and irrational is this belief that state medical societies are spending large amounts of money and time to try to end homebirth by stopping direct-entry midwives. Lee Stewart, co-director of NAPSAC, confirmed for us that "midwives are under fire in many states. A new wave of problems is starting because state medical organizations are using their resources to go to state legislators to get medical practice acts rewritten to make direct-entry midwifery illegal."

A "safe birth" is attended by an obstetrician. Accepting the assumption that birth is a dangerous procedure that must be actively managed with risky interventions, you can understand why obstetricians feel they—not midwives or family practitioners—are the only ones qualified to attend the birth.

While a number of hospitals have certified nurse-midwives on their staffs, and growing numbers of health-care activists are lobbying hospitals to give certified nurse-midwives delivery privileges, many obstetricians are unaware of the high quality of care given by midwives. They are aware of the economic threat that the growing numbers of certified nurse-midwives present to their livelihood. In her article in *Medical Economics*, "How Fast Are Patients Abandoning Doctors for Midwives?", Laura Clark reports that the twenty-three nurse-midwives at Group Health Association in Washington, D.C., are seeing more women than the twenty-six ob/gyns in the group practice. She notes Kenneth Bell's research at the Kaiser Permanente Medical Center in Anaheim, California. Bell, medical director of the center, found that 75 percent of the women there chose a nurse-midwife or did not prefer an obstetrician. Clark quotes Ruth Lubic, director of the Maternity Center in New York City, to explain women's preference for midwives: "We're willing to share the control of the birth with the parents. I don't know a lot of doctors who are."

Clark notes that independent nurse-midwives will increasingly become competitive with obstetricians as women seek midwife care and as third-party payers recognize the lower costs of maternity care with midwives. ACOG is unhappy with that possibility, since ACOG policy supports "nurse-midwives when it is practiced as part of an OBG led team, but opposes CNMs going into independent practice."

Obstetricians feel uneasy about family practitioners, too. In the United States today, 75 percent of births are attended by obstetricians, 15 percent by family practitioners. In fact, the percentage of babies delivered by family practitioners has been steadily decreasing—down from 1968, when they delivered 31 percent of the babies born in the United States. Believing that the care that they give is superior to that of other birth attendants, obstetricians are passing around a catchy phrase that best describes their feelings toward family practitioners and midwives: "Why settle for a Ford when you can have a Cadillac?"

A "safe birlh" is measured solely in terms of whether or nol there is a live mother and a live baby. We all certainly agree with doctors that a live mother and baby are the foremost concern. When everything reasonable has been done and death still occurs, there is some solace in knowing that every safety precaution was followed. That's the reason we are going to the doctor in the first place. Obstetricians, however, justify their interventive measures on the basis of improved maternal and perinatal mortality rates. "It has been the sophisticated medical technology afforded by the fetal monitor and the cesarean section that has vaulted this country's [perinatal] mortality rate to the best in the world," said obstetrician William A. Cook. Proclaimed Clayton T. Beecham, at a Philadelphia meeting of ACOG: "By tolerating or encouraging 'natural childbirth' methods and the escalating use of midwives, American gynecologists and obstetricians could jeopardize the impressive decline in maternal mortality rates achieved in the past fifty years, which is directly linked to the spread of modern medical techniques in childbearing."

The obstetricians' keys to a "safe birth" (i.e., the birth is managed, predictable, and controlled by them; takes place in a hospital; and is attended by an obstetrician) are all justified because obstetricians believe their technology and interventions are the reasons for improved maternal and perinatal mortality rates—their overriding concern, their measure of success, and the justification for their belief in their activity as scientific. Let's closely examine that claim.

Maternal and Perinatal Mortality

Reasons for the Decrease

The maternal mortality rate is measured by the number of deaths of women per 100,000 live births. The maternal mortality rate has declined steadily since the beginning of this century, when more than 700 women died out of every 100,000 live births.

Year	Maternal Deaths per 100,000
1940	376
1950	83.1
1970	21.4
1980	9.2
1989	7.9

Perinatal mortality includes the deaths of fetuses from seven months of pregnancy through birth and to seven days of age of the baby. In other words, perinatal mortality measures deaths of babies around the time of birth. Perinatal mortality is so much higher than maternal mortality that it is measured per 1,000 births.

Year	Perinatal Deaths per 1,000
1960	28.9
1970	23.2
1980	12.8
1988	9.7

Obstetricians tend to claim most of the credit for the steadily decreasing maternal and perinatal mortality rates. Because the decreasing death rates are so impressive, obstetricians feeling that "what I'm doing must be the reason" might be easy to accept. But it's just not that simple.

The falling rates are due to complex interrelated factors having little to do with what obstetricians believe are the keys to a safe birth. For example, dramatic falls in the maternal mortality rates in the 1940s were aided by the development of antibiotics, which controlled infection, and by the development of blood banks, which allowed needed transfusions for the mother to survive a severe postpartum hemorrhage. It wasn't until 1950, according to Herbert Ratner, former director of public health in Chicago, that birthing women were free from pelvic bone abnormalities caused by rickets, which had been a major problem complicating births. With better nutrition—especially the addition of vitamin D to milk, which started in the 1930s—this was the first generation of women who could give birth without the complications of rickets and other diseases of malnutrition.

In those years, too, obstetricians were in the forefront of changing maternity care. Then, as now, most births were normal, that is, uncomplicated vaginal deliveries. Then, as now, complicated births (both vaginal and cesarean deliveries) resulted in the highest rates of maternal and perinatal mortality. Obstetricians made a major contribution to reducing mortality rates by starting to use—and by setting high standards for training in the use of—drugs, anesthetics, forceps, and IVs in the care of those complicated births. Ratner paints a dramatic picture of the obstetrician's role in reducing maternal mortality: "The actual fact is, and it must not be forgotten, that if it weren't for the contribution of obstetrical specialists, some of your mothers, and some of your grandmothers, would have died in childbirth and some of you in this audience would not be here today.... These specialists played an important role in the continuing reduction of preventable maternal deaths by reforming correctable professional and hospital practices." Obstetricians took the lead, and still do, in changing the care of complicated deliveries to make them safer for women.

Right up to the present many factors having nothing to do with labor and delivery affect maternal mortality rates, such as falling birthrates and the availability of family planning. "Some may argue that the improved statistics are due more to improved availability of family planning and abortion services," says Richard Aubry, co-director of the Perinatal Center, State University of New York, Syracuse. "However, it should be noted that a major part of the reduction in maternal mortality occurred before effective family planning was widely available [the sixties] and clearly well before the availability of abortion services [the seventies]." That's right. As shown in the maternal deaths chart, the giant drop occurred in the forties—long before the spread of technological interventions came to the ob floor.

The drop in perinatal mortality is also complex. The greatest cause of perinatal mortality in the United States today is the same as it has always been: respiratory distress syndrome, most often found in premature or low-birth-weight babies. Specialized pediatricians, called perinatologists, have reduced perinatal mortality by saving more babies born with complications and by saving smaller and smaller babies. "That newborn intensive care can lower mortality in low-birth-weight infants is widely accepted," reported Nigel Paneth, et al. in a special article for the *New England Journal of Medicine* in 1982. Over the rest of the 1980s other studies supported the idea that newborn intensive care is the important factor in the reduction of perinatal mortality.

Low birth weight remains the most significant factor, rising above all others affecting perinatal mortality. The major reasons for perinatal mortality in the United States were traced by researchers J. David Erickson and Tor Bjerkedal, who compared perinatal mortality in Norway and the United States and reported their findings in 1982. A high number of low-birth-weight babies born into economically deprived families is the major reason for the United States' perinatal mortality rate, "poor" in relation to Norway's, said the authors. They concluded that any major improvement in the U.S. rate will await a reduction in the births of low-birth-weight babies. A decade later the

United States continues to lag badly in reducing the numbers of low-birth-weight babies.

International Comparisons

Many factors affect mortality rates, so the rates alone can't be used to justify the way a baby is delivered. The mortality rates are useful in looking at differences in obstetrical care between countries.

The infant mortality rate is a different measure from perinatal mortality. Infant mortality measures the death of a live-born baby within the first year of life. For international comparisons it is the measure commonly used. The relative standing of the United States in comparison to other countries tells us how well we are doing. Though the infant-death rate for 1991 in the United States was the lowest in history—8.9 deaths per 1,000 live births—population experts call the rate high for an industrialized nation. The United States rate was higher than rates in most Western European countries.

One cultural group of Americans with little prenatal care, Hispanics, have a much lower infant mortality rate than African-Americans, who often lack prenatal care as well. Hispanic infant mortality is even slightly lower than that of white Americans, in a report from the National Center for Health Statistics (NCHS). Hispanic-Americans are the third-largest minority group in the United States. Despite a high rate of poverty and low use of prenatal care, their infant mortality rate for 1990 was nine deaths per 1,000 live births. Social support among members of the Hispanic community may be the reason, according to Joel Kleinman, analyst with the NCHS. Social support may be as simple as help with work and child care or emotional and financial assistance from family members and friends.

A program at the University of Rochester Medical School showed that fewer low-birth-weight babies were born to women with low income when they were given social support. Registered nurses visited pregnant women at home, gave them information on prenatal care, and helped them get the community services they needed. The nurses also helped each woman develop a supportive relationship with a friend or relative, and they continued their visits after birth. Not only were the babies born heavier, but their mothers were less likely to abuse or neglect them.

The U.S. Commission to Prevent Infant Mortality invited Marsden Wagner, European office representative of the World Health

Organization, to testify in 1988. Wagner outlined for the commission the WHO's major findings regarding the successful efforts of those European countries with the best record for lowering infant mortality.

Universal access to prenatal care is one of the four interrelated findings. The two factors during pregnancy most associated with low birth weight are smoking and a lack of social support for the woman. When prenatal care includes help for these factors, perinatal mortality is improved. Maternity protection is the next element in pregnancy and birth care in Europe. Protection includes pre- and postnatal paid maternity leave, regulations regarding working conditions, and nursing breaks for breastfeeding mothers.

Obstetrical interventions are far fewer in the countries with the best records. Wagner quoted other WHO officials: "Countries with some of the lowest perinatal mortality rates in the world have cesarean rates less than 10 percent." He noted that "the excess cesarean sections in the U.S." mean that "the U.S. is paying a considerable human price."

The final link in lowering infant mortality is midwifery. "In every European country practicing midwives far outnumber obstetricians," he testified. "Fundamental to the entire perinatal care system is that midwives provide the majority of pre-and postnatal care as well as being the principal birth attendant at uncomplicated births." The midwife has "a more social, non-interventionist, supportive approach. The physician's role is more interventionist and medical in nature. These two styles nicely complement each other."

Wagner summarized, "What is needed is less money spent on medically oriented prenatal care, more resources shifted to social and financial support and maternity benefits for families, far less money spent on interventionist obstetrical care and more resources put into building up a large, strong, independent midwifery profession."

Randomized Controlled Trials

What we know from looking at mortality rates is that obstetricians can't measure what they do in labor and delivery by using mortality rates (called "crude mortality rates"). They cannot say the dropping maternal and perinatal mortality rates are due to interventions such as using fetal monitors, Pitocin, cesareans, or other procedures. The active management of all births is an invention of the seventies, long after the greatest decreases began and continued in maternal mortality. Perinatal mortality was decreasing before the seventies too, and the decrease has many different reasons behind it. Current research clearly shows, however, that any major decreases in perinatal mortality will now come from prevention—reducing the large numbers of low-birth-weight babies in the United States.

Obstetricians call their tools beneficial, but can they prove it? They need to show the benefits, risks, and safety of each intervention by testing it separately. Much more research is needed to evaluate the interventions of obstetricians on the basis of whether the interventions are better for the mother and baby than when they are not used.

In 1977 Iain Chalmers and Martin Richards, British medical researchers, examined the tendency of obstetricians to claim their activities cause the falling maternal and perinatal mortality rates:

> One is left wondering how a profession which has always thought of itself as scientific could have remained complacent in the face of such haphazard changes in practice. Certainly the relative research design has been available for many years: Johnston and Sidall in 1922 allocated alternate women to experimental and control groups in a prospective study which failed to demonstrate any beneficial effect of perineal shaving prior to labor. The fact that these findings, although confirmed by subsequent research in 1965, do not seem to have a major impact on actual practice, raises the question of whether well-conducted research influences practice to a greater extent than opinion and anecdote.

The evaluation that the authors refer to is called "randomized controlled trial" (RCT), which shows whether a new way is better than the old way, and whether doing nothing is better than either the old or new way.

In the example given, women were assigned on a chance, or random, basis to either of two groups. In the first, "the experimental group," the women's perineal areas were shaved. In the second, "the control group," the women were not shaved. Although the reason usually given for the perineal shaving is that it reduces infection, there was a slightly higher infection rate for the experimental group (with perineum shaved). From several RCTs involving thousands of women, we know perineal shaving does not reduce infection.

The use of RCTs for the various interventions of the obstetrician would tell us whether any one intervention was of any benefit and what the risks were. A doctor can only claim to be scientific if he uses the scientific method in his practice; if he either carries out research using RCTs, or in his practice uses only those interventions that have been evaluated and proven beneficial. "What constitutes science is the use of scientific method and not the status or the hopes of its practitioners," says author M. D. Riley in *The Benefits and Hazards of the New Obstetrics*.

Diony Young, editor of *Birth* journal, reports, "In 1979 Archie Cochrane, former Director of the MRC Epidemiological Research Unit in Cardiff (Great Britain), threw down the gauntlet by giving the 'wooden spoon award' to obstetrics as the specialty that he believed demonstrated the worst use of randomized, controlled trials for evaluating the effectiveness of patient care and treatment."

An international team of researchers, Iain Chalmers, Murray Enkin, and Marc J. N. C. Keirse, took the challenge and spent ten years reviewing research to judge the effectiveness and safety of maternity care and practice. The team evaluated the best 3,000 clinical research studies from a complete review of sixty key journals published from 1950 on. They also wrote to 40,000 obstetricians and pediatricians in eighteen countries to find unpublished research. With many others' help, in 1989 the team put together an encyclopedia, *Effective Care in Pregnancy and Childbirth*.

A Guide to Effective Care In Pregnancy and Childbirth by Enkin, Keirse, and Chalmers, is a summary of the larger work, without references. Reviewer Henci Goer wrote, "You may be shocked to find what little evidence exists in support of most obstetric practices, and by how much of this evidence favors non- or at least cautiously-interventive management."

The authors give a list of types of care that should be abandoned based on the complete review of the obstetric literature. "Failing to involve women in decisions about their care" heads the list. Some others to abandon are: involving doctors in the care of all women during pregnancy; involving obstetricians in the care of all women during pregnancy; and insisting on universal institutional confinement (hospital birth). The obstetrician's beliefs about a safe birth are contradicted by the research evidence. (We will make other references to the guide as we show you that what obstetricians do is not scientific.)

7

The Obstetrician's Black Bag of Interventions

Jenny and Dick talked eagerly about their first baby due in a week. "It seems like we've waited so long for this," Jenny said. "We were married two years when we decided to have a baby, then it seemed to take forever to get pregnant!" she added, blushing now. "We've finished our Lamaze course," Dick broke in with a sparkle in his eyes. "I know we can use everything we learned." Jenny seemed to be reminding Dick when she said quietly, "Our teacher emphasized that this is not natural childbirth, and I shouldn't be a martyr. She said just enjoy it, and do whatever is best for the safe delivery of the baby."

As the days went by, and the due date came and went, Jenny became discouraged; it seemed so difficult to move around now. One week after her due date, she awakened slowly, aware that what woke her was a heaviness, a tensing in her lower abdomen that had come and gone several times before she was fully awake. Was this it? She glanced at the clock and saw that it was almost time to get up anyway, so she sat up and started timing her contractions. Disappointed, she noticed there wasn't much of a pattern—first ten minutes, then eight minutes, then twelve minutes. By now Dick was waking up, and he asked what she was doing. When he found out she was timing contractions, he jumped up and scurried around nervously getting ready. Jenny told him she didn't think it was labor. But within an hour the contractions had settled into a fairly regular pattern of every eight minutes, and she decided to call her doctor. He told her to come in since he was already at the hospital (it was seven A.M.). It sounded to him like she was probably in labor. Now they both really got excited. This was the big day! By the time they got to the hospital, it was eight o'clock. Jenny missed Dick, who had gone to sign her in, but she was busy undressing to get into bed. She was disappointed to find out from the nurse's examination that she was only two centimeters dilated. The contractions were already hard to handle, especially without Dick there.

Before the years of high-technology births, mothers-to-be were often sent back home if they came to the hospital in very early labor, as Jenny had. But sending a mother home once she comes to the hospital—even in very early labor—is now almost unheard of.

Laboring in Bed

The trouble began the moment we arrived. I was in very early labor so I wanted to keep walking and take a shower. The nurse told us that walking would slow labor and the best place for me was bed. I refused her advice and kept walking and took a shower.

—Colorado

This misinformed nurse doesn't know about the benefits of an upright position for labor. In most countries women in labor are encouraged to walk around or stay upright rather than go to bed. The false belief that women are safer in bed is common in North America.

No research shows any benefit in putting the laboring woman to bed. On the contrary, research shows a danger to the fetus when a mother labors on her back, and the benefits of a side-lying, upright, or walking position in labor. A world authority on the supine (or flat-on-the-back) labor and delivery position is Roberto Caldeyro-Barcia, director of the Latin American Center for Perinatology and Human Development of the World Health Organization (WHO) in Montevideo, Uruguay. He and later researchers, using randomized controlled trials, discovered that the supine position is the *worst* one for labor and delivery. It has the disadvantage of "adversely affecting pain and comfort, uterine activity and maintenance of normal blood pressure," says Frederic Ettner in *21st Century Obstetrics Now!* A drop in the mother's blood pressure affects the circulation of blood within the uterus, resulting in poor oxygen supply for the unborn baby. Caldeyro-Barcia states, "Except for being hanged by the feet, the supine position is the worst conceivable position for labor and delivery."

The upright position, with the assistance of gravity, increases the strength of contractions and dilates the cervix faster. Women report less pain in the upright position. There is also less need to use drugs to speed up labor, or relieve pain, and babies are in better condition at birth. Finally, women *like* being upright. According to Caldeyro-Barcia, 95 percent of women given a choice choose to be upright.

Nurse-midwife Katherine Camacho Carr reviewed the medical and cross-cultural literature on a woman's position in labor and birth. When the upright position is used, labor is much shorter than in the supine position. Standing, strolling, sitting, kneeling, or on hands and knees are the ways for a woman to labor upright. In terms of efficiency of contractions and shortening of labor, Carr's review concludes there is an order from best to worst for labor position:

1. Walking or standing
2. Side-lying
3. Sitting
4. Lying down or lying in a semi-sitting, propped position

Joyce Roberts, *et al.* reviewed the literature for randomized controlled trials of labor positions and concluded that changing position throughout labor is as important for good contractions as using the upright or side-lying position. Childbirth educator Janet Balaskas was one of a group of British women who, recognizing the benefits of active birth in upright positions, founded the Active Birth Movement in 1982. Putting her experience and wisdom into print, Balaskas wrote *Active Birth*, in which she explains the benefits and how-to's of active birth using movement and upright positions.

> *By now Dick was back with Jenny, trying to get her back in control, helping her with her slow breathing, encouraging her to relax. At this point the nurse came in with some equipment and asked Dick to leave. Jenny felt miserable and embarrassed as she submitted to the prep and enema and the procedure to put an IV opening in the back of her left hand—"just in case," the nurse said. Jenny realized that her contractions were not regular at all now, sometimes very mild, sometimes a little uncomfortable. Jenny was still at two centimeters dilation.*

All About IVs

In most other industrialized countries, a normal laboring woman is allowed to eat and drink lightly. In the United States, however, most laboring women are forbidden any nourishment during labor. The woman is required to fast "just in case" of an emergency that would require general anesthesia. Unconscious under the anesthesia, this thinking goes, she may vomit and inhale the fluids—and may die. However, the responsibility for observing the unconscious woman rests with the anesthesiologist sitting at her head, who can quickly turn her head if she vomits, thus avoiding any peril.

An IV, or intravenous pathway, is inserted in a laboring woman's arm. This gives a quick means of giving anesthesia, drugs, or blood during emergency surgical intervention. Fluids may also be given through the IV to sustain a woman fasting through a long labor. The most common use of the IV, however, is for giving Pitocin, either to induce labor or to speed it up.

No research shows that an IV needs to be used before an emergency or that having an IV in place in a normal laboring woman has made a difference in an emergency. Hospital ob nurses and birth attendants know how to start an IV quickly when needed. Also, an IV has risks. It ties the woman down during her labor when she needs to be active. She may develop an infection from the IV. Either IV fluids or the "nothing by mouth" rule for a laboring woman can lead to abnormal blood chemistry, a condition that puts the unborn baby at risk.

More U.S. hospital staffs are recognizing the benefits of encouraging a woman with a normal labor to drink and eat lightly, according to Charlotte Elsberry, director of Midwifery Services at North Central Bronx Hospital. This hospital's policy is longstanding in allowing self-regulation of nourishment during a normal labor, Elsberry told us. In a demonstration review of this policy in 1989, Elsberry reported that those women who nourished themselves at home during labor were likely to come to the hospital in more active labor than women who did not take nourishment. Women who do self-regulate their nourishment know what, or if, they need to eat and drink during labor, she told us.

Preps

A prep is the shaving of the perineal or pubic area, a procedure that more than half of American women giving birth routinely undergo as part of being admitted to the hospital. When women question the use of a prep they are told that it reduces infection. Research in the 1960s, using randomized controlled trials involving 7,600 women giving birth, showed that the infection rate was lower among those who were *not* shaved, however.

Enemas

Although enemas are still a routine part of hospital admissions for over half of laboring women, no research proves any medical benefits. Many mothers experience a natural bowel cleansing in labor; they may have several bowel movements over a period of minutes or hours as the baby moves down in the pelvis. Some birth attendants believe this cleansing gives the baby more room in the mother's pelvis. If a mother does not have this natural diarrhea, she may feel more comfortable having an enema. Also a fear of passing feces with pushing contractions may inhibit some women who have not had an enema. These possible benefits suggest the choice of an enema should be left up to the laboring woman. "Shaving the perineum routinely prior to delivery and administering enemas or suppositories routinely during labor are forms of care that should be abandoned in light of the available evidence," say Enkin, Keirse, and Chalmers, authors of *Effective Care in Pregnancy and Childbirth*.

Jenny had now been at the hospital two hours, and her contractions were becoming weak and irregular. The doctor examined her for the first time and found she was still at two centimeters dilation. He said he was going to break the amniotic sac "to get things moving." Jenny didn't feel anything, just a little wetness between her legs. However, within minutes, her contractions became strong again, and she needed Dick to help her with her breathing. Dick, feeling anxious now that he was doing the real thing and not just practicing, worked with Jenny, reminding her to take her cleansing breath at the beginning and end of the contractions.

Amniotomy

Amniotomy is the deliberate breaking of the bag of waters surrounding the baby. The nurse or doctor uses a blunt, sterile instrument that looks like a long crochet hook to puncture the amniotic sac. Amniotomy is so common in laboring women in hospitals that few nurses and doctors have ever seen a laboring woman with a bag of waters intact during late labor or delivery.

Amniotomy is done to speed up labor, to induce labor (usually accompanied by Pitocin), to get the bag of waters out of the way to apply the electrode to the fetal scalp, necessary when using an internal fetal monitor, and to test the fluid. Early research showed that amniotomy may reduce labor time by half an hour to an hour. In 1991 the only randomized control trial done showed no evidence that amniotomy reduced labor time. Until we can get much more research, the benefits of an intact bag of waters are significant.

Before rupture, the bag of waters provides a cushion of even pressure from contractions, and protection from excessive molding of the head as the baby moves through the mother's pelvis. After rupture, the pressures on the baby's head during contractions are direct and uneven. Also, the umbilical cord can be compressed, sometimes denying the baby necessary oxygen.

Levy *et al.* studied 29,960 deliveries at the University of Colorado Health Sciences Center. The authors were concerned that out of 79 cases of cord prolapse (when a loop of cord emerges before the baby does), ten happened because of amniotomy. Although cord prolapse is uncommon, it is a serious complication. The added risk of cord prolapse from amniotomy led the authors to caution caregivers about this intervention. "I didn't know, when I was an intern, about the literature showing that the amniotic fluid protects the head," a family practitioner told us. "To me it was just something that was in the way, and the sooner you ruptured the membranes, the better off you were."

When the bag of waters is not ruptured artificially, 95 percent of women who start labor spontaneously at full term, and have uncomplicated, unmedicated labors, will have the bag of waters intact until very late in labor or even during delivery. This provides a significant measure of protection to the baby and to the baby's lifeline, the umbilical cord. Most women who have their bag of waters rupture naturally—even in early labor—can have normal labor and deliveries. However, whenever possible, it seems reasonable to allow the extra margin of safety the intact bag of waters provides. There is a direct benefit to the mother, too, since the longer her bag of waters is intact, the lower her risk of infection is. "Avoiding amniotomy would probably reduce many of the abnormal factors seen so often in labors, including severe drops in fetal pH, cord compression, infections, and increased numbers of cesarean sections," says Katherine Camacho Carr, reviewing obstetric practices that protect the unborn baby during labor and birth in the journal *Birth*.

Within a few minutes of the amniotomy, two nurses came in pushing a large machine, the electronic fetal monitor. They had Jenny spread her legs again so they could screw the electrode to the baby's scalp. Dick was fascinated by the machine, by the colors and sounds—the winking and blinking of the lights. He felt they certainly were receiving the best in care. The only problem Jenny noticed was that whenever the nurse came into the room, she went straight to the fetal monitor as if Jenny were no longer there. The nurse didn't ask anymore how Jenny felt.

Electronic Fetal Monitoring

Fetal monitoring is keeping track of the baby's heartbeat as a means of measuring how the baby is doing and showing a possible need for intervention. Traditionally, the nurse listened to the baby's heartbeat with a stethoscope (auscultation). In the seventies a substitute for auscultation came into use. Originally intended for high-risk laboring women, electronic fetal monitoring (EFM) is now used almost universally in the United States.

There are two kinds of EFM, external and internal. *External* electronic monitoring is indirect monitoring that picks up the fetal heart rate by the use of constant ultrasound waves. The external monitor is considered less accurate than the internal monitor in measuring the fetal heart rate.

The *internal* fetal monitor measures the fetal heart rate directly by an electrode inserted in the baby's scalp, and measures the mother's uterine contractions by a catheter placed just inside the uterus. Electronic fetal monitoring is high technology with beeps and readouts that seduce you into believing you're getting useful information. For some onlookers, the machine is mesmerizing. "It is almost like watching television to stand in a labor room and watch this monitor," says Madeleine Shearer in *Birth* journal. "The paper comes out and lies in folds in the drawer of the cabinet upon which the machine is set. A lighted green window up on the left of the monitor has an oscilloscope display of the fetal heart pattern. Then right next to that is a digital display in red, the numbers constantly flickering with each beat of the heart. I stand and watch and think to myself, 'How could I possibly question this advanced technological breakthrough in obstetrics?' Just the added information alone must be worth the effort."

Many, if not most, obstetricians wholeheartedly believe in EFM. They see EFM as useful, proven, and therefore essential for assessing fetal well-being. EFM definitely gives a much more accurate measure of the fetal heart rate. The problem is the interpretation of all that data.

One extensive study comparing universal EFM with selective use of EFM, and eight randomized controlled trials of EFM versus auscultation, give clear answers. The use of EFM does not reduce perinatal mortality, reduce the number of low Apgar scores, or reduce admissions to intensive care nurseries. The use of EFM does increase the use of operative delivery, either by forceps or cesarean, and in some studies greatly increases cesareans.

Commenting on his own coauthorized study of 34,995 women in Dallas, Kenneth Leveno said in 1986, "With electronic monitoring, we were identifying more abnormal heart rates that led to more cesarean sections, and the result was that the babies' outcome was no different." The problem was that the fetal monitors "do not precisely identify the baby in distress all the time. Most children with abnormal fetal heart rates are really in good condition."

In their summary of the monitoring trials reported in *Lancet* in 1987, A. Prentice and T. Lind agreed with this assessment: "Interpretation of the wealth of information is still difficult and many mothers will have operative deliveries for 'distressed' babies who show no such distress at birth." They noted that van den Berg *et al.* reported that 71 to 95 percent of babies diagnosed as distressed during labor did not have that diagnosis confirmed at birth. The good condition of the babies at birth means that the original reading of fetal distress ("positive reading") was a "false positive": The fetuses were diagnosed as distressed when they were not. Most of those babies in such good condition at birth were born by cesarean when they could have been born vaginally.

Originally intended for high-risk labors, particularly premature labors, EFM was finally studied in that group. Kirkwood Shy *et al.* compared EFM to auscultation in premature infants in a multicenter, randomized controlled trial. The authors reported that "electronic fetal monitoring does not result in improved neurologic development in children born prematurely."

Fetal scalp sampling is encouraged by some obstetricians to verify a monitor's readout of fetal distress. This involves taking a sample of blood from the unborn baby's scalp. If the sample is normal, the obstetrician can have confidence the baby is not distressed. Fetal scalp sampling has reduced the problem of using EFM alone. But researchers have shown the same problems with fetal scalp sampling as with EFM: Sometimes there is indication of a distressed fetus when the baby is normal. Writing in the *New England Journal of Medicine*, Emanuel Friedman concluded, "The promise of such major technological advances as continuous electronic monitoring of the fetal heart rate and fetal-scalp blood sampling has not been fulfilled."

Bowing to the avalanche of data, the American College of Obstetricians and Gynecologists recognized that auscultation is as effective as EFM in monitoring low- or high-risk labors. For high-risk labors, ACOG recommends auscultation every fifteen minutes during the first stage of labor and every five minutes during the delivery stage. For low-risk labors, the recommendation is auscultation every thirty minutes during the first stage and every fifteen minutes during delivery.

Doctors do not believe there are enough nurses in hospitals to give the one-to-one care necessary to regularly monitor the baby's heartbeat with a fetoscope. Researcher Judith Lumley of Queen Victoria Medical Center in Melbourne, Australia, described it as "sobering" that the United States, "the richest country in the world [is] unable to provide women giving birth with the necessary one-to-one care."

The widespread use of EFM in the United States is the best example of the unscientific nature of American obstetrics. Auscultation will be discouraged because doctors and hospitals have decided to use and promote EFM, and they have the power, according to Lumley. In her article, "The Irresistible Rise of Electronic Fetal Monitoring," she quotes another writer describing the stages of medical innovation: "The success of an innovation has little to do with its intrinsic worth (whether it is measurably effective as determined by controlled experimentation) but is dependent upon the power of the interests that sponsor and maintain it, despite the absence or inadequacy of empirical support."

The risks of *external* monitoring to the baby involve the unknown effects of the use of constant ultrasound. The risks to the mother include intervention in a normal labor because of the unreliability of the reading or because of a "false positive" reading. She is put to bed and told to lie quietly when freedom of movement is important to a normal laboring woman. If you feel you cannot avoid the external monitor, lie on your side during use and *ask* if you can have the monitor removed after a normal reading is established in ten to twenty minutes.

The risks to the baby of the *internal* monitor include the loss of protection of the bag of waters because of amniotomy, as well as injuries from misplacing the scalp electrode, infections, and (rarely) death due directly to infection from the scalp electrode. The mother has a risk of greater infection rates, possibly from early amniotomy (required for the internal monitor) or increased internal examinations. She, too, loses her freedom of movement, feeling tethered to the bed. In addition are the problems of starting her on the road to active medical management of labor and delivery, and an increased likelihood of having a cesarean.

"Fetal distress" (often a false positive reading) is not the only likely cause for a cesarean in women who use internal fetal monitors; "failure to progress" in labor is the most common reason for a cesarean when EFM is used ("fetal distress" is second), according to Havercamp *et al.* in 1979, and Minkoff and Schwarz in 1980.

The two diagnoses of failure to progress and fetal distress are very important in the increasing rate of cesareans (see next chapter). Because of this, and because auscultation is as good or better than EFM, you need to find out if your chosen birthplace can give you the recommended nurse fetal monitoring. This demands a high degree of one-to-one nurse-patient contact for laboring women in hospitals, and many hospitals do not have adequate staff to do that. If your hospital is understaffed, consider hiring a private-duty nurse (a monitrice) to give you the nursing care you need.

At noon, when the nurse came in to check the fetal monitor, she also gave Jenny another exam and remarked, "You certainly are not cranked up yet; you're just three centimeters." Those had to be about the most discouraging words Jenny had ever heard. When the doctor suggested that a "little" Pitocin would make Jenny's labor more normal, Jenny readily agreed. The nurse pulled in a stand with a bottle on a six-foot pole and quickly got the "Pit" going since the IV was already in place. Jenny felt an immediate change in the contractions. They seemed much closer and more intense. Dick redoubled his efforts to help her stay in control, massaging her arms and legs, and lightly stroking her tummy. Soon the contractions were three minutes apart and sixty seconds long, and getting harder to cope with. Jenny switched to accelerated breathing. The nurse came in about every fifteen minutes now, and several times made an adjustment in the IV that increased the Pitocin drops flowing into Jenny's hand.

Induction and Augmentation of Labor

Induction of labor means to start labor artificially. Augmentation of labor means to speed up a labor that has started naturally. "I have seen hundreds of deliveries screwed up because of unnecessary intervention," said one nurse interviewed by writer Judith Glassman. "In many hospitals 60 percent of labors are chemically induced or stimulated even though Pitocin often causes overly strong contractions, as well as blood pressure problems in both mother and child. It's just easier for the doctor to administer Pitocin than to supply emotional support."

In the medical management of labor and delivery, the usual way to artificially begin labor is to break the bag of waters and start the intravenous administration of Pitocin. Many doctors believe induction should be done only when the risk of continuing the pregnancy is greater than the risk of inducing labor and delivery. The conditions where continuing the pregnancy presents a threat to the life or well-being of mother and baby include severe blood incompatibility between mother and fetus, some severe diabetics, severe preeclampsia, severe high blood pressure, kidney disease, and an overdue pregnancy (postmaturity) where a danger to the fetus has been *proven*. If induction of labor were carried out only when these conditions were present, Caldeyro-Barcia estimates that, at most, 3 percent of births would be induced. Iain Chalmers and Martin Richards, writing in *The Benefits and Hazards of the New Obstetrics*, concluded, "It has not been possible to demonstrate any striking advantage or disadvantage of a widened use of the induction of labor. The truth of the matter is that we are ignorant about the circumstances in which the benefits of induction outweigh the disadvantages and are likely to remain so using the research techniques employed so far."

Intervening to speed up a labor begun naturally is much more common than induction. Estimates of augmentation range up to 60 percent of all labors that start spontaneously. "We used to have women laboring twenty-four, forty-eight, and even seventy-two hours!" an obstetrician told us. "We won't allow that anymore. I don't think augmentation is overused." Speeding up the labor goes along with the belief that the states of normal labor must fit within a carefully defined standard of time. "Shortening the phases of normal labor when there is no sign of fetal distress has not been shown to improve infant outcome," says Doris Haire, president of the American Foundation of Maternal and Child Health.

Pitocin is a synthetic version of the hormone oxytocin, which is produced in the body of the laboring woman and is one factor in the progress of her labor. Pitocin is usually (but not always) highly effective in beginning or speeding up labor, as many of you reading this book can testify. If Pitocin must be used, administration through an IV is preferred, because it offers the best means to control the dosage over a period of time.

However, even the most careful administration of Pitocin simply does not duplicate naturally occurring labor. This is because the progress of labor is under the dual control of the baby and the mother. The complex chemical and hormonal interrelationship of the mother and baby in starting and continuing labor is still not clearly understood; but we do know that it is impossible to reproduce normal labor. Mothers given Pitocin often describe the contractions as being longer and stronger, and with a shorter period between contractions, than those they experienced in unaugmented labor.

> I tried to put a good face on it and handle the contractions, but my body was being forced to do something it just wasn't ready to do. I kept wondering what was wrong with me that I felt totally out of control. It never occurred to me until recently that there was nothing wrong with me...that it was the Pitocin and that my body couldn't handle it because my body wasn't *doing* it.
>
> —New Hampshire

During both normal and induced or augmented labor the blood supply to the uterus (and therefore the oxygen supply to the baby) is temporarily reduced. With normal contractions, however, there is time between contractions to allow the baby's blood to be well oxygenated, to enable him to "hold his breath," so to speak, during the next contraction. In induced or stimulated labor, the baby's oxygen supply can be shortchanged in two ways. The time between contractions is shorter; there is less time to oxygenate his blood between contractions. Also, the contractions are longer; the fetus goes for a longer period of time before he receives a full supply of oxygen. For the unborn baby, it can be like being pushed into a swimming pool before he has had a chance to catch his breath, and then having someone push him down deeper, just when he had bobbed to the surface for much-needed air. This possibility of an inadequate oxygen supply for the baby is one reason that all induced or augmented labors are considered at risk for developing complications.

Research shows the most significant risks of either induction or augmentation of labor to be:

For mother:
- Higher rate of complicated labors and deliveries

- More use of analgesia or anesthesia because of the intensity of the contractions
- Postpartum hemorrhage (induction only; there has been no research to determine if hemorrhage is associated with augmentation of labor)
- Higher rate of ruptured uterus and placental separation, which may lead to the death of the mother or baby

For baby:
- Fetal distress
- Higher rate of jaundice in the newborn
- Greater chance of a premature baby (induction only; why all induced labors are "high risk")
- Low Apgar scores at five minutes
- Permanent central nervous system or brain damage
- Fetal death

In "An American Warning," which she wrote for a British childbirth journal, Doris Haire asks why the U.S. Food and Drug Administration has ignored the lack of studies on the long-term consequences of Pitocin and other obstetric drugs. She suggests a link between Pitocin use during a woman's labor and later problems in her child. "Our U.S. Department of Health and Human Services estimates that one out of every nine American children is significantly learning disabled despite having normal intelligence. 75% of these children are born at full term into middle and upper class families. Our National Institutes of Health estimates that 75% to 85% of all disabled children in the U.S. were born within the normal range of birth weight and gestational age and had no familial or sociological predisposing factors," she writes.

While there is consensus that the risks of Pitocin are worth taking when continuing the pregnancy would be life threatening, there is no evidence that benefits outweigh risks in the vast majority of inductions and augmentations being done. "The timing of spontaneous delivery is controlled by complex mechanisms which are still incompletely understood . . . and which have as their end point the delivery [of the baby when] survival of the newborn is most likely," said an editor of *Lancet*.

Enkin, Keirse, and Chalmers, in *A Guide to Effective Care in Pregnancy and Childbirth*, say, "From the data thus far, it does not appear that liberal use of oxytocin augmentation in labor is of benefit to the women and babies so treated. Simple measures, such as allowing the woman freedom to move around, and to eat and drink as she pleases, may be at least as effective and certainly more pleasant for a sizable proportion of women considered to be in need of augmentation of labor."

The first randomized control trial (RCT) of Pitocin versus the upright position was finally done in 1980 at the Los Angeles County/University of Southern California Medical Center. This RCT studied the effectiveness of Pitocin versus the upright position in reviving stalled labors. Women whose labors had slowed were randomly assigned to one of two groups. In the first, women were given the usual routine of Pitocin. In the second group, women were not given Pitocin; instead, they stayed out of bed, either walking, standing, or sitting. The study showed stimulation of labor was more effective by using the upright position than by using Pitocin.

> *Jenny, scared, began to complain about the contractions. They were more overwhelming than painful. The tremendous sensations she felt in her lower body were unlike anything she had ever felt before. It seemed to take too much effort to stay in control, to work with her body; otherwise there was pain. "I wish there was more time in between. It seems like only a few seconds from the time one is over until another one starts. They hurt." At this point the nurse returned to check Jenny and said that things seemed to be on track now, that she had dilated a centimeter in the last hour and was now four centimeters dilated. Jenny's contractions were now every two minutes and she thought, "I think I need the anesthesia now, I can't take this if it's going to get worse than this." She told Dick she needed something, and he rang for the nurse. The nurse said, "I'll let the doctor know." A half hour later the doctor arrived to give Jenny an epidural injection, remarking, "If I were having a baby, I'd want an epidural as soon as I could." He added, however, that four centimeters was about the earliest he felt he could give an epidural. Within fifteen minutes, Jenny became talkative and could hardly feel the pain. She felt good about being able to talk coherently to her husband now without grimacing with discomfort.*

Pain Control

Enkin, Keirse, and Chalmers describe many comfort and pain-control measures for the laboring woman that are harmless to her baby. Maternal movement and position change, touch and massage, use of heat or cold, baths and showers, acupressure, visualization, self-hypnosis, music, and more—all are listed as potential aids to reducing pain. In *Easing Labor Pain*, Adrienne Lieberman gives the reader clear information on how to use each of these comfort measures. Most of our readers have used one or more for their births and have found that the comfort measures assisted their labors.

> I was stuck at six centimeters after more than twelve hours of labor. I had been given Pitocin and amniotomy already, so they were talking c/section. My doula arrived and we asked the nurses to leave to have privacy. She led me in a 45-minute meditation and visualization and gave me some acupressure. When the nurses came back to check me, I was nine-plus centimeters dilated. They were so impressed they offered to leave again.
>
> —Colorado

Drug control of pain is the overwhelming method offered in hospitals. Obstetric pain medications for labor are drugs given by mouth or injection. Anesthetics are drugs administered by injection to obliterate sensation. *Analgesia* is a medical term covering any drug administered for pain. Epidurals are sometimes called "epidural analgesia."

Obstetric drug use in the United States is very widespread. National data of use are incomplete, but comprehensive reports from many hospitals indicate that almost all (80 to 98 percent of birthing women, depending on the hospital) receive medication, anesthesia, or both. Even taking into account the very high cesarean rate in hospitals, that compares very unfavorably to freestanding birth centers where drug analgesia is used sparingly and women are very satisfied with their care.

Almost all birth attendants agree that in complicated deliveries, whether vaginal or cesarean, drug use is beneficial because it sedates or anesthetizes a woman so that essential interventions can be carried out. The disagreement comes in deciding whether the birth attendant may, by intervening, be *causing* complications. In hospital settings the complication, intervention, and drug-use rates are much higher than in alternative settings. The excellent outcomes for mother and baby in alternative settings show us that complications—and the need for intervention—can be avoided in most births.

The evidence suggests that for normal mothers and their babies, the risks of heavy medication and any anesthesia outweigh the only benefit—pain control for the mother—especially when harmless comfort measures have not been tried. The comfort measures require time and effort, often of someone other than the woman's partner. The high-tech management of birth gives priority to drug use, and the ready availability and marketing of epidural anesthesia is probably the reason it is now used in almost every hospital birth with twenty-four-hour anesthesia coverage.

Epidural Anesthesia

"Epidural anesthesia has become a valuable marketing tool for hospitals trying to lure pregnant women to their facility to deliver their children," says Margery Simchak, a childbirth educator who has made herself an expert in understanding epidurals. Responding to obstetricians' demands for twenty-four-hour anesthesia availability, many hospital administrators hired anesthesiologists. "To staff a unit 24 hours a day, the hospital usually needed at least three doctors," reports Simchak. "Administrators soon discovered that three doctors' salaries plus the cost of their liability insurance created a negative cash flow if the doctors administered epidurals only for cesareans. Thus the marketing began."

The marketing is directed at the pregnant woman, and "in many cases it is carried out through hospital-based childbirth classes," Simchak confirms. "The educator is sometimes required to include in the class series an anesthesiologist who explains the wonders of epidurals. Some hospitals send epidural booklets to pre-registered women hailing the advantages of the procedure and minimizing its side effects."

> I have launched into a quest to discover why it is I was brainwashed into not trusting the way God created my body to birth. Women are taught that childbearing is *dangerous*. Hospital "birth class" was a $50, six-week session designed to scare women into submitting to the staff's intervention. The class was very slanted. Epidurals were prearranged, as well as mild pressure not to nurse. After all, "most women want to sleep, not to feed the first few days."
>
> —Michigan

The anesthesiologist's power and the pressure on nurses to conform is huge. Emily Aldrich, a childbirth activist in Connecticut, reports that as she talks to women about epidurals, they tell her no nurse wanted to risk telling the truth about the anesthesia. "The women would ask the nurses about the risks and the nurses wouldn't answer," Aldrich told us.

A nurse volunteered to us that another nurse in her hospital was "let go" because of pressure on the administration by anesthesiologists incensed that she publicized information critical of epidurals. Doctors feel that only they are qualified to discuss epidurals, but the information given is slanted to encourage the use of epidurals for their own and the hospital's benefit.

A childbirth educator told us that when she speaks to nurses at workshops, she frequently finds that they have never heard of the effects of medications and anesthesia on the infant, in particular of epidurals. They don't know that the drugs in an epidural cross the placenta to the baby.

Most nurses readily encourage epidurals because they make their jobs easier. James Thorp, a researcher in obstetrics, described in *Birth* journal the part nurses play in encouraging epidural use. "It is quite alarming to see how nurses and physicians rely on epidural analgesia in labor. Many nurses who practice in institutions where it is the preferred analgesia have lost their clinical ability to coach and assist a patient through labor without an epidural, and become noticeably uncomfortable when asked to do so. It is much easier for a nurse to call anesthesia and see the patient smiling during labor than it is for her to stay at the woman's bedside and help her through an uncomfortable labor. At many institutions the rule rather than the exception is a call from the nurse in early labor asking, 'Doctor, *when* can I call anesthesia for Mrs. Smith's epidural?'"

In general, women believe epidurals are safe for their babies. They hear it or read it in the media. Television personalities talk of being assured by their obstetricians that epidural drugs will not reach or harm their babies, report Doris Haire and Trisha Thompson. David Stewart of NAPSAC suggests that when offered drugs of any kind in labor, women should ask:

- What is it for?
- Will it hurt me or my baby?
- If not, please put that in writing.
- If yes, what warrants such a risk to the baby?

Iain Chalmers faults women, the media, and doctors for the use of epidural anesthesia without adequate research. "The introduction of epidural block for pain relief during labor provides an example of an intervention that, before adequate evaluation of its effects, was actively sought by many women, actively promoted by the media, and willingly provided by many doctors. Like the introduction of twilight sleep in the 1920s and 1930s, epidural anesthesia was introduced into obstetrics as a massive and poorly controlled experiment," he wrote in 1991 in *Birth* journal. "Unfortunately, because of the manner in which women and professionals adopted epidural block in obstetrics, we have almost no properly controlled evidence to address these important uncertainties about its effects."

Here is most of what we do know about epidurals from the obstetrical literature.

- For nearly all women, they obliterate the sensations of labor and delivery. Occasionally the block is incomplete.
- Continuous electronic fetal monitoring is almost always used.
- An IV must be used.
- The woman must stay in bed, losing her ability to be active and limiting the positions she may assume.
- Pitocin is frequently given at the same time for slowed labors.
- They can lower the woman's blood pressure and put the woman and infant at risk.
- The relaxation of the woman's pelvic muscles that epidurals bring may prevent those muscles from assisting in the usual rotation of the fetus as it moves to a normal birth position.
- The urge and ability to push may be reduced or extinguished.
- They more than double the use of instrument delivery and more than triple the use of midforceps delivery because the baby has not rotated normally or the mother cannot push (Kaminski *et al., Obstetrics and Gynecology* 69:770 [1987]).
- They increase the cesarean likelihood due to "failure to progress" in women giving birth for the first time at least two- to threefold; cesareans are at least six times more common for failure to progress in women giving birth for the first time if the epidural is given before 5 centimeters of dilation and the woman's dilation is slower than average (Thorp *et al.,* presentation at 1989 *Birth* journal conference).
- Failure to progress is the most common reason for a first-time cesarean.

- Persistent, chronic backache is significantly greater among women who have epidurals during labor (MacArthur *et al.*, *British Medical Journal* 301:9–12 [1990]).
- Serious, nonfatal complications (cardiac arrest, spinal damage, toxic reactions, and prolonged severe headache) associated with epidural anesthesia in women occur in the range of one per 10,000 deliveries (Scott and Hibbard, *British Journal of Anesthesiology* 64:537–41 [1990]).
- Narcotics are now being given at the same time to strengthen its effect.
- Narcotics are known to cause breathing problems in infants when given within several hours of birth.
- All drugs cross the placenta and affect the baby.
- When the cord is cut, the infant is left with trace amounts of any drugs that were being given to the mother at the time of birth.
- The infant's immature organs must detoxify the drugs.
- The infant's immature brain can be affected by his mother's drug use in labor and delivery.

We don't know the short- and long-term effects of the epidural on the infant. In the past, those of us who had babies born with and without drugs were sure we saw differences in the muscle control, responsiveness, and sucking of our drugged and undrugged babies; nurses and doctors have told us they have seen these differences, too. Chele Marmet, coordinator of the UCLA Clinic Lactation Program at the Department of Pediatrics and director of the Lactation Institute, has seen an increase in sucking problems in newborns. "I suspect one of the reasons we see so many babies today with sucking problems is because of the frequent use of epidural anesthesia," she told us. "I would like to see research into this problem."

Oxytocin naturally produced in a woman's body increases during labor, "reaching a peak just before the expulsive stage in both the mother and fetus," reported psychologist Niles Newton in her talk, "Oxytocin, the Hormone of Love," at the 1991 La Leche League International Conference. Oxytocin is crucial to the progress of labor, to the pushing stage, and in the attachment process between mother and baby after birth, she said. She called for immediate research to study the possibility that epidural anesthesia reduces oxytocin production in the mother, and she referred to an animal study that showed the animals did not bond well to their babies immediately after birth when epidural anesthesia was given more than ten minutes before delivery. Animal research has also shown a reduction in oxytocin levels in animals given an episiotomy (which reduces the stretching of the vagina). Newton linked these animal studies to raise the question of whether epidurals and episiotomies also reduce oxytocin levels in humans.

Selma Taffel *et al.*, researchers with the National Center for Health Statistics, reported in *Birth* journal in 1989 that "there has been a steady decline in one minute Apgar" scores of 9 or 10 in the United States in the past decade, and it is suspected that this may be associated with the concomitant increase in the number of cesarean sections performed." When we spoke with Taffel, she said the decline in Apgar scores is certain, but no one knows why. We would like to see research to find the cause of the decline and to determine whether epidurals, Pitocin, and cesareans, all of which show dramatic increases in use in that decade, are to blame.

Long-Term Drug Effects on Infants

The results of older research on the effects of drugs, either medications or anesthesia, on the newborn are frightening. Yvonne Brackbill and her associates have done the most comprehensive research on the short- and long-term effects on infants whose mothers were given drugs during labor and delivery. Esther Conway and Brackbill, working through the University of Denver, showed that obstetric drugs impaired the muscular, visual, and neural development of the baby two to five days postpartum.

Later, Brackbill, then research professor of psychology and obstetrics and gynecology at the University of Florida, reported on the lasting behavioral effects of obstetric drugs on children to the Food and Drug Administration. Brackbill reviewed forty-one studies on obstetric drugs and infant/child behavior. All but two of the studies found significant drug effect. Brackbill reported four key findings from the studies. First, obstetric drugs affect the child's behavior negatively (they interfere with normal function). Second, the behavioral effects are dose related; that is, the stronger the drug and the larger the dose, the greater the behavioral effect. Third, "At all ages,

---

*A measurement of baby's health in the minutes following birth, with 1 being poor health and 10 being excellent.

the effects are more clearly visible when the tasks are difficult, that is, when they require the child to exert itself to make an effort to cope with problems." And fourth, the behavioral effects of obstetrical drugs persist for years.

Working with Sarah Broman, a psychologist at the National Institutes of Health, Brackbill analyzed data from a study of 53,000 women who gave birth at twelve different teaching hospitals from 1959 through 1966. Broman and Brackbill studied the data on the 3,500 women in the project who were the *healthiest* and who had the *most uncomplicated* pregnancies, labors, and deliveries, trying to rule out the possibility that any results showing damage to the babies would be due to complicated pregnancies or deliveries. In this select, healthy group, they found that obstetrical drugs affect the children's behavior at least through seven years of age. Among the older children whose mothers had received drugs during labor and delivery, there were lower reading and spelling scores, and lower scores on a visual-monitor test.

Some doctors are concerned, however, that if women have full information on the risks of brain damage to their unborn babies when drugs are used, they will be frightened away from using them when needed. This issue came up when Brackbill presented her findings. Brackbill's reply was, "I see evidence everywhere I turn that women are capable of making risk-benefit decisions."

Many of us believe that the Food and Drug Administration would not allow unsafe drugs to be used in obstetrics. In a study of this issue, Doris Haire reports that the dictionary definition of *safe* ("free from harm or injury") is not the definition used by the FDA; in fact, the FDA has no definition of what "safe" is. In a letter to Haire, the FDA director said that the FDA does not guarantee the safety of any drug, even those drugs that it approves as "safe." Furthermore, the FDA does not require the drug given to a woman during labor or delivery to be proven safe for the unborn baby. Says Haire, "There is no doubt in my mind, and in the minds of many other individuals working with brain-injured children, that a large proportion of brain-injured and learning disabled children are the result of obstetric drugs administered to women to relieve discomfort or pain, or to induce or stimulate their labor. Most women are unaware that obstetric drugs diminish the supply of oxygen to the unborn baby's brain and can result in brain damage."

The American Academy of Pediatrics discourages the use of drugs for the laboring woman and states that no drug has been found safe for the baby *in utero*.

In the next hour and a half, Jenny and Dick chatted. They even became a little bored. Jenny felt hungry, but knew she couldn't eat. Her sense of smell seemed very sharp; everything reminded her of food. She hadn't eaten since last night's dinner, and it was almost twenty-four hours since then. Jenny felt nothing from the top of her tummy down, but she could, strangely, feel the baby moving around. At 3:30 P.M. she became aware the epidural was wearing off. About that time the nurse came in for a check and told her she was six centimeters dilated and doing fine, but the nurse helped her turn on her side because her blood pressure was "a little low."

Jenny wasn't so sure that she was doing fine. She was afraid of feeling the overwhelming contractions again. She asked Dick what she should do. He suggested they start timing the contractions again, and get back with the breathing. By 4:30 she was eight centimeters dilated and feeling unable to handle the contractions again. She rang for the nurse to come back. "Please, I need something now!" She felt she didn't do very well the next half hour waiting for the doctor, losing her breathing rhythm, even though Dick was now breathing along with her with each contraction. Nothing seemed to be working. At 5:00 the doctor arrived, found she was at nine centimeters dilation, and gave her a second injection of epidural anesthesia. As the sensations of labor began to disappear (much to her relief), she overheard her doctor talking to the nurse outside her door. "If I could have talked her into waiting another half hour or so for the first one, I probably wouldn't have had to repeat it." By 5:30 Jenny was feeling nothing and became very excited when the nurse coming in to check her told her she was nearly fully dilated and almost ready to push.

A few minutes later the doctor returned to check her and confirmed she could now push. Dick and the nurse helped Jenny round her back and grab her knees. "Push as long as you can!" the nurse encouraged. After about twenty to thirty minutes the stretcher was wheeled in for the move to the delivery room.

Delivery Position

The usual position for a North American woman giving birth in a delivery room is on her back, with her legs in stirrups—the lithotomy position. "Maybe the position is undignified for the mother," one doctor said, "but it's convenient for me." And that's the only good thing about it. There are no benefits and several serious drawbacks for the mother and baby.

In *The Cultural Warping of Childbirth*, Doris Haire summarized the literature indicating the problems in the lithotomy position for delivery.

1. It adversely affects the mother's blood pressure and the blood supply to her heart and lungs.
2. It decreases the normal intensity of contractions.
3. It makes it difficult for the mother to push the baby out and, therefore, increases the need for forceps. (You feel as though and you are, in fact, pushing the baby *uphill*.)
4. It makes it difficult for her to expel the placenta, which increases the need for procedures such as pulling on the cord, which put her at risk of hemorrhage.
5. Because the mother's legs are pulled wider apart than is normal for an easy delivery, and the baby's head presses against the back of the perineum, there is an increased need for an episiotomy to prevent tearing.

Many mothers find delivery not only safer but far easier curled on their side, or in a semisitting position with the soles of their feet on the bed, with a comfortable, relaxed spread of their legs. However, there are five upright positions that use gravity to assist the woman in delivery: sitting, squatting, on hands and knees, kneeling, and fully supported standing.

> When I moved to the delivery table, my contractions weakened. I was allowed to get up and walk. I sat on a bedpan and did my best pushing there. On and off the table three or four more times. It was the Michel Odent technique of a standing squat, hanging on my husband while I pushed, that finally moved the baby down. Back on the table and the baby slipped back. Off the table and more standing squat, hanging on my husband and pushing. The baby moved down again, and this time on the table he didn't slip back. *It was such a triumph to get out of the stalled second stage.* By the way, our son weighed 10 lbs., 9 oz.
>
> —Alberta

Jenny liked the idea of moving to the delivery room. Now she knew her baby was almost here. As the nurse and Dick helped her slide onto the delivery table, she felt another contraction coming, a tightening of her tummy with no other sensation. "I need to push!" she exclaimed. But she had to wait while her legs were positioned in the stirrups, and the sterile draping carefully arranged around her legs and stomach. Dick placed himself at her head. The nurse put a pillow under Jenny's shoulders. For another twenty minutes, Dick and the nurse encouraged her to push fully with each contraction. Finally the doctor told her he was going to help her with forceps and "a little cut." She'd probably feel some pressure in her back, he mentioned. As he worked positioning the forceps, he said, "This one is staying in one spot, so push hard. It's pretty tight...okay, now we're moving, just lie back and let me do the rest." An eight-pound girl slid into the world at 6:18 P.M. The nurse took the baby from the doctor, who cut the cord immediately. The nurse brought the baby around to Jenny and Dick for a brief look. Jenny and Dick were thrilled to see their new daughter. Both had seen the delivery in the overhead mirror with feelings of awe from watching the miracle of birth. The nurse took the baby over to check and clean up. Within a few minutes the nurse brought the baby to Dick and asked if he'd like to take his new daughter to the nursery "while the doctor finished up here." The doctor explained that Jenny had torn, even with the episiotomy, since the baby was in there "awfully tight," and he'd had to go a little higher with the forceps than usual.

Episiotomy

Episiotomy is a cut made with scissors at the lower end of the vagina—a slice made through the skin and underlying muscle to enlarge the birth opening. It is the Western way of genital mutilation.

—Sheila Kitzinger, *Mothering* magazine

The practice of episiotomy is so widespread that today there is hardly a North American woman who has given birth vaginally who has not had one. Kitzinger, a British anthropologist, author, and childbirth educator, reports from her personal research that "9 out of 10 American women having their first babies in a hospital get an episiotomy.... In the Netherlands, as few as 2 or 3 out of 10 first-time mothers are cut." This kind of information leads one to believe that it is not women's perineums that are different from country to country, but medical fads.

Enkin, Keirse, and Chalmers found three reasons given for the frequent use of episiotomy. First, an episiotomy substitutes a straight incision for a tear. The incision is easier to repair, better for healing, and prevents damage to the anus and rectum from deep tears, called third- and fourth-degree lacerations. Second, an episiotomy prevents "trauma to the fetal head." Third, an episiotomy prevents "serious damage to the muscles of the pelvic floor." In their complete review of the world literature, the authors found *no research* to support *any* of these beliefs. In fact, the "liberal use of episiotomy is associated with higher overall rates of perineal trauma."

In 1989, the same year that Enkin, Keirse and Chalmers published their findings, James M. Thorp and Watson Bowes, Jr. reported their review of the literature on episiotomy. They summarized twenty-five studies of how often third- and fourth-degree tears happened. In nearly 50,000 women who had episiotomies, 6.5 percent had third- or fourth-degree tears. In nearly 39,000 women who did not have episiotomies, 1.4 percent had similar tears. Women with episiotomies had almost five times as many severe tears as women without episiotomies. Thorp and Bowes concluded that routine episiotomy is not supported by the evidence, and "may well increase the incidence of third- and fourth-degree lacerations."

The high rate of episiotomies and the many severe lacerations in hospital deliveries occur because (1) obstetricians simply are not trained to ease out the baby's head any other way than to enlarge the opening with an episiotomy, (2) the lithotomy position is nearly universal for hospital delivery, and (3) large numbers of deliveries are done with forceps.

If your birth attendant is not familiar with, or unwilling to try, a delivery without an episiotomy, you can increase your chance of avoiding an episiotomy and tears by:

1. Choosing an upright or side-lying position (with a curved back like a spoon) for delivery.

2. Avoiding anesthesia.

3. Pushing only when you feel the need, for five to six seconds at a time.

4. Stopping pushing for one or two contractions when you feel a burning sensation.

5. Asking your doctor to use a gentle massage with warmed olive oil to stretch the perineum during the pushing stage.

6. Preparing your perineum with the Kegel exercise and massage.

7. Asking your doctor to avoid forceps if at all possible.

Instrument Delivery

Forceps, in use since the 1500s, are a metal device placed around the baby's head to lead it through the birth canal. A newer device, the vacuum extractor, uses a plastic cup on the baby's head and a suction tube. Both devices apply traction to the baby's head to shorten delivery. The textbook *Williams Obstetrics* describes "elective low forceps" as forceps used when "the obstetrician elects to interfere knowing that it is not absolutely necessary, for spontaneous delivery may normally be expected within approximately fifteen minutes. The vast majority of forceps operations performed in this country [United States] today are elective low forceps. One reason is that all methods of analgesia interfere to a certain extent with the mother's voluntary expulsive efforts."

The elective use of low forceps is sometimes called preventive use of forceps (meaning "to make delivery easier") and is widely used in the United States. Instrument delivery is used in 25 percent of all hospital deliveries, according to data from the National Center for Health Statistics. This contrasts with freestanding birth centers, where less than one percent of women have instrument delivery.

There is no research to support the elective use of forceps. Forceps are being used without a scientific basis, in normal deliveries, when there is no need to hurry. The risks to the infant are of hemorrhage within the head and damage to nerves serving the face and arms. For the mother, episiotomies almost always accompany the use of forceps. In spite of this, severe lacerations of the mother's perineum are more frequent when forceps and episiotomies are used. Using a vacuum extractor lessens the risk of trauma to the mother's perineum that forceps cause.

Summary

Obstetricians are not scientific in their practice. None of the ob's interventions has been evaluated and proven better than avoiding the interventions for the 80 to 95 percent of women who could have normal labors and deliveries, and most of the interventions have substantial risks. Research indicates which of the obstetrician's interventions are the most dangerous to you and your baby: continuous electronic fetal monitoring, Pitocin use, narcotics and anesthesia, the lithotomy position for delivery, and the use of forceps. The risks are to the health of the mother and baby and extend to long-term problems. Testifying before a 1978 Senate Health Subcommittee hearing on obstetric interventions, Doris Haire said she believed "that at least a large percentage of learning disabled and handicapped children result from obstetric practices which interfere with normal biochemical checks and balances provided by nature to assure the normal progression of labor and a good maternal and infant outcome."

It has been as scary for us to write about the unproven interventions of the obstetrician as it is for you to read it. We are afraid of the risks being taken with the lives and health of women and their babies when those risks are unjustified in normal births. We can hear women who are reading this book say, "Why are you telling me this? It's only making me frightened of what might happen."

The management of normal labors and deliveries is new in the history of childbirth. As recently as the early to mid-1970s, several of the obstetrician's interventions were used only in complicated cases of labor and delivery, where the health and welfare of the woman or her baby justified them. Now the technology is being used on most women in labor whether the labor is normal or not. *It will probably be used on you if you don't negotiate to prevent its use.*

Usually when complications arise in childbirth, the birth will still result in a live mother and a live baby. Perinatology (the care of the unborn and the newborn) has resulted in the greatest saving of babies in trouble. If your baby is two pounds or more, it is more likely than ever that your baby will live, regardless of what kind of childbirth you have.

But technology not only is unsafe for normal birth, it also changes the experience of childbirth for women and babies, with far-reaching results. What have we lost? Janice Raymond, a family practitioner in British Columbia, Canada, says, "Childbearing provides a potentially empowering process for women to realize the natural creative powers of their own bodies as they star in their own birthing drama. High technology, by its very nature, robs women of this empowerment.... Technology confers power and control to those who own, apply and interpret the technology." The mother becomes a spectator at her own baby's birth. And if interventions lead to intensive care for the infant, then the mother and baby are separated at birth.

What we are losing here is the experience of childbirth at its best: an exuberant experience of enormous courage, effort, and incredible pleasure. We are losing the kind of childbirth experience that empowers us, makes us feel better about ourselves as women, helps us grow and develop as mothers, and is important in the attachment process with our babies. More than that, the active management of labor and delivery is leading to an epidemic of cesarean births at great costs to women and their children.

8

The Cesarean Epidemic

The most common cause of cesareans today is not fetal distress or maternal distress, but obstetrician distress.

—Gerald Stober,
New York City Obstetrician

Typically, a laboring woman does not see her doctor in the hours before birth. Then he strides in, takes charge, and accomplishes an efficient, quick delivery. But she has been on his mind from the time the hospital nurse notified him of her arrival. He has been on call for her, all the while seeing other patients in his office or offices. In his mind, the danger is mostly to the baby. He has never lost a mother, but no matter how hard he has tried, he has had a "poor outcome" for a baby several times in his career. The constant anxiety in his mind is, Am I going to get a healthy baby? The uncertainties of labor's progress result in more anxiety than almost any obstetrician can handle. He usually gets in there and does something.

Belief, Training, and Money Are Behind the Epidemic

When physicians are asked why cesareans have increased, the most frequent reason they give is the threat of a malpractice suit. Helen Marieskind, a Seattle public-health specialist who interviewed physicians and evaluated cesareans for the federal government, was the first to report this belief. In the interviews, physicians called cesareans "defensive medicine" and said that, even if a baby was "less than perfect," if a cesarean had been performed, they were covered.

Acknowledging this widespread belief, Lynn Silver and Sidney Wolfe of the Public Citizen's Health Research Group reported that

132

doctors and the public "commonly perceived that the threat of malpractice is a major cause of the increasing c-section rate." In their report, *Unnecessary Cesarean Sections: How to Cure a National Epidemic,* Silver and Wolfe reviewed the relationship between states' cesarean rates and malpractice premium rates: "Variations in malpractice premiums were unable to explain the enormous variations between hospitals and physicians in the use of this surgery. In fact, there is no empiric evidence demonstrating that the performance of unnecessary cesarean sections lessens the legal risk for an obstetrician."

"Cesarean sections mean better babies" is another important belief causing the dramatic rise in cesareans.

- "You get pregnant to have a healthy baby, not a vaginal delivery."
- "We are looking for a neurologically and psychologically sound human being."
- "Now, in an advanced country, we expect a baby to survive."

The above comments were made by medical experts interviewed by Silvia Feldman. Until the 1960s, the obstetrician's emphasis was on saving the mother, since maternal death rates had been so high. When maternal mortality rates dropped dramatically, the emphasis shifted to the baby.

Women now find themselves faced with the ultimate intervention—a cesarean—because the doctor believes cesareans result in fewer damaged or dead babies. For years obstetricians linked the falling perinatal mortality rates with the increasing cesarean rates. That belief was shown false with the publication of a study by O'Driscoll and Foley in 1983. The authors reported on 108,987 infants born in National Maternity Hospital, Dublin, from 1965 to 1980. The perinatal mortality rate plummeted in Dublin just as it was doing in the United States, but the cesarean section rate remained below 5 percent. Throughout Europe, cesarean rates remain far below U.S. rates with as good or better perinatal mortality.

The evidence is growing that cesareans do not produce "better babies" and may be resulting in more damaged babies. For example, Roberta Haynes de Regt, *et al.* reported in 1986 on 65,647 deliveries in Brooklyn over a five-year period, comparing cesarean rates and outcomes for clinic patients versus private patients. The clinic patients had higher risk factors, and their babies had lower birth weights. Yet their babies did better than the private patients' babies. Private patients, who had a significantly higher rate of cesareans, had a significantly greater number of babies with poor outcomes: birth injuries or low Apgar scores (a measure of condition at birth). Silver and Wolfe summarize, "Surgery is more likely to make the infant or his mother ill, rather than perfect and whole. The myth of the perfect cesarean baby should be laid to rest."

Despite the evidence, the widespread belief that a cesarean is better for the baby persists among obstetricians and the public. It is often given to a mother in labor as a persuasive reason to undergo a cesarean. And certainly, told that something might happen to her baby if she goes ahead with a vaginal delivery, a woman is unwilling to take that risk. But the public needs to know that we cannot always expect a baby to be whole or to survive. "Most fetal death and damage is unpreventable, in that it is related to events or factors before delivery, over which physicians have no control," wrote Emanuel Friedman in the *New England Journal of Medicine*. "It is unrealistic, therefore, to expect every delivery to result in a living, healthy, unaffected child."

"Infants were stillborn not because of delayed diagnosis or delivery, but because the severity of fetal distress was so great that it precluded saving the babies," said Leveno and Cunningham, commenting on their study of selective and universal electronic fetal monitoring in 34,995 pregnancies in Dallas. "This may be our most important result, since the expectations of patients, obstetricians, and more recently, attorneys are such that all fetal deaths in labor units are considered preventable. They are not."

An obstetrician's training contributes to his anxiety about the dangers of childbirth and to his urge to resort to a cesarean delivery. "I believe the present high-risk childbirth model is creating more anxiety than obstetric personnel can handle, and the increasing cesarean rate is in part a manifestation of this anxiety," says obstetrician Philip Sumner, coauthor of *Birthing Rooms*. Many doctors recognize the problem that obstetrical training emphasizes high-risk care. Doctors get little or no training in normal obstetrics, and are, therefore, poorly prepared to handle normal labors, according to Marieskind in her cesarean evaluation study and in her 1989 update. Residents receive little or no training in normal birth and are not prepared to handle labor and delivery unless they use interventions and surgery. By contrast, they receive extensive training in the use of technology in labor and delivery: in the use of electronic fetal monitoring, ultrasound, scalp sampling, anesthesia, forceps, and surgical deliveries. Obstetricians are more likely to perform cesareans when they are trained according to this high-risk model.

In addition to the obstetrician's belief and training, there is a financial and time-management incentive behind the increasing cesarean rates. Physicians are paid more for a cesarean delivery than for a vaginal one. Silver and Wolfe refer to studies showing that "patients with the best-paying insurance plans have the highest c-section rate. While physicians may or may not be deliberately or consciously performing c-sections for financial reasons, these findings, which have been replicated in studies in the U.S. and other countries, clearly show that financial factors probably are associated with a physician's decision to perform a c-section."

Changing the incentive can lower cesarean rates. Silver and Wolfe report that "one health maintenance organization, Total Health Care, Kansas, was able to rapidly lower its cesarean rate from 28.7 percent to 13.5 percent in one year simply by changing to the same reimbursement whether the woman had a cesarean or a normal delivery."

"Time is a *dear* commodity," said Richard Porreco, director of AMI/Saint Luke's Perinatal Program in Denver, speaking at a *Birth* journal conference. He went on to explain how time management spurs cesareans: "With out-patient and in-patient surgery and several offices in which to see patients, the doctor has little time for expectant management of labor. The influence of time is seductive. The doctor doesn't think about time determining whether he does a c-section, but it does."

Obstetrician Joseph Nouhan from St. Louis agrees that time management affects the way a doctor practices. Nouhan prefers low-intervention obstetrics, and gives a copy of this book to each pregnant woman coming to him, saying, "This is my philosophy of childbirth; read it and tell me what you want." He observes, "My practice is run the way I like, but it takes time to be with women in labor and help them have a natural birth. I see how the other obs work and it's easier for them. Usually they don't go to the hospital during a woman's labor, but call in an order for the anesthesiologist to give an epidural. Epidurals slow labor, and even if the woman is pushing, they know they will have time to make the delivery."

Evidence of unnecessary cesareans for convenience comes from several different reports. Susan Doering, a research scientist at Johns Hopkins University, found that 80 percent of a small sample of emergency cesareans were performed during the day rather than randomly around the clock. She also reported on unpublished research of L.K. Gibbons, showing that 58 percent of cesareans on first-time mothers, supposedly in emergency situations, were done during the day, and only 42 percent were done at night. Similar results were found in a third study, a survey of five New York City hospitals by personnel with the state's Maternal and Child Health office. In women having their first babies, 62 percent of emergency cesarean deliveries were performed during the working day, and only 38 percent were performed at night.

Cesarean Rates Differ Among Doctors and Hospitals

Whether you have a cesarean depends much more on the hospital you choose—and the doctors who practice there—than on you. Among the ten hospitals with the most deliveries covered in the Baltimore COMA Survey, cesarean rates ranged from 12 percent to 32 percent. Among the eleven physicians in our survey (who delivered most of the babies) the cesarean rate ranged from 5 to 23 percent. This wide variation among hospitals and doctors was confirmed by Public Citizen's Health Research Group studies.

Silver and Wolfe's 1989 report on unnecessary cesareans brought together current available national data on cesarean section rates. In 1992 Ingrid Van Tuinen and Sidney Wolfe updated the cesarean rates by hospital and state. Throughout the country cesarean rates showed extraordinary variation among hospitals, with no correlation to the rate of high-risk deliveries. The rates ranged from nearly 60 percent cesareans to near zero.

Few hospitals have low cesarean rates. Out of several thousand hospitals listed, only one in eight had cesarean rates of 15 percent or less. In Ohio, only four hospitals had cesarean rates of 15 percent or less, but ten hospitals had rates of 35 percent or more. Ohio is used here as an example. Your state is likely to have the same wide variation.

The reports list over 100 hospitals on "the cutting edge"—those hospitals with cesarean rates over one in three deliveries. In these hospitals you are more than likely to have the kind of completely managed birth described on page 36. Over half of the hospitals on this "cutting edge" list had cesarean rates of 40 percent or higher. All types of hospitals have excessive rates. The "cutting edge" list includes small and large hospitals, medical centers and Humana hospitals, and community and general hospitals. Obstetrical teaching hospitals sometimes are isolated islands of low cesarean rates. For example, Louisiana's University Medical Center in Lafayette has a 5.4 percent cesarean rate for 1990 in a state that has seventeen hospitals on the "cutting edge" list.

Dramatic variations occur within cities. In Missouri, for example, St. Louis Regional Medical Center, with over 3,500 births, had a 10.0 percent cesarean rate; St. John's Hospital, Creve Coeur, with almost 6,000 births, had a cesarean rate of 28.9 percent. If you chose St. John's rather than St. Louis Regional you nearly tripled your chance of a cesarean.

Hospitals do not perform cesareans; doctors do. Silver and Wolfe reported on all doctors in the state of Maryland delivering more than twenty babies a year in 1987. The differences are startling. Variations among doctors were as great as among hospitals. Rates for individual doctors varied from no cesareans to 57 percent. Of the 484 physicians studied, nearly half had personal cesarean rates of 30 percent or more. Forty-three doctors had rates of 40 percent or more. Only twelve doctors (one out of forty) had personal rates at or below 10 percent, "although many Maryland physicians practice low-risk obstetrics," report Silver and Wolfe.

Within each Maryland hospital, rates among doctors often vary hugely. Frederick Memorial Hospital staff had the greatest differences—from zero to 42 percent cesarean sections. Three of the doctors there, with rates of zero to one percent, stand in dramatic contrast to the rest of the staff. More typically, most hospitals had a few doctors with low cesarean rates, most doctors with high rates from 20 to 40 percent, and one or two doctors with a cesarean rate of 40 percent or more. Maryland hospitals overall showed a decrease from 26.4 percent cesareans for 1987 to 24.4 percent in 1990.

"The data in this report make it crystal clear that much more than the size of a woman's pelvis or the health of her baby, the factor which is most likely to decide how she delivers her baby is the practice style of her obstetrician," report Silver and Wolfe. "Differences in c-section rates can only be accounted for by different policies that physicians use to manage their patients."

Depending on the doctor you choose, your chance of a cesarean can vary from nearly nonexistent to one chance in two. "While hospitals have tremendous variability in their overall rates, in many hospitals this variation can be accounted for by a few physicians who dramatically abuse cesarean surgery," conclude the authors.

How do you find a hospital and doctor with low cesarean rates? You can get a copy of the reports from the Public Citizen's Health

Research Group (see Appendix D) to identify rates for individual hospitals. Some states give you access to the information. Massachusetts became the first state to pass a cesarean disclosure law through the efforts of a consumer group, Cesarean Support, Education and Concern (C/Sec, Inc.). Every hospital there is required to give women its cesarean rate and rates of other common maternity practices. As of this printing New York and Rhode Island are the only other states with similar disclosure laws.

Although New York hospitals are required to offer women leaflets giving specific rates of interventions, you will probably have great difficulty getting this legally mandated information, asserts a *Consumer Reports* writer; half the hospitals contacted by the reporter never gave out the information. If you live in New York state, you have "another more practical alternative," according to Diony Young, editor of *Birth* journal.

The New York State Department of Health offers *Your Guide to a Healthy Birth*, which "discusses the rights of the parents, pros and cons of various routines, and C-section rates for every hospital in New York state," writes Deborah Amis, childbirth educator. In general, according to Diony Young and to *Consumer Reports*, New York health provider groups (hospitals and doctors) opposed making the information public, while women's health and other consumer groups intensely lobbied for the information.

We believe women can fully understand information on interventions and make their own choices in health care (why else would we write this book?). In 1989 a new standard birth certificate in all states enabled state officials to have detailed information on cesarean rates and other maternity practices by hospital and physician. Because of the experience in New York, where most hospitals resist complying with the law, your state health department is the best place for publishing this information. Call your local health department—and your state legislator—and demand that the information be made public if it hasn't already. Make the health department's job easier: Get them a copy of New York's *Your Guide to a Healthy Birth* ("Healthy Babies," Box 2000, Albany, NY 12220). Maybe you can get your health department to include individual doctors' cesarean rates—information they have on hand.

Finally, simply ask hospital administrators and doctors for their cesarean rates. "When I began suggesting that my students ask their obstetricians about their cesarean section rates, I supposed that physicians with high rates would hedge, or at least be embarrassed," wrote childbirth educator Henci Goer. "I couldn't have been more wrong. Doctors seem proud to tell patients that their cesarean rate is 20 percent or more."

The Epidemic

An epidemic is an outbreak of anything that spreads or increases rapidly. We certainly have an epidemic of cesareans by that definition. The cesarean birth rate was 3 percent in the decade before 1970 when doctors looked at a cesarean as a last resort, a life-saving measure for the woman or her baby. Increasing just over one percent a year, cesareans soared from 5.5 percent of all births in 1970 to 23.5 percent of all births by 1990, report Paul Placek and Selma Taffel of the National Center for Health Statistics. Nearly one-fourth of all births today are by cesarean delivery.

A cesarean rate of 23.5 percent of all births is so high that healthcare providers separate cesareans into two groups: those that are primary, or first-time, cesareans, and those that are repeat operations—operations for another birth after a previous cesarean. More than one-third of all cesareans are repeats, and just under two-thirds are primary cesareans. The primary cesarean rate of 16.8 percent is the percentage of cesareans among women giving birth with no previous cesarean. Before 1970, when doctors were extremely cautious in doing a first-time cesarean, the primary rate was a small 1.5 percent. If you are having your first baby, or you have never had a cesarean and are having another baby, your chances of having a cesarean delivery today are eleven times greater than before 1970. That's an alarming change in the way babies are delivered and represents a fundamental and widespread change in medical practice.

Taffel reports that over 980,000 cesareans a year are now being performed, making it the most common major surgery in the United States (650,000 hysterectomies a year is the second most common major surgery, also done by ob/gyns). The cesarean epidemic has not gone unnoticed by the popular press, government officials, or doctors. In the 1980s Canada and the United States each had a national consensus conference to review the world literature and to discuss and come to agreement on clear and strong recommendations to reduce cesareans. These recommendations by the U.S. National Institutes of Health (NIH) task force and the Canadian National Consensus Conference were published in major obstetrical journals. The cesarean rates continued to soar, however, going up by 50 percent in the eighties. Most obstetricians failed to use the guidelines.

"The majority of American physicians, hospitals and third-party payors have continued to stick their heads in the sand and ignore over 10 years worth of overwhelming evidence that American women are being subjected to an onslaught of unnecessary and dangerous surgery," conclude Silver and Wolfe in their national report on unnecessary cesareans.

What is an appropriate cesarean rate? You decide. Edward Quilligan, dean of the School of Medicine at the University of California at Irvine, reviewed the literature and suggested an 8 percent national rate. European rates range from under 5 percent to 12 percent. Richard Porreco reports a 6 percent cesarean rate for the clinic he directs at AMI/Saint Luke's, Denver. Obstetrics department head Norbert Gleicher coauthored the report of a successful program that lowered the cesarean rate to 11.5 percent for all deliveries, private and clinic, at Mount Sinai Hospital in Chicago. Using worldwide data, Silver and Wolfe estimate a target rate of 12 percent.

These rates are all far below almost all hospital and doctor rates and the U.S. rate. Using the target rate of 12 percent, Silver and Wolfe estimate at least half, or 500,000 of the cesareans in the United States annually, are unnecessary. Using our estimate of an additional $3,000 for a cesarean delivery over a vaginal delivery, these unnecessary cesareans cost $1.5 billion each year. What price can we put on the human cost in injury, illness, and death to women and babies for these unnecessary cesareans?

Epidemic Worse for First Births, Older Women

We need to make a distinction between women laboring for the first time (called primiparas) and women who have already had babies (called multiparas).

Obstetrician William Cook describes his view of the difference:

> The fact that a first childbirth is usually so different from subsequent births as to be almost unrelated is of such prime importance that it should be emphasized by every childbirth instructor and author (but isn't)....The effect of much childbirth education is to blur the distinction between the often long labor and difficult delivery of the first child and the shorter and easier labor and delivery of subsequent births.

The cesarean birth rate is much higher in primiparas than in multiparas who have never had a cesarean—three to eight times higher, according to a Massachusetts Department of Public Health study. The risk of cesarean birth has increased for everyone, but the risk is much greater than it used to be for a first-time mother. The typically longer labor of a primipara is an important factor in the cesarean epidemic. (See the section "Abnormal Labor" later in this chapter.)

The most common age for a woman to have a baby is in her twenties. However, a shift in the timing of births has resulted in many more women having babies in their thirties than in the past, according to the National Center for Health Statistics. More than one-fourth of all births are to women over thirty. Steady increases in first births to women in their thirties and forties is another trend reported by the center. The risk of a cesarean delivery goes up as the age of the mother increases from the teens to age forty or more. A woman in her early twenties has one chance in eight of having a primary cesarean; a woman thirty-five years old or older has one chance in four.

Phyllis Mansfield, a specialist on age and childbirth, reviewed the scientific literature and found little reason for obstetricians to continue in their belief that older women, especially older women having first babies, are at high risk. She found "the vast majority of the 109 studies on age and childbirth so flawed as to be totally useless." The only clear risk of older women is for a Down's syndrome baby, a genetic deviation linked with mental retardation.

University of British Columbia researchers, reporting in the medical journal *Lancet,* analyzed 500,000 live births to conclude that no association exists between birth defects and increasing age of the mother (with the exception of genetic defects). More than three-quarters of all birth defects result from unknown causes. Women over thirty-five years of age who have fetuses with no detectable genetic disorder are not at any greater risk for birth defects than younger women, reported study team leader Patricia Baird.

The higher cesarean rate of older women is not related to any evidence that women age thirty-five or older or their babies benefit from a cesarean rather than a vaginal birth. "Premium baby" is a term obstetricians have coined for any baby especially desired by the mother—particularly the older, first-time mother. The need to "guarantee the product" (so to speak) results in increased cesareans for these premium babies. Look for a birth attendant who will see you as the healthy, normal pregnant woman you are.

Why the Epidemic?

A doctor is legally required to give a specific medical reason for performing a cesarean. "The fear of a malpractice suit," "a premium baby," "first birth," or " I don't know how to do a vaginal breech birth" are not reasons obstetricians write on medical records. Until the 1970s the most likely medical indications for cesarean delivery were different from what they are today. The primary cesarean, viewed as an emergency lifesaving event for mother or baby, was done for such medical complications as life-threatening maternal bleeding (hemorrhage), placenta blocking the birth canal (placenta previa), or baby's head too large to pass through the pelvis (severe cephalopelvic disproportion, or CPD). There were other, quite rare, reasons, too—including a repeat cesarean, always done, but still unusual, because there were so few women with previous cesareans.

Four reasons account for over 80 percent of cesareans today:

- Repeat cesarean birth
- Abnormal labor
- Fetal distress
- Breech position of baby

Repeat Cesarean Births

"Once a cesarean, always a cesarean," has been a strong belief in American obstetrical care since the early 1900s. The practice of requiring repeat cesareans was started to avoid the risk of uterine rupture at the scar site, a life-threatening situation.

Even today, any uterine scar may rupture (a rare, serious, sudden bursting of the scar) or separate before or during labor. However, a change in the kind of incision done in cesareans has resulted in a greatly reduced possibility of separation or rupture, and a greatly reduced threat to the lives of the mother and baby. The "classical" cesarean operation was performed through a long vertical incision from the navel to the pubic hair, and then a similar vertical incision in the uterus. However, today's preferred method for cesarean delivery is a low horizontal incision in the uterus, after first cutting a similar low skin incision. Over 90 percent of cesarean deliveries are now done this way. The skin incision is called a "bikini cut," implying that it won't be visible when you wear next summer's bikini. This widely accepted, newer technique has greatly reduced the risk of separation or rupture of the uterus in subsequent pregnancies or labors—to far less than one percent.

Even then, more than 90 percent of the problems consist of a partial separation of the old scar with no dangerous results to mother or baby. A partial separation can heal on its own or is easily repaired. A rupture of a low horizontal cesarean scar is exceedingly rare and less serious than a rupture of a classical uterine scar. "Mortality fears for mother and infant due to rupture of the uterus in trial of labor are unjustified by present statistical data," said Luella Klein, then president of the American College of Obstetricians and Gynecologists.

Most countries do not have a policy of repeat cesareans. Trials of labor and successful vaginal deliveries following cesareans are common. Over three decades many studies in the United States with tens of thousands of women in different medical centers have shown that most repeat cesareans are unnecessary. Both national consensus commissions documented that vaginal birth after a previous cesarean (VBAC) is as safe for the baby and safer for the mother. ACOG's review of the literature showed that maternal mortality is at least twice as high for repeat cesareans as for VBACs. ACOG set out guidelines to encourage vaginal delivery after a cesarean.

Most practicing obstetricians are simply not listening. In 1990 four out of five United States women who had cesareans and gave birth again had repeat cesareans. Although the proportion of VBACs is increasing fast, we have a long way to go to stop unnecessary repeat cesareans. (See page 176 for additional information on vaginal birth after cesarean.)

Abnormal Labor

The diagnosis of abnormal labor is the most prevalent reason for a primary cesarean, accounting for well over 40 percent of all first-time cesareans. When the diagnosis is made, it is almost always a first birth, too, so women having their first babies are at particular risk of having this label put on their labors. When counting all cesareans, abnormal labor is number two behind repeat cesareans.

Dystocia (pronounced dis-toe-sha) is the medical term for abnormal labor. Dystocia means there is difficulty in the progress of the labor ("failure to progress"), for any of three reasons: weak contractions ("uterine inertia"), a poor position of the fetus, or an abnormal size pelvis that prevents the baby descending or passing through the mother's birth canal (cephalopelvic disproportion, or CPD).

Banta and Thacker, in their literature review on fetal monitoring for the U.S. Department of Health, Education and Welfare, reported that although true CPD occurs rarely (in 2 percent of first-time labors), it is a common reason given for cesareans. Obstetrician Richard Hausknecht went even further in the NIH task force report, noting the "indiscriminate overuse of the wastebasket term, 'dystocia.'" The task force found that when the diagnosis of dystocia or failure to progress is made, cesareans did not improve infant outcome compared to vaginal birth.

> There is no magic number of hours beyond which labor should not continue.
>
> —Emanuel A. Friedman
> Developer of "Friedman Curves"

Doctors use the "Friedman curves" to decide whether a labor is abnormal. Friedman analyzed the progress of labor, averaged the time for many normal labors, and drew graphs to show the average labor. He describes two stages of labor, latent and active. The latent phase is early labor, the period of time when the cervix becomes effaced (thinned out) but dilates slowly, up to three to four centimeters. A normal latent phase, according to Friedman, can last up to twenty hours in a first-time mother, and up to fourteen hours in a woman who has already had a baby, but averages nine hours. The active phase of labor (sometimes called "true labor"), when the cervix dilates faster and steadily, is from four to ten centimeters of dilation. The average time for the active phase is four to six hours.

Doctors misuse the Friedman curves, according to Friedman himself. At the "Crisis in Obstetrics—Management of Labor" conference, reports Diony Young, "He asserted that the Friedman labor curve 'is being abused more than it is being used appropriately' and that to intervene with a cesarean for prolonged labor is 'unthinkable.'"

"We've forgotten that most women deliver in time," said Edward H. Hon at the same conference. "If you allow twenty-four hours to elapse before intervening, you wouldn't have the high cesarean rate." Doctors misuse the Friedman curves when they equate slow progress with abnormal progress. They tend to forget that the graphs are based on averaging many labors of widely varying lengths. Most obstetricians view a normal labor (to full dilation of the cervix) as lasting no more than a total of twelve to fourteen hours for early and active labor. Yet twelve to fourteen hours is the length of the *average* first labor, according to the Friedman curves. Many perfectly normal labors will last longer than that, some much longer.

"People should recognize that because America thinks of itself as a can-do society, doctors emphasize the risk of doing nothing and tend to minimize the risk of doing something," said Lynn Payer, author of *Medicine and Culture*, to writer Joanne Silberner. "Try asking your doctors, 'What do I risk if I don't do anything at all?' Sometimes you'll be surprised, because if they are honest, they may say that you don't risk much. Sometimes they will try to scare you, and this is the point where you should get a second opinion."

Very prolonged labor (over twenty-four hours) is associated with increased perinatal mortality. That is, according to the research, in very long labors there is a small increased risk that the infant will not survive. However, according to Hellman and Pritchard, authors of *Williams Obstetrics*, the textbook used to train obstetricians, we don't know if the increased perinatal mortality is the result of the longer labor itself or if it is because of the complications from the interventions that the doctors use to speed up or end labor.

Researchers implicate anesthesia as a cause of many cesareans for dystocia. Friedman found that the use of medications or regional anesthesia (such as epidural, caudal, or spinal anesthesia) given before the mother has gone into active labor often results in a prolonged latent (early) phase of labor. At the 1989 *Birth* journal conference obstetrician James Thorp described an association between epidural anesthesia in first labors and an increased risk of cesarean for dystocia. The studies at the University of Houston medical school showed two to three times more cesareans for dystocia in first labors in the epidural group than in the group of women without anesthesia. If the epidural was given before five centimeters of dilation to the women with slower labors, they had a six times greater risk of cesarean section for dystocia than women with slow labors but no anesthesia.

Pitocin to speed slowed labors helped to reduce the cesarean rate in the Mount Sinai Hospital experiment in Chicago. Where Pitocin use has been successful in slowed labor, it is used only when labor is clearly established. Hellman and Pritchard warn that "one of the most common mistakes in obstetrics is to try to stimulate labor in patients who have not been in labor at all." They direct doctors to consider Pitocin only when the woman is in active labor.

Pitocin, primarily for first-time labors, is also considered an important part of Dublin's National Maternity Hospital's very low cesarean rate. Other factors include sending a woman home when she is in latent labor and giving continuous one-to-one labor support by a midwife. Some observers believe the labor support is as important as the Pitocin. (See doula research in Chapter 1.)

Water is being discovered as an assist to slowed and painful labors. Michel Odent reported in *Lancet* on the use of a warm-water pool for women experiencing painful contractions and labor not progressing at five centimeters dilation. "In most cases, the cervix becomes fully dilated within 1 to 2 hours of immersion in the pool, especially if the lights are dimmed," wrote Odent. In the 100 births under water reported, there were no complications and no infections.

In the hundreds of water births at the Family Birthing Center near Los Angeles, Michael Rosenthal also reports no complications and one minor infection. "About half the women choose to get in the water at some time during the labor process, and half of those stay there and deliver in the water," said Rosenthal in the video *Water Baby: Experiences of Water Birth* by Karil Daniels.

Using birth pools helps the caregivers, too, says Sheila Kitzinger, by subtly changing their behavior: "Instead of 'managing labor,' they learn to watch and wait, and to support the physiological process by nurturing the mother."

Odent believes the water helps women to let go and become instinctive in giving birth. "When labor stalls, you must do what your intuition tells you feels right," say Beverly Savage and Diana Simkin in *Preparation for Birth*. "This may mean removing the monitor and going for a walk, having a snack, taking a shower, calling a friend, yelling out or having a good cry. Surprisingly, loss of control can help, because tears produce a tremendous release of tension, which will allow labor to proceed."

The second stage of labor is the pushing stage, the time from full dilation until the woman pushes her baby out. Epidural anesthesia can increase cesarean section for dystocia in the second stage as well, reported Thorp at the *Birth* journal conference. An epidural interferes with the woman's ability to push and also, by relaxing a woman's pelvic floor, prevents the natural rotation and progress of the fetus through the birth canal. Anytime epidurals are given, instrumental delivery is two and a half times more frequent than without the epidural, report H. M. Kaminski *et al*. The instrumental delivery might be even higher, but because of fear of malpractice suits, "the obstetrician is less likely to intervene with forceps, and therefore, an increased incidence of cesarean for dystocia could result," said Thorp.

Most obstetricians allow one or at most two hours for the pushing stage, believing that longer than that is dangerous for the baby. They seem unaware of a 1976 Harvard Medical School study of the pushing stage of 4,403 first-time mothers by Wayne Cohen. The study shows "no adverse influence of a long second stage on perinatal or neonatal mortality in nulliparas [first-time mothers]. The elective termination of labor simply because an arbitrary period of time has elapsed in the second stage is clearly not warranted."

"Cesarean section for dystocia in nulliparas represents the single most important factor in the cesarean epidemic," reports Thorp. Because most doctors do repeat cesareans, the large number of women given cesareans for dystocia usually will have a cesarean for their next birth, magnifying the effect of the first cesarean

What can you do to avoid the "abnormal labor" tag? The NIH task force noted that "failure to progress may, in fact, be false labor or prodromal labor or otherwise not abnormal." False labor is the "practice" contractions of the last few weeks (for many first-time mothers) or the last few months (for many subsequent pregnancies). Prodromal labor is very early labor or, some would say, the contractions that signal that labor may come soon (hours or a few days away). If you are in very early labor, stay home.

Especially if this is your first baby, think about staying home from the hospital as long as possible in labor. Hospital staff tend to measure the length of your labor from the time you arrive at the hospital. Because first labors tend to be longer and often harder for the woman to handle (she's never experienced this before, and her cervix is opening for the first time), staff distress goes up. You are likely to avoid the diagnosis of abnormal labor if you stay home until you are *sure* you are in active labor and that you really don't want to stay home any longer.

By staying home in early labor, you can drink, eat, rest, or sleep (all important in a long labor) when you want to, without feeling any pressure to have your labor fit the hospital's standard of how fast you should be dilating. Consider having a doula with you (see Chapter 11) to help you and your partner relax with a long early labor at home. Or have a trained labor-support person with you who can examine you, tell you where you are in your labor, and help you.

"What is wrong with a woman waiting until it is time for her to deliver, coming into the hospital, staying two to eight hours and taking her baby home?" said Paul Wexler, chairman of the Department of Obstetrics and Gynecology of Rose Medical Center, Denver.

If you are in active labor and have been diagnosed as failing to progress, Diony Young recommends trying the following alternatives:

- Asking for more time.
- Trying position changes, particularly upright ones; use one position for a while, then try another—maybe what you need is variety.
- Walking.
- A warm shower or bath.
- Loving encouragement (tell your helpers you need their encouragement in words and touch).
- Change in environment (ask if you can leave the hospital for a walk in the park—or at least try the early-labor lounge or lobby).
- Privacy with one's partner (shoo everyone else out, leave a guard at the door, and you and your mate can cuddle, kiss, massage, or whatever you need—maybe talk!).
- Breast and nipple stimulation. Remember, breast and nipple stimulation can make the uterus contract and can work for those women who have enjoyed it as part of lovemaking and either are uninhibited in a hospital setting or can arrange for the privacy they need—or use a breast pump.
- Removal of persons who cause stress (be honest).
- Letting the anesthetic wear off and allowing the labor to develop normally.

To avoid failure to progress in the second stage of labor, use one of the efficient delivery positions discussed in Chapter 12. If you have no choice but to use the delivery table, you can help your second stage in several ways, most of which need to be agreed on ahead of time.

- Have the delivery table tilted down at a slight angle; you won't feel you are pushing uphill as much.
- Avoid stirrups. They can quickly be swung into place if needed. Your legs should be relaxed and spread apart so you are comfortable. This position allows you to relax your perineum, so your pushes are more effective. It also protects your perineum from tears and episiotomy, because there is no tension holding back the birth.
- If you must use stirrups, have the nurse adjust them for you in an upright, supported sitting position, so you are not forced to lie flat because the stirrups are fixed for that position.
- With each pushing contraction, have your helpers lift you to

an upright position; round your back, hold on to your knees, but don't pull on them (causes perineum tension); relax your perineum, and push, using your abdominal muscles.
* Have a stack of pillows behind your head and shoulders so you can relax between contractions without lying flat.

Fetal Distress

The diagnosis of fetal distress accounts for 10 percent of all cesareans. Fetal distress is most often defined by variations in the fetal heart rate, which are considered abnormal. The difficulty is in telling whether the fetus is simply normally distressed or is in true distress needing intervention.

Researchers in Sweden, Great Britain, and the United States have identified what is happening in normal birth to cause unnecessary cesareans for fetal distress. Most infants diagnosed as distressed during labor are in excellent condition at birth after a cesarean. The process of labor does stress an infant, resulting in a release of stress hormones (catecholamines, pronounced "cat-a-cola-means") that are crucial for the protection and good health of the fetus.

Catecholamines cause vital processes in the fetus which help it survive and adapt at birth, according to researchers Hugo Lagercrantz and Theodore Slotkin. The effects of the catecholamines on a fetus, which include a *slowing* of the heart rate, protect it from less oxygen during contractions. (In adults catecholamines *increase* the heart rate, part of the "fight or flight" response.) The slowed heart rate may be diagnosed as fetal distress needing a cesarean, when it is a sign of the fetus adapting beautifully to the stress of labor.

The stress hormones do other good things. The lungs are stimulated to change in several ways, including absorbing amniotic fluids so the baby can breathe at birth. Blood flow increases to the heart and brain, protecting these vital organs. The fetus is put into a highly alert state that researchers believe may help in mother and infant attachment at birth.

The fetus has several means for increasing catecholamines. One of the best is the compression of the fetal head during the pushing stage of labor, conclude Lagercrantz and Slotkin. They say this may be the reason infants born by cesarean after labor have a much higher rate of breathing difficulties (and lower measured catecholamine levels) than babies born vaginally. Repeat cesareans where the fetus experiences no labor also show breathing problems and the lowest levels of catecholamines.

The electronic fetal monitor (EFM) is almost universally used to measure the fetal heart rate. In Chapter 7 we discussed the problems of the EFM in showing fetal distress and increasing the risk of cesarean birth without any better outcome for the baby.

Obstetrician, researcher, and professor Edward H. Hon is the inventor of EFM. "Most women in labor are much better off at home than in the hospital with the electronic fetal monitor," he said at the "Crisis in Obstetrics—Management Labor" conference, reported by Diony Young. He believes that "most obstetricians don't understand the monitor. They're dropping the knife with each drop in the fetal heart rate. The cesarean section is considered as a rescue mission of the baby by the white Knight, but actually you've assaulted the mother."

In their comprehensive review of the literature, the NIH task force summarized the most common suggestions for reversing fetal distress without resorting to surgery:

- Give the mother oxygen.
- Change the mother's position.
- Give intravenous fluids (hydration).
- Turn Pitocin off if it is being used.

A simple means of preventing the overdiagnosis of fetal distress is to use a nurse to regularly monitor the baby's heart rate. In addition, the widespread use of Pitocin needs careful evaluation. Pitocin can intensify natural contractions, reducing the oxygen supply to the baby and triggering fetal distress. Because this is so well known, women receiving Pitocin are placed in the high-risk category. So another way to prevent a diagnosis of fetal distress would be to avoid Pitocin in the first place. Try other means of stimulating labor, such as having the mother walk.

Breech Presentation

Ten percent of cesarean delivery rates are due to the decision to deliver almost all breech presentations by cesarean. Most babies are born head first. In a breech birth, the baby's bottom comes first, called a frank or complete breech presentation or, rarely, the baby's feet come first, called a footling breech presentation. Breech presentation happens in 3 to 4 percent of deliveries. The labor lasts no longer than the average headfirst presentation. Breech position is nine times more common earlier in pregnancy than at term, which means that most breech babies naturally rotate to a head-down position before the end of pregnancy.

Perinatal mortality and complication rates are higher in breech presentations than in headfirst presentations. There are often other problems, such as prematurity and placenta previa, along with the breech presentation. However, even when problems such as these are not present at breech deliveries, the outcome for the baby in a breech presentation may not always be as good as for headfirst presentation. Because of this, there has been a shift to cesarean delivery of most breech births. Some obstetricians will not deliver any breech presentations vaginally (and some of them have not had any training in vaginal breech deliveries either).

The trend toward cesarean delivery of breech presentation is a major area of controversy among obstetricians, however. The reason for the controversy is that cesarean birth increased from 12 percent of all breech presentations in 1970 to 84 percent in 1989. In spite of the greatly increased use of cesarean delivery, there is no evidence of a better outcome for the baby: There was no overall decrease in mortality for breech presentations during that period, and no evidence of better health in breech newborns.

Studies from different medical centers and hospitals report successful vaginal deliveries with term and premature breech presentations, now adding up to thousands of births. In United States medical centers at least 50 percent of breech presentations are now delivered vaginally. At National Maternity Hospital in Dublin, where the cesarean rate has remained very low, nearly 80 percent of breech presentations are delivered vaginally. Several older, experienced obstetricians told us, "So, what's new? I've always delivered most breech babies vaginally." Obstetricians Michel Odent and Leo Sorger use the supported standing or squatting position for breech presentation because of gravity's assist, more pelvic room for the fetus, and faster delivery.

The consensus is no longer to assume a cesarean simply because of fetal position. The new consensus is represented in the Canadian commission's report that "a cesarean section should not be performed for breech presentation unless it can be shown to be justified." Obstetricians can use the recommendations, widely publicized in their journals, for vaginal delivery of breech fetuses.

Another solution to reducing cesareans for breech is to get the baby in a headfirst position. *External version* is a term used to describe gentle manipulation by the doctor of the mother's abdomen during the last month of pregnancy to turn the baby from a breech to a headfirst position. "The three randomized trials of external cephalic version at term that have been published all show that the external cephalic version significantly reduces the incidence of breech presentation at birth, and that the rate of cesarean section may be halved," sum up Enkin, Keirse, and Chalmers in *Effective Care in Pregnancy and Childbirth*.

No medical procedure such as external version is without risks. Two nonmedical exercises to turn breech presentation are the tilt position and the knee-chest position. The tilt position was originated by Juliet De Sa Souza at Grant Medical College in Bombay, India. If, by the beginning of the eighth month of pregnancy, the baby is still in a breech position, the mother lies in the tilt position for ten minutes twice a day. With an empty stomach, lying on her back on the floor, knees bent so that her feet are flat on the floor, the mother puts three good-sized pillows under her bottom. De Sa Souza reported in 1977 that 89 percent of 744 babies in breech presentations turned to a headfirst position with this exercise, most within two to three weeks. Once the baby has turned from a breech to a head-down position, discontinue the tilt exercise.

The knee-chest position is assumed by kneeling and leaning forward until your head rests on your folded arms (your head will be lower than your bottom). You'll find that you have to spread your knees to accommodate your late-pregnancy abdomen. Starting at the thirty-seventh week of pregnancy, assume this position for fifteen minutes three times a day, the first time before arising in the morning and preferably with a full bladder. (The slight weight of the full bladder is thought to encourage the fetus to turn.) Do the exercise for seven days. Both of these exercises have yet to be tested in randomized controlled trials with sufficient numbers to know whether they are really helpful or whether fetuses turned because they often do anyway.

Other Reasons for the Epidemic

A wide variety of reasons account for the remaining 17 percent of all cesareans: increased "elective" (by choice, not emergency) cesareans for mothers at high risk (for example, for some mothers with serious kidney disease); increased elective cesareans for babies at high risk (for example, multiple birth, or cesareans when *active* genital herpes in the mother is confirmed); or cesareans for prolonged pregnancy or premature rupture of membranes. Many of these are widely accepted as necessary, but others have no evidence of better outcome. For example, twins may be delivered by cesarean, or the first is delivered vaginally and the second by cesarean, with no evidence of better outcome for the babies than a vaginal birth for both babies. Neither do cesareans help very-low-weight babies survive.

Premature Rupture of Membranes

PROM, as it is called, does not refer to the old high school dance. The letters stand for premature rupture of membranes, meaning that the mother's bag of waters has broken before labor begins. It is one of the most common complications in pregnancy and can result in a cesarean, often unnecessarily. You can lessen the chance you will have PROM.

The routine weekly pelvic examination usually done in the month before your due date is "associated with a significantly higher incidence of PROM," according to J. P. Lenihan, reporting in *Obstetrics and Gynecology*. A pelvic examination is when the doctor puts his gloved fingers in your vagina to examine your cervix, the opening to your uterus. Lenihan recommends no pelvis examinations during the last three months of pregnancy unless there is a valid medical reason for examining the cervix. Discuss this recommendation with your birth attendant to lessen your risk of PROM.

There is strong controversy among obstetricians over what to do when the membranes rupture before labor. Some argue for immediate delivery to reduce the risk of infection in the mother and the baby. Others say that because PROM is often associated with a pregnancy not yet at term, that is with prematurity, nothing should be done. These two approaches are termed "aggressive" and "conservative." The aggressive approach means delivery within twenty-four hours of ruptured membranes by induction or cesarean if necessary. The conservative approach means waiting with close attention for either spontaneous labor or signs of infection.

More and more, obstetricians are coming around to believe that it is better for the baby to take the conservative approach with PROM, if delivery is going to mean a premature baby. In *Effective Care in Pregnancy and Childbirth*, Enkin, Keirse, and Chalmers' review of the world literature on PROM not yet at term can be summarized: Two controlled trials show no protective effect including no less infection in mothers or babies when the mother is given aggressive treatment for PROM. "On the whole the tendency is for most outcomes to be less favorable in the group with pre-emptive delivery," say the authors.

Most obstetricians, however, still believe that if PROM happens in a term pregnancy, and spontaneous labor does not begin within a few hours, they must induce labor or do a cesarean to make sure the baby is born within twenty-four hours. The research does not support them in this belief. "The evidence thus suggests that a policy of induction of labour for prelabour rupture of the membranes at term exposes the mother not only to a higher risk of cesarean section and infectious morbidity, but also to a longer and probably less comfortable labour, without any demonstrable benefit," state Enkin, Keirse, and Chalmers.

If doctors will simply wait, most women with PROM at term go into labor and deliver, "almost 90 percent within 48 hours," report Enkin, Keirse, and Chalmers. Ninety-five percent will deliver within 72 hours. The world literature shows that patience is the best treatment for PROM. "For the woman who is not in labour, is not infected, and shows no evidence of fetal distress or other fetal or maternal pathology, continuation of the pregnancy is more likely to be beneficial than harmful," explain Enkin, Keirse, and Chalmers. "The limited evidence that is available suggests that measures to effect delivery do more harm than good." The key reason doctors give for the aggressive approach—infection—is often the iatrogenic (doctor-caused) result of pelvic examinations after membranes have ruptured.

The placenta continues to manufacture amniotic fluid and sometimes the tear in membranes seals over. If PROM happens to you, talk to your doctor about the research. Try to negotiate for those precious forty-eight hours to start labor on your own. If you get the extra time, are nearing the end of the forty-eight hours, and haven't started labor, try natural labor induction: nipple stimulation or castor oil (see "Prolonged Pregnancy" in this chapter). Most of the following common-sense measures suggest how to avoid getting an infection:

- Allow *no* pelvic examinations.
- Avoid intercourse.
- Avoid sitting in water; take showers instead.

- Stay home until labor starts.
- Avoid contacts outside the family (alien germs).
- Watch for signs of infection, such as an elevated temperature and pain or tenderness in the abdomen.
- Drink plenty of fluids.
- Keep in touch with your doctor.
- Wait for spontaneous labor to begin.
- If you have active genital herpes and PROM, you will need a cesarean within six hours to avoid the possibility of infecting your baby.

Active Genital Herpes

Genital herpes is a viral venereal disease. The Centers for Disease Control in Atlanta estimate that 25 million men and women have genital herpes, with as many as 500,000 new cases each year. Genital herpes is an incurable disease that becomes latent (without symptoms) but can reappear in the infected person. Usually, the first infection, called primary genital herpes, is the most uncomfortable and lasts about three weeks. Recurrences are usually milder and last nine or ten days.

If a baby contracts herpes from the mother at the time of delivery, it is a very serious disease for the baby. The risk of death or chance of the infant becoming abnormal as a result of the disease is very high. Researchers believe that only mothers with active lesions in their genital area at the time of delivery are at risk of passing the virus on to their babies. Even then, the risk of the baby contracting the disease is low if the active lesions are from a repeating infection. The risk is very high if the lesions are from a first-time or primary infection of the mother.

An automatic cesarean for every woman with herpes is *not* necessary. "Thousands of babies are born every day to women with genital herpes," says Lawrence Corey of the University of Washington School of Medicine in Seattle. "Vaginal deliveries are usually possible, and the babies are perfectly normal. Even abdominal delivery is not foolproof. Neonatal herpes infections have occurred after abdominal delivery."

Charles Prober *et al.* at Stanford University School of Medicine studied the risk of infection in babies exposed to the active virus during delivery to women who had histories of repeating herpes infections. None of the infants got herpes. The researchers believe the risk of a baby acquiring an infection from a mother with a repeating infection at delivery is low. The mother passes resistance to the disease (antibodies) to the fetus.

However, because of the seriousness of the disease in infants, the researchers recommend a cesarean if a woman with recurrent herpes has visible lesions when she goes into labor. If the woman has no symptoms, they do not recommend a cesarean because the chance of passing on the virus to the baby is very low. They conclude that the baby of a woman having her first herpes attack at the time of delivery has a very high risk of contracting herpes and should be delivered by cesarean.

A special risk to the baby of a woman with a history of herpes in her or her mate is the use of the internal fetal monitor. Edward Kaye and Elizabeth Dooling of Boston City Hospital reported on neonatal herpes associated with fetal scalp electrodes. Other reported cases of infants contracting herpes from mothers via the internal fetal monitor are reported by Zane Brown *et al.* at the University of Washington. In the cases reported, the mothers had no signs of active herpes, but their babies contracted herpes at the site of the insertion of the electrode. Because of this reported risk, a woman with a history of or suspicion of past genital herpes in her or her mate should strongly consider refusing the use of the internal fetal monitor. "We have shown that neonatal herpes simplex virus must be considered an added risk of fetal monitoring," say Kaye and Dooling, who question the use of internal fetal monitoring in low-risk labors because of the added danger.

Prolonged Pregnancy

When nine months pregnant, some of us feel as if our pregnancy is prolonged. When we go much past the "due date" everyone asks, "Haven't you had your baby *yet?*" Think about adding a week to the due date you tell everyone.

The due date is estimated by counting 280 days forward from the first day of your last period. Forty weeks is the average "term" pregnancy, and later than forty-two weeks is considered prolonged. The problem with this average due date, of course, is that you may not be average. Your menstrual cycle may not be average (twenty-eight days). Or maybe it is normal for you to have a forty-three week pregnancy for *this baby*.

The time-honored method of estimating due dates may be plain wrong. Harvard School of Public Health researchers found that for middle-class whites, first-time pregnancies will have a due date of 288 days, or forty-one weeks—eight days longer than the old figure. A woman who has given birth before will have a due date of 283 days, or three days longer than the old figure. "What we're saying is maybe the real due date for whites is a week later, and this will certainly have implications for the post-term infant," explained Robert Mittendorf, one of the researchers. Obstetricians who routinely induce two weeks past the old figure for a due date may be inducing an infant well within normal limits of pregnancy. We are hearing of obstetricians advocating induction at forty weeks, a position supported by no research at all and likely to place infants at great risk of prematurity.

In 1965 an obstetrician wrote, "There is less than a 50 percent chance that labor will ensue within a week of the estimated date (early or late). I emphasize the word 'estimate.' Relax and be patient. Enjoy your pregnancy secure in the knowledge that your baby will be born when it has completed its normal growth and development in the uterus." Although you may get the impression from your obstetrician that he is sure of your due date, and he must induce you at forty-one weeks or forty-two weeks or whatever, nothing has changed. Due dates are still estimates, and women still start labor when they are ready.

True prolonged pregnancy (no mistake in dates) has an increased risk of perinatal mortality (death of the fetus before or during birth). Perinatal mortality is low at term and beyond, but it is higher at forty-two weeks (three fetal deaths per 1,000 births) and at forty-three weeks (four per 1,000) than at forty weeks (2.3 per 1,000), report Mary Halperin and Murray Enkin in *ICEA Review*. Though this increased risk is widely known, no one really knows what should be done about it.

"All studies since 1978 on the management of postterm pregnancy have found no benefit, or increased risks, with routine termination of pregnancy at 42 weeks of gestation," report Madeleine Shearer and Milton Estes in *Birth* journal. Routine induction leads to delivery of some premature infants because of mistaken due dates. Almost all reports agreed that about 50 percent of pregnancies called prolonged are not past term but reflect mistaken due dates. The use of sonograms (ultrasound) in estimating due dates was "remarkably misleading," wrote the authors. It led to "marked escalation in other tests, interventions in labor, and cesarean sections." The authors found it "disturbing that women's own due date calculations seemed to carry less weight than did sonograms in managing these pregnancies."

Even with some certainty that a pregnancy is prolonged, current tests for fetal well-being are not a great help in determining which pregnancy is at risk. The authors reviewed the literature for all current tests and found only fetal movement counting (FMC) of possible benefit. (FMC is having the mother count the number of fetal movements in a certain time period.)

The nonstress test (NST) and contraction stress test (CST) are both commonly used today in pregnancies past forty to forty-two weeks. Both use the external fetal monitor. The NST simply notes the fetal heart response when the mother indicates the fetus has moved. The CST measures the fetal heart response to a challenge of induced contractions, either with Pitocin or nipple stimulation. Shearer and Estes report Grant and Mohide's analysis of four randomized controlled trials of these two tests. In all the trials all women received NSTs and CSTs, but only half of the women had the test results revealed to their doctors. Grant and Mohide found that "in each of the four trials, there were [significantly] *more* deaths in the group for which clinicians had access to the test results ('revealed') than in the 'concealed' group." Having the information from the tests resulted in worse outcomes for the babies.

"Unfortunately, the available clinical tools have not had adequate evaluation to determine reliably whether or not they do more harm than good," writes Kirkwood Shy of the University of Washington School of Medicine. "I believe that we have promised patients too much with obstetric testing. Under almost all circumstances, including postdatism, outcomes are overwhelmingly good, and we credit ourselves and 'modern medicine' with these results."

"It is hard to accept that a baby should die so close to the beginning of a whole life, which is now denied to her," writes Marc Keirse, professor of obstetrics. "Such events should not occur, yet they do, and they will probably continue to do so for a long time to come. Should we avoid them? Yes. Can we avoid them? No."

"Prolonged pregnancy, in most cases, probably represents a variant of normal, and is associated with good outcome, regardless of the form of care given," say Enkin, Keirse, and Chalmers.

You may find yourself with a true prolonged pregnancy and a doctor pressuring you to accept induction. If you don't want to change doctors, and you are ready to give in to the pressure, try natural induction first. In order from most fun to least fun:

- Sexual intercourse with orgasm
- Nipple stimulation by you, your mate, a baby, or a breast pump
- Castor oil

"Prostaglandins, A Time Honored Method of Labor Induction," is the title of Ina May Gaskin's article in *The Birth Gazette*. Gaskin, a midwife, suggests lovemaking to her couples when she finds the woman past the due date with "an unripe cervix, tightly closed and thick around the opening. Prostaglandins occur in highest concentration in the body in seminal fluid," explains Gaskin in the article. The obstetric literature confirms that prostaglandins put in the vagina as a medical procedure are effective at inducing labor if the woman is at term. In unprotected sexual intercourse the man's seminal fluid, full of prostaglandins, is deposited on the woman's cervix. Researchers "left it to me and other midwives to devise the most pleasant and practical method of administration," humorously concluded Gaskin.

None of these natural induction methods work if your body is not ready for labor, but they are much less risky than Pitocin induction. Castor oil irritates the intestines, causing diarrhea and stimulating contractions. Midwife Anne Frye of Informed Homebirth suggests, "Take two ounces castor oil, two ounces orange juice and two ounces hard liquor. Take a hot shower. One hour later, take the same formula (sans liquor) and a high enema. One hour later take the same formula (castor oil and orange juice) and another hot shower. The idea is the liquor loosens up any psychological reservations the mother may have to labor beginning. I've seen labor start after the first dose!" Drink a lot of water so you don't get dehydrated from the diarrhea.

Cesarean Surgery

"A cesarean section has become less a matter of last resort and truly simply another method of delivery," said Basil Maloney, discussing breech delivery at a West Coast ob/gyn meeting. What most physicians don't know, and might even be shocked to discover, is that most women don't take cesareans quite as casually as they do. The aftereffects and recovery from a cesarean birth, for some women, are about as close to hell as they choose to get. For others, it can be less dramatic, but still traumatic.

The surgery itself, however, *is* an easy, quick, and usually safe procedure. Because cutting into the abdominal wall is involved, all cesareans are major surgery. In preparation for surgery, a catheter is put into a woman's bladder, the abdomen and perineum are shaved, and an IV is inserted in the back of her hand. The IV and catheter remain in place for about twenty-four hours after the surgery. Regional anesthesia (a spinal or epidural), which allows the mother to be awake but without feeling below her waist, is administered. In an emergency situation, a general anesthesia (gas) can be used. The advantage to gas is that it takes effect immediately, in preference to the fifteen to twenty minutes taken by regional anesthesia. A drape is placed at about chest level, to keep the woman from observing the surgery. Then the abdomen is sterilized with a cold anesthetic solution.

The first incision is made in the abdomen, usually a four- to six-inch "bikini cut" just above the pubic hair line. The bladder is separated from the uterus and pushed down out of the way before another horizontal incision is made in the lowest part of the uterus. The baby is lifted out of the uterus within ten minutes from the beginning of surgery. The afterbirth is removed, the uterus is sutured, the bladder is stitched back into place, and the abdominal incision is closed. The total surgery takes about an hour, with most of the time spent in sewing up the incisions.

How Safe Is "Safe"?

Well, why not have a cesarean? With the cesarean section rate so high, your chances of having one are pretty good, one in four in fact. Why fight the system? It's an easy, simple, safe operation for the doctor to perform, and if he says, "I think you need a cesarean," isn't it easier to just go along? Yes, it is. And if you do have a cesarean, the chances are excellent that you will survive, and so will your baby.

Risks to Baby

Although cesareans are safe today, they are certainly not as safe as vaginal deliveries, either for the mother or the baby. A baby is always considered at high risk for complications when born by cesarean section. Madeleine Shearer, in *Birth* journal, reviewed the literature and summarized the four most frequent complications of cesarean to the infant, in order of their frequency:

- Jaundice
- Fewer quiet alert periods after birth
- Respiratory distress
- Drug effects

Jaundice is an overdiagnosed, overtreated problem in more than half of all newborns and is a recognized risk of cesarean delivery. Why is not known. Newborn jaundice sometimes requires putting the infant under bilirubin lights. Having a blindfold placed over his or her eyes for nearly twenty-four hours a day for several days can be uncomfortable, frustrating, and perhaps even terrifying for the infant. Certainly, the treatment interferes with early contact between mother and her baby.

Infants born by cesarean section have fewer quiet alert periods after birth, the time when the infant is most likely to respond to its mother. Mothers and babies need all the help they can get in the early time they are getting acquainted with each other. A cesarean-born baby has fewer of these ideal times, when he is neither sleeping nor crying, but awake and taking in his surroundings—most importantly, his mother.

Breathing difficulty or respiratory distress is the most feared of the frequent complications of a cesarean baby. "Babies delivered by cesarean section are at a considerable disadvantage during the first few days of life," reported British researchers John Brice and Colin Walker, studying respiratory distress. Breathing difficulty may be temporary or may be the much more serious respiratory distress syndrome (RDS). This disease varies from mild to severe, and often requires mechanical assistance for the baby to breathe.

Studying how doctors cause RDS, R. L. Goldberg *et al.* observed that a major factor in RDS was a misjudgment of the actual length of pregnancy and a too-early ending of the pregnancy by induction or cesarean. "The ill-advised timing [by doctors] of cesarean sections is threatening to become the leading cause of respiratory distress, or hyaline membrane disease in infants," said researcher Lewis Gluck of the University of California Medical Center in San Diego.

However, several studies found an increased risk of RDS from the cesarean section, not only from poor timing. At all gestational ages, more babies had RDS when delivered by cesarean than vaginally, reported M. Douglas Jones, Jr., *et al.* in their study of 16,485 birth records at University Hospital in Denver. Researchers at the University of Washington in Seattle identified two important factors in RDS and their relation to cesarean surgery. Labor (preventing RDS) and lung fluids (causing RDS) were found by E. White *et al.* to be significant factors linking cesareans and RDS.

These findings fit with the research on catecholamines (see page 149). Naturally produced by the infant in reaction to the stress of labor and delivery, catecholamines help the fetus by clearing the lungs of amniotic fluid so the baby can breathe at birth. Babies born by cesarean section do not have the high levels of catecholamines of vaginally born infants.

Drug effects on the cesarean infant can be noticeable and are the fourth most common complication. The infant may appear to be drugged, or slowed down, because of medications or anesthesia given the mother during labor and delivery. The baby may also have an elevated blood pressure from drugs given to the mother to correct her *low* blood pressure as a complication of the anesthesia. Drug effects may be contributing to increased sucking problems observed after epidural use.

In addition to these four common complications the medical literature shows babies born from *planned repeat* cesareans (cesareans done before labor begins) are at risk from two additional complications: They are more likely than babies born vaginally to have abnormal neurological responses, and more likely to have these abnormal neurological responses still present when the babies are a year old. Abnormal neurological responses are a rare complication in repeat cesareans performed after labor starts.

Risks to Mother

A vaginal delivery is safer for the mother almost all the time. Regional anesthesia, availability of blood transfusions, a horizontal uterine incision, and antibiotics have made cesareans safer for mothers than ever before. Yet the maternal death rate after a cesarean is *still* higher than it is for a vaginal delivery. Some controversy exists about how great the difference is. Maternal mortality for vaginal deliveries is placed at less than one death for every 10,000 live births. Obstetricians generally quote maternal mortality for primary cesareans four to six times higher than for vaginal births.

Some suggest that the maternal death rate after cesareans is even higher. From his review of the literature, obstetrician Richard Porreco reported a sevenfold increase in maternal mortality after cesareans, but a much higher increase when the mother is unhealthy before birth. He also reported no additional risk to waiting for labor before a repeat cesarean rather than scheduling a repeat cesarean.

Cesarean maternal mortalities were also higher than commonly reported according to a study by George Rubin et al. of the Centers for Disease Control. If a cesarean mother dies after she leaves the hospital (from a pulmonary embolism, for example) her death is not likely to be recorded as a "maternal mortality." Comparing death certificates of women with birth certificates of babies born up to sixty days before a woman's death, the authors found a maternal death rate of 9.7 per 100,000 live births (or one per 10,000) for vaginal deliveries, but a rate of 105 maternal deaths per 100,000 live cesarean deliveries (or slightly more than ten per 10,000). The cesarean mothers were more than ten times likelier to die than the mothers who gave birth vaginally. The authors consider these mortality figures low because they limited their search to sixty days before the women's deaths and they excluded maternal deaths associated with stillbirth.

In this study, half the maternal deaths after a cesarean were directly caused by the operation, from pulmonary embolism (a blood clot migrating from the surgical incision to the lungs) or from complications of the anesthesia. At about the same time, other researchers were also finding that half the maternal deaths associated with cesarean sections are directly caused by the operation itself. Death from pulmonary embolism and complications of anesthesia are "an inevitable risk of any pelvic operative procedure," say authors Iain Chalmers and Martin Richards in *Benefits and Hazards of the New Obstetrics*. In a study of cesarean section deaths in England and Wales, these authors found that half the maternal deaths following a cesarean section were caused by these two complications. "Earlier studies have underestimated the risks of cesarean sections," concludes Rubin. "Physicians should carefully assess the risks whenever they are considering performing cesarean sections."

The true cesarean maternal death rate, or the odds of a mother dying after a cesarean delivery, are about one per 1,000. Certainly this relatively high rate, compared to vaginal delivery, should be a strong reason for caution when the question of cesarean comes up.

Other reasons for caution are the complications, the physical problems, that cesarean mothers have: severe pain from the operation itself, pain from the intestinal gas resulting from shock to the intestines, and possible future cesareans. Hospital stays are longer, costs are much higher, and the physical recovery from the surgery and birth takes much longer than the recovery from a vaginal birth. The woman who has a cesarean may also find she no longer has maternity insurance coverage for her next birth. Industry-wide, the usual policy is to terminate maternity coverage after a cesarean delivery for a woman with an individual insurance policy or a group policy that has a small number of employees (ten or less). Fertility problems are another reported risk following cesareans, as are increased complications in subsequent pregnancies and births.

Almost half of cesarean mothers have serious complications from the surgery, some complications more easily treated than others. The three most frequent serious complications are infection, hemorrhage, and internal problems from scarring or injury to other organs, according to Madeleine Shearer's review of the literature. Women who are internally monitored during labor, and then have a cesarean, have more uterine infections than cesarean mothers not internally monitored. Overall, the cesarean uterine infection rate is fourteen to forty-five times higher than uterine infections following vaginal deliveries. The cesarean mother is at greater risk than the vaginal mother of developing other infections too, for example, in her bladder and in her abdomen.

Use Caution

If you are advised to have a cesarean, you must be ready to ask, "Is this really necessary?" It's probable that this crucial question must be asked by your husband or your doula to protect you, because you are likely to have been laboring for hours, to be tiring, to be vulnerable and open to any suggestions around you.

Most doctors will not like your questioning their decision. Because no evidence exists that cesareans improve infant outcome when the diagnosis of abnormal labor is made, you and your doctor will have to relearn toleration of a long labor. You may have to remind your doctor to try other measures to reverse fetal distress, such as those recommended by the NIH task force. Knowing that vaginal birth is possible in place of a repeat cesarean or for a breech presentation, you have to doctor-shop during your pregnancy to get what you want. Finding Dr. Right is still your best bet for a vaginal birth.

Emotional Pain

Almost all cesarean mothers survive the surgery, and their wounds eventually heal. However, the emotional pain can be much harder to heal, and this is an area physicians pay little, if any, attention to. Whatever the reason for the cesarean, it tends to promote a poor self-image for the newly delivered mother: "My body screwed up," is the common complaint. If a woman has had a vaginal birth before this cesarean delivery, the feelings about herself may not be as poor. But most women need to try to understand what happened, why *they* couldn't give birth vaginally. Yet many women complain that their doctors leave them with little or no lasting understanding of all the medical concerns leading up to the cesarean.

Another emotional problem can occur with maternal-infant attachment, which may be difficult because of the inevitable separation during the first hours or day following delivery, when the mother is in so much pain. Some mothers who have been given regional anesthesia for the surgery and no drugs to knock them out have found they can take advantage of the first hour in the recovery room before the anesthesia wears off. They are not yet feeling the pain of the incision and can respond to their babies. But maternal-infant attachment can be affected by the surgery. "We are finding that mothers are upset with their babies because they had to have surgery," said nurse Debbie Pile, interviewed for a television documentary on cesareans. Pile says the mothers feel toward the baby that "it's your fault I had to have the cesarean. I was relaxing and breathing and it was you who developed fetal distress."

All new mothers are vulnerable and need loving care from those around them so that they can learn to love their babies. Cesarean mothers need more loving nurturing and for a longer period of time after birth. Many decide they just won't go through it again and make sure of that by having themselves sterilized. Postpartum sterilization is far more common for cesarean mothers at all ages, according to the U.S. Public Health Service.

The physical pain and emotional trauma of the cesarean experience has been much overlooked by doctors. Our next chapter gives one mother's story.

9

Having a Cesarean Is Having a Baby

With my first baby, I was in labor for nineteen hours before my doctor decided a cesarean was indicated. I was very, very upset, and my husband was very frightened. All the rules of the game had been changed on me. I had totally lost control. I had never had surgery, and I was angry and frightened at the thought of it. The abruptness of it all shocked me, and then, of course, there is always the underlying threat that maybe things will not come out well. It was very traumatic.

The anesthesiologist on call preferred to give gas, and my doctor recommended I go along with his specialty. They put me out and then it was over. When I finally woke up—after five hours of fading in and out—everything ached. I was intensely sore where they had cut. I wasn't inclined to move, to hold my baby, or to breastfeed her—which broke my heart and disappointed my husband greatly! My body just hurt too much.

The physical pain was one thing, but the emotional and psychological pain was, I think, worse. Sometime before I finally woke up, they had shaken me awake, and told me three times that I had a girl. I felt very empty, very empty, very detached from the whole experience. They said, "Hey, take a look at this," and I thought, "Big deal." I did feel my husband's presence in the room when I would wake up for a minute before falling back to sleep. I would see him sitting in the chair holding the baby, and there was a great deal of comfort in that. When I finally unfogged enough to talk to my husband and my sister, who is an obstetrical nurse, I felt good that they were there and that they were taking care of the baby; at least the baby was in the hands of the people that I loved.

One of the things that upset me most in my first cesarean was that neither physician, neither my family practice doctor nor my ob, asked me anything about how I felt about the cesarean. There was no emotional support or concern from either of them. There I was feeling,

Okay, now here you are, you have this pain in your belly. You have this baby you feel detached from. You have what was supposed to have been a wonderful experience all turned upside down.

You do need someone to talk to after a cesarean, regardless of whether it's a traumatic one or not. My sister was there for me, and we talked continuously for hours. She also got after me to start walking really soon. It was very painful to get up and walk around. It almost didn't hurt too much if you lay still and didn't move, but moving—changing your position in bed, or trying to get up—was enormously painful. I didn't want to do that. But she told me that the sooner you start walking, the sooner you start passing gas, which means that the intestines have begun working again, and you are beginning to recover. That was the magic word!

I had wanted to nurse my baby as soon after birth as possible. Well, that was a joke. I knew that nursing helps the uterus to contract, but I was so fearful of any additional pain, I wasn't going to let that baby anywhere near me. My sister knew my fears and told me that, because this was my first baby, I probably would not feel the uterus contracting, especially because there was so much pain down there anyway. She very gently kept urging me to nurse, and with her help I did it. She helped me get the baby on the breast, and I discovered that there was no additional pain...just a wonderful joy.

After that, I felt emotionally very good for the rest of my three-day hospital stay, because I had my sister, my husband, and my baby all rooming in with me. My sister acted as my advocate after the surgery, and it was wonderful for both me and my husband to have her around. Together, she and my husband made me feel good about everything—about the baby and the experience—and I felt optimistic about the future. So, all in all, I would describe my first cesarean as a positive experience, because I felt so cared for during my hospital stay (by my family), and later, when I went home. I felt emotionally high for months afterward.

After my second cesarean I was extremely depressed. As high as I was with my first, I was that depressed with my second. We had a trial of labor, sort of as an experiment, because a vaginal birth after a cesarean had only been done three or four times at my hospital. I was four centimeters dilated when they decided to do a cesarean. I thought they were pretty quick to jump in as soon as they saw that the labor wasn't going fast.

I realize now that I was very apprehensive about another cesarean, and I would have been willing to labor forever to avoid surgery. I should have talked out my fears long before the labor. My worst fear was the overwhelming remembrance of the pain. That, and remembering the recovery, remembering just how complicated the whole thing is, emotionally and physically.

I had decided beforehand to have an epidural if a cesarean were needed, so that I could stay conscious and have my husband with me. He had to wait outside while I was given the epidural, and I felt alone and frightened. I had to curl up into the fetal position, which was difficult for me because of my big belly. The better fetal position you get into, the better chance the anesthesiologist has of hitting the epidural space. My back was numbed, but he had to poke around several times. I was afraid, thinking, "What are they doing behind me?"

Later, as I lay on the table holding my husband's hand, I barely knew he was there. I kept thinking, "They are going to cut me up again, dammit." I felt that the anesthesiologist was moving too fast. Everything was moving too fast, and no one cared how I felt. People were bustling about in the delivery room, and I was feeling very helpless. My second chance at a vaginal delivery was shot. Once again I had lost all control over the situation. Why the hell was this happening to me again?

Once the surgery started, it happened within minutes. They were taking the baby out, but I didn't know it. I was still thinking, "When are you going to start?" I was holding my husband's hand, just looking at him, trying to block everything else out, frightened to death. My sister, who was with me again, all of a sudden said to me, "It's a girl," and I didn't know that they were cutting me open yet.

They showed the baby to me just briefly. I started crying and shaking a little bit, and they said later, "Oh, Sandy was so touched, it was such a euphoric experience because she was crying." I was crying because I thought, "God, it's another girl, and I have to go through this one more time to have a boy, and I can't do it. I can't do it again." My sister went down with the baby to the nursery. They called back over the intercom to say she weighed ten pounds. That's the one positive, happy feeling I will have from the whole experience—the utter astonishment I felt at having such a large baby.

I was so cold in the delivery room and shaking with chills. I shook more and more until I was out of control—apparently because I had hemorrhaged so badly, and my body was compensating for the loss of fluids. That really frustrated me. The anesthesiologist gave me something, and I went out. It was all over. Once again, I didn't have a chance to be with my baby after the delivery.

The pain after my second cesarean was more intense, because my emotions were so negative, I believe. It was also made worse by my getting a spinal headache. The anesthesiologist was not able to get into the epidural space well enough; and the epidural had turned into a spinal. It was complicated by a tightening of all the muscles in my back, which was more painful to me than the headache. Two days later they ended the headache and muscle spasms when they did a "blood patch"—injecting some blood from my arm into the epidural space. Because of the headache, though, I hadn't been able to get up and move around to help my recovery. Also I didn't have the same kind of support in the hospital as I did the first time. At the last minute the person I had lined up to care for my two-year-old couldn't come, and my sister went home to take care of her.

Emotionally I was a mess. My baby was in the nursery more than she was with me—no rooming in this time. I was feeling very negative that I had had another painful experience, and I didn't have anyone in the hospital to help me. When I got home, my sister did not have the physical energy she had the first time to sit and talk with me, to empathize. She was too busy keeping up with the two-year-old, the cooking, and the rest. My husband was involved with his work, so he wasn't available very much. So I felt alone, and it was very stressful for me. After three months my belly was still hurting every day, all the time, because every time I lifted my two-year-old, I pulled on my incision.

I finally figured out that the physical part would have been barely noticeable if I had felt good emotionally. But I was mad at everything. I was mostly mad at my husband. Yet there was no way he could have been what I wanted him to be. I wanted him to make it all go away, and he couldn't. I was mad that I had no energy, and every little stress became impossible to cope with. I was mad at my physicians, and it wasn't until weeks later, at the urging of a friend, that I actually even acknowledged that I was mad as hell at the anesthesiologist for knocking me out after the delivery, and for screwing up my recovery with a spinal headache. I was even mad about having hemorrhoids.

I am still angry about the whole experience, and I still haven't talked to anybody about it. My poor husband is afraid to bring it up; he's just trying to keep his head above water to keep me from biting it off all the time. He can't begin to understand my anger, and I'm just now beginning to accept that he never will, and it's not his fault. I've alternated from thinking I am going to get a stress-related disease, because I'm not coping well, to my marriage is going to break up because I've turned into such an unhappy shrew. What alternatives!

After my first cesarean I felt I was physically recovered after three *weeks, although it was three months before I felt that all the fog was out of my head. But I was feeling very high, and very well loved, and very excited about the first baby. This second time I didn't have the gas, which I am grateful for, but I have an awful lot of anger bottled up. There were even times when I have felt suicidal in the last four months. After three months I began feeling better because I went home for Christmas and let other people take care of the baby (except for breastfeeding) and I just slept and relaxed, so I broke the fatigue and self-pity cycle. Once or twice since then, I have regressed and have felt like I was going back to the old depressed mode. It's now four months postpartum. I announced to my husband a week ago that my incision didn't hurt anymore. But, then, after spending a whole day painting my daughter's bedroom, it began hurting again, and it's been hurting ever since. Nothing to run to the doctor about, but just enough pain to annoy me.*

Finally, after four months, I am feeling more in control of my life again—but I'm working at it damned hard. The phrase that I often use when I think about the difference in the cesareans is that the first time I was surrounded by "a love bath," that is, love, concern, and security coming from my mother and my mother-in-law (who were both there to help when I came home from the hospital); my sister, who took care of my emotional needs and taught me how to care for my new baby; and my husband, who was just thrilled with the new baby. I felt good about myself and about my baby. After the second cesarean, there was no love bath. It just didn't happen. For some reason I just felt all alone and negative—about myself, the experience, and especially about my future.

Some people would say, "Just give me a cesarean and forget the pain of labor." Well I don't think there is a comparison between the pain of a cesarean and the pain of labor. Labor is a transitory pain. It's over when it's over. Labor pain is a physical thing. With a cesarean, however, there are so many other factors involved besides the physical: the emotional pain of apprehension and fear, the resentment and the anger, and the feeling of having lost all control—first over your body in pregnancy and in surgery, but also over your life. That's why—unless there is enormous support to make it a positive experience—the pain of a cesarean is really so much worse. When labor is over, the pain is over. When the cesarean is over, I don't think the pain is ever over—unless it was nipped in the bud by some very energetic, loving people.

Sandy is every cesarean mother. She is also a real person, though her name has been changed to protect her privacy. The fear, the disappointment, the anger, and the relief are almost universal feelings of cesarean mothers—albeit to different degrees. Support groups have sprung up across the country just for women who have had cesareans, so every cesarean mother can have the chance to express her intense feelings about her baby's birth, and to feel the support and understanding of other women who have had the same experience.

Where do these incredibly deep and intense feelings come from? Almost all women know how babies grow and how they are born. Nearly every woman grows up believing that some day she will become pregnant and give birth. A woman's monthly menstrual cycle is a regular reminder of her fertility and how her body is made to bear children. A woman's very image of herself, carried with her for years, is shattered when she must have a cesarean delivery. "I felt like a terrible failure," said one mother, Jane Richardson. "It was like training for the Olympics, then falling down the stairs. I had practiced so hard. I did nine months for this delivery. I know other women who feel guilty too, and they say, 'If only I had breathed better and tried harder.' I felt disappointed, cheated, deprived, ugly, and angry."

The feeling of failure is intensified in women who prepare for childbirth. They are prepared to be in control, to participate in the delivery of their child, to experience the joy of giving birth vaginally. Suddenly all that is taken away. They lose the support of their partner when they need him the most, and they lose the moment of becoming acquainted with their newborn baby after birth, a time they have looked forward to as the culmination of their pregnancy. Cesarean mothers have suffered a loss of the very image of themselves as able to give birth vaginally. Grief is the normal human response to loss. Knowing that a cesarean was done for the sake of their baby is a great comfort to cesarean mothers, but it does not make up for the sense of loss and need to understand, "Why me?" Cesarean mothers need a long time to heal emotionally.

In spite of what they have been through—the major surgery, the physical pain, the grieving—cesarean mothers cope. They learn to mother their babies. They heal and often go on to have another baby, even though it often means another cesarean. Cesarean mothers nurture, touch, and breastfeed their babies just the same as mothers who give birth vaginally. However, cesarean mothers need more comfort, more understanding, more help after their babies are born. They also could use a lot more respect for their incredible courage in immediately putting their baby's needs first, and readily giving up the kind of birth experience for which they have waited so long.

> Every birth is a perfect experience in its own way. It takes pro-found courage for a laboring woman to confront complica-tions and to willingly open her already open self even further to include unfamiliar people and procedures into her experience. Monks spend lifetimes in soggy caves trying to achieve this state of humility that women are able to experience through giving birth, being then vessels through which the ultimate cre-ative impulse is served and manifest. There is truth to be gotten and beauty to be seen in all births. Who is to say if one set of circumstances is more perfect than another, and who is to say that the mother whose child is taken from her at birth did not "bond" with the child?
>
> —Kate Botlos,
> Assistant Editor, *Mothering*

"Grapefruit are sectioned but women give birth," is a phrase cesarean mothers have come up with to remind doctors that ce-sarean mothers, too, need family-centered births. By using the infor-mation we've assembled, you the reader can greatly reduce your chances of having a cesarean. But mothers sometimes really do need cesareans. You may have done all you can to reduce your risk of ce-sarean, and then find yourself in labor with the necessity to have an abdominal delivery.

Because the possibility is there for all women, you need to know what you can do to make your baby's cesarean delivery as good an experience for you, your husband, and your baby as it can be.

What Cesarean Mothers Want

> In my experience a cesarean can be a wonderful and positive experience. I never felt I was excluded from the decision-making process and was treated with respect throughout my stay. I believe the secrets to making a cesarean a positive experience are: Choose a doctor you can communicate with, who allows fathers in the operating room. Choose a hospital where the staff is not overloaded with work. Have your baby brought to you and your husband in the recovery room. Arrange for plenty of pain relief; you want to enjoy your baby.
>
> —Arizona

Women who have had cesareans are very sure about what is important to them. In the surveys cesarean mothers' opinions were stronger and more unanimous than those women who had vaginal deliveries. Because of what they have been through, they are much more sure about the importance of their partner's presence and about having contact with their babies. Cesarean mothers want hospitals and doctors who will give them the following options:

- To be awake, if possible
- To have their partner with them during and after surgery
- To see the baby immediately after it is born
- To hold the baby when surgery is completed
- To be encouraged to hold and care for the baby if it must be in a special nursery
- To care for the "well" baby in their room whenever they want

Every mother needs to have her care individualized. Because almost all cesarean mothers want these options, doctors need to support their patients in getting them. Hospitals also need to change their policies so that family-centered maternity care is as strongly supported for cesarean mothers as for mothers who deliver vaginally. The care a cesarean mother receives needs even more sensitivity to her preferences, however. For example, while almost all cesarean mothers have a lot of pain following surgery, they will vary greatly in what they are willing to try to do—walk the first day, nurse their babies, have rooming in, or have visitors.

Most cesarean mothers want to be awake. Although any kind of anesthesia has its risk, the National Institutes of Health's task force recommended that women have the option of receiving regional anesthesia when they have a cesarean.

Women want to have their partners with them during and after surgery. A woman's fear and anxiety when a cesarean is recommended is high enough without having her key support person denied her. Partners also are reassured by staying with their mates. Many hospitals are easing their policies to allow partners to be present for a scheduled or repeat cesarean. It's unusual, however, to find a hospital that will allow partners to stay in an emergency—a sudden cesarean that is decided on during labor. It is unlikely, in most emergency cesareans, that the need for the cesarean is so urgent that a staff member cannot take the time to include the partner in the preparations, allowing him or her to change into a scrub suit and stand by the mother. Emergency cesareans allow plenty of time for careful preparation, explanation, and some choices on the part of the parents if the baby is not in acute fetal distress. Having the partners with them is so important to cesarean mothers that it should be the exception, not the rule, when partners are asked to wait outside during an emergency cesarean.

> My husband was there in the operating room and a day or two later I asked him to write down *everything* that happened to me, and especially to our son, up to when I came to. Those papers are precious to me and help me feel more a part of the birth. I would strongly suggest a cesarean father do that for his wife if she is under general anesthesia. The father's own words and feelings are more important than a tape of the birth.
>
> —Wisconsin

If your partner is with you, he or she will not be able to see the surgery, just as you will not. The cesarean mother lies on her back on the delivery table. A drape is raised above her midsection, so she cannot see beyond that point. She does not see her baby born through the abdominal incision, and neither does the partner seated next to her head (unless he or she chooses to look over the drape). If the doctor keeps up a running commentary on what he's doing, however, the parents can participate in the excitement of the few minutes before the baby is born. Then the baby should be carried around the drape for them to see. If the baby is not in breathing distress, there is no reason why the partner cannot carry the newborn to the nursery for an examination while the doctor closes the incisions on the mother. If the partner does accompany the infant to the nursery, the new mother may prefer to have a familiar person stay with her—the doula, perhaps.

Women who have had cesareans are keenly aware of what a difference it can make in their feelings toward their baby if they are given the chance to view her immediately after she is born, and, then, when surgery is completed, to hold her and bond with her in the recovery area before the anesthesia has worn off. For many women it may be the only chance they have to get acquainted with their babies for another twenty-four to forty-eight hours because of the pain following surgery.

Women want both parents to be encouraged to hold and care for the baby if she must be in a special-care nursery. Klaus and Kennell's research strongly supports this preference because many women who are separated from their babies may have difficulty developing a normal mother-baby relationship.

Women want to care for their "well" baby in their room whenever they wish. The pace of each mother's recovery will vary, but after the first day or so she will have the strength and inclination to begin to care for her baby. If the partner and doula take over the baby's care for the first day, the mother can, as Sandy did, gain great comfort from knowing her baby is being watched over and cared for by those she loves. Having the partner and doula remain with the mother for much of her hospital stay gives her the extra care and assistance she needs.

Negotiating Cesarean Birth

To have your own kind of cesarean birth you must negotiate during your pregnancy. If you have had a cesarean and *may* be having another cesarean, you are more likely to have strong preferences for your next. If you have not had a cesarean, your chance of having one today is high enough that if you want it to be as family centered as possible, you must negotiate for this ahead of time. Although most of you are not anticipating a cesarean delivery, you should negotiate for your kind of cesarean birth, just in case. Remember: Negotiation is your tool for getting what you want. (Review Chapter 5.) Decide what you *may* want (you can change your mind later) and get that insurance policy in writing, just as you did for the other options you want for your vaginal delivery.

Many hospitals have eased their policies to make cesarean birth more family centered, but allowing partners to attend emergency cesarean deliveries is unusual. If the hospital and doctor you have chosen allow partners to be present for planned cesareans, the next step is to persuade them to permit your partner to be with you for an emergency cesarean. To do this you need to find out the position each hospital anesthesiologist takes on letting partners in to the surgery, since he can veto your doctor—and often does.

The anesthesiologist is *the boss* in the operating room. He decides whether your partner and doula can be there; he decides on the anesthesia for surgery; and he decides the drugs routinely given "pre- and post-op" (before and after surgery). Because your doctor will know which anesthesiologist may be flexible and go along with your preferences, he can often handle the negotiations for you. But if your doctor can't "put it in writing," you may want to negotiate in person by scheduling an appointment for you and your partner with the anesthesiologist. A personal interview may be the only way to convince the anesthesiologist that you want *him* to be on call for you, so you can avoid pre- and post-op sedation (until the anesthesia wears off) and so you can have the regional anesthesia.

Depending on how important cesarean delivery options are to you, if you cannot negotiate for what you want, remember you can change doctors during your pregnancy. You'll feel discouraged if you have to start your search over again for the hospital and Dr. Right. And you'll have to overcome the natural feelings of dependency in pregnancy. But having your baby *your* way is the reason you are going to all this trouble, remember?

If your cesarean-born baby must be in a special-care nursery after birth, you will need to negotiate with the pediatrician so you and your partner can have as much contact with the baby as possible.

Vaginal Birth after Cesarean (VBAC)

"The best way to reduce the number of cesareans is to be sure the *first* one is necessary," says Gerald Stober, New York City obstetrician. But for the nearly one million women who are given cesareans every year in the United States, the advice comes too late. Many of these women are looking to the future, not the past, and want to have a vaginal delivery for their next baby. If you are one of these women, scientific evidence strongly supports your having a vaginal birth after a cesarean.

Experts now agree that routine repeat cesareans are not acceptable because vaginal delivery is safer for a woman and her newborn. If a woman has had a previous cesarean with a low horizontal uterine incision ("bikini cut"), a vaginal birth is strongly recommended, assuming no current specific medical reason for a cesarean.

Reports are accumulating of vaginal births for women with two, three, and four previous cesareans. Women with two or more previous cesareans "should not be discouraged from attempting a vaginal delivery," according to the guidelines issued by the American College of Obstetricians and Gynecologists. In an attempt to affect the cesarean rate, ACOG endorsed VBAC (pronounced vee-back). ACOG's guidelines for VBAC are the same as for any other vaginal birth: The hospital should be able to respond to an emergency during labor. "No hospital that considers itself capable of handling any childbirth emergency could claim to be unable to meet ACOG's guidelines for VBAC," says Beth Shearer of C/Sec, Inc.

So far, most obstetricians have been ignoring recommendations for VBAC. In 1990 four out of five women with a previous cesarean had a repeat cesarean. More and more obstetricians are willing, even eager, to try a VBAC, but you may have to search for them (a family practitioner backed by an obstetrician can also give you a VBAC). Christiana Syed wrote to La Leche League International to tell them of her efforts resulting in a VBAC:

> For a few weeks after Eric's birth, it was easiest and most comfortable for me to believe that my cesarean (first birth) was necessary. But then I started to question, and to read, and then through friends in my La Leche League group, to get in touch with people who helped me come to terms with my cesarean and myself. I've always thought it terrible that in this culture we have to do so much work during pregnancy—soul-searching, reading, talking, careful thinking, searching for the right health-care provider and birthplace, making birth plans, and confronting doctors. All this to assure the birth experience that ought to be every mother and child's uncontested right! Now, however, I am very glad to have done this work, and I urge other women to do the same. Only by doing so can we be certain, whatever the outcome of our births, that we have done the best for ourselves and our babies, and only by doing so can we hope for a future in which no woman will have her self-trust, her strength, and her faith in her own body and her mothering undermined by dangerous and unnecessary interventions.

Your choice of birth attendant can make a difference in whether or not you have that vaginal delivery. Just as cesarean section rates vary among doctors and hospitals, so, too, do the rates of vaginal delivery following cesarean. Success rates of 50 to 90 percent vaginal delivery after previous cesarean are reported in the medical literature. So ask what your doctor's success rate is.

You can be misled by a doctor who says he is in favor of VBAC. One doctor we know has been allowing labor trials for almost all of his patients who had previous cesareans, but only 30 percent of them deliver vaginally. His low rate of success seems to come from his belief (as told to another physician) that he can tell during the first hour of labor whether a woman can deliver vaginally after a previous cesarean.

The two most common reasons for a repeat cesarean after a trial of labor are "Failure to Progress" and "Fetal Distress." Review these sections in Chapter 8 for suggestions to prevent or resolve these problems. Staying home until you are well established in labor is a tactic used by many women who have VBACs.

"Women wanting a VBAC should go to the hospital when a normally laboring woman would," Richard Porreco, director of Maternal Fetal Medicine at AMI/Saint Luke's Hospital in Denver, told us. He considers the attending doctor's attitude a key factor in whether a woman will have a VBAC: "Success is related to the doctor's enthusiasm for VBAC. You can't treat her like a time bomb." Over seven years and 1,000 VBACs later, Porreco remains convinced that unless a new reason for a cesarean is present, a trial of labor is "the best and safest form of obstetric management." One hundred percent of his clinic patients with previous cesareans start labor, and 90 percent have VBACs. To insure a high success rate, "Pitocin and regional anesthesia ought to be used for the same indications as for any other laboring women."

Porreco finds "increasing enthusiasm around the country for [women to have VBACs with] vertical and classical scars." He reminds couples that "in the unlikely event" of scar separation during birth, there is not enough data to assure them that the fetus will be saved.

Caroline Sufrin-Disler, writing in the *ICEA Review*, listed a variety of conditions in the medical literature which did not prevent many women having VBACs: prolonged pregnancy, breech position of baby, large baby (over 4,000 grams or eight and a half pounds), twins (and one set of triplets), previous preterm cesarean, low vertical uterine scar, and unknown uterine scar.

Sufrin-Disler reported that "the National Association of Childbearing Centers has recommended that VBAC mothers be supported in birth centers since VBACs 'are safe and should be treated as normal births if the type of uterine incision is documented as low transverse and adequate physician/institutional backup is available in the unlikely event of an obstetric emergency.'" Her conclusion states, "A mother who has had a previous cesarean section should not 'attempt a VBAC.' She should simply labor and give birth, like any other normal pregnant woman."

Unless you discuss the issue with your doctor ahead of time, you may find that after your VBAC, your doctor carries out a manual examination of your previous scar, an experience many women find extremely painful. "No studies have shown any benefit from routine manual exploration of the uterus in women who have had a previous cesarean section," assert Enkin, Keirse, and Chalmers in *Effective Care in Pregnancy and Childbirth*. These researchers report excess risk of uterine infection and risk of turning a slight scar separation into a rupture with routine manual examination of the uterus.

Even with all the research on your side, you may find you need more than reading to have a VBAC. Childbirth education and support groups are particularly important to women wanting VBACs. "The uterus works the same whether it has a scar on it or not," wrote childbirth educator Elizabeth Conner Shearer, commenting on the similarity of educating VBAC women and others. "Effective preparation for childbirth helps women accept the pain of birth, to appreciate it as a sign of how strong and well their bodies work, quite different from the pain that signals injury or illness." The special difference for VBAC parents, Shearer said, is "to know, trust, and rely on their bodies to give birth...when their bodies did not 'work right' the first time." She says parents need to understand the reason for the previous cesarean to be realistic about their chances for vaginal birth after cesarean.

Shearer was a member of the NIH task force on cesarean birth. She makes special note of "how unscientific 'CPD' and 'failure to progress' are as diagnoses. All 'CPD' means is that *the baby did not get out in the time the doctor thought s/he should*" (Shearer's italics).

The International Cesarean Awareness Network (ICAN) offers support groups and help all over the United States. In 1982 a small group of dedicated women, recognizing the need for an organization to give practical help to women in the face of the cesarean epidemic, founded ICAN. The national ICAN office receives up to 200 calls and letters a week from women wishing to avoid a cesarean or to have a VBAC, according to Esther Zorn, president of ICAN. Not only pregnant women call. "We've had mothers of pregnant daughters call us for information to help their daughters avoid a cesarean," Zorn told us.

C/Sec, Inc., was the first cesarean support group for parents. Writing in the C/Sec, Inc., newsletter, Zorn noted, "The medical profession is finding it difficult, if not impossible, in some areas of the country, to listen to their own medical reports...and make steps to correct medical practices which are leading to unnecessary major surgery on pregnant women.... It will take time for women to understand and then act on their understanding that birthing is their responsibility, not to be handed over 'carte blanche' to an 'expert' who has learned about birth from a textbook and as an onlooker."

Finally, there is some evidence that your belief in your own ability to give birth naturally is important to a vaginal birth after a previous cesarean (it's important in any vaginal birth). "As you consider your decision to have a VBAC, you will probably have to deal with some fears," write Marianne Brorup Weston *et al.* in the article "Vaginal Birth After Cesarean." "The unknown is always scary and you may find yourself afraid of pain, of a long labor, of possible complications, of trying something new and unusual, of failure, of another cesarean.... The list goes on and on."

"Two things are most important for a woman about to have a VBAC," says Nancy Wainer Cohen, a VBAC counselor, in the video, *Once a Cesarean: Vaginal Birth after Cesarean.* "One is absolute confidence in herself and her ability to give birth to this baby, a feeling that her body is designed to give birth to this baby, that she is going to be fine, that the process is safe. The second is to have wonderful support people around her, people who believe in her and who believe in the process of birth, who are patient, kind, loving and knowledgeable, and who are not going to pressure her or very subtly make it more difficult for her to have this baby."

Cohen coined the term *VBAC*. Following a cesarean delivery with her first child, she had two vaginal births (the last one at home). She has counseled hundreds of women in VBAC. Among the more than 90 percent who had VBACs are women who had more than one previous cesarean, women who had breech presentations, women with vertical and classical uterine scars, women who delivered babies weighing over ten pounds when they had cesareans for CPD with five-pound babies, and three women who had twins through VBAC. Cohen explained to us why she thought these women were so likely to have a VBAC: "They are free to have the same labor as anyone else. They have no IVs, no electronic fetal monitor. They walk in labor. They eat or drink as they desire. They have confidence in their body, and they have loving support during labor. They have no time limit on their labors." Cohen added that some of the women had very long labors of up to forty hours, some at home before going to the hospital for the birth, and some in the hospital.

In her literature review, Sufrin-Disler reports that two different studies found that the labor pattern of a VBAC is different from what might be expected. When a woman is in labor after previously giving birth only by cesarean, she is very likely to labor like a first-time mother. The researchers felt this was particularly important information for birth attendants who need to be patient and wait longer, six to eight hours longer than for a woman who has previously given birth vaginally.

"I am finding it common to see VBAC mothers experience what I have termed 'emotional dystocia' at some point during labor," wrote childbirth educator and monitrice Polly Perez. "To get past this point requires infinite patience on the part of the caregiver as well as the ability to work with the mother toward resolution of the emotional block.... Much time has been spent in labor discussing fears and anxieties that she was not able to confront until that time. I am awed by the strength of these women to complete not only the physically but emotionally demanding tasks of labor and birth."

Having a VBAC is unusual in many places in the United States. Just as it took time for family-centered maternity care to become widely accepted, it will take time for most doctors to feel comfortable with VBAC. Having VBAC is a pioneer effort in many places. "I am convinced that the best preparation for birth involves choosing caregivers who understand the emotional as well as the physical components of birth, the grieving and healing prior to labor, and the importance of trusting in one's body and baby," wrote Perez. You'll need persistence and determination to find a willing birth attendant. Just as important for you, you'll need to have people around you who are loving, caring, and supportive of your labor.

What if you end up needing another cesarean? Counselors who help women prepare for a VBAC say that every woman is glad she made the effort, for she had the labor, she knew it was the best time for her baby to be born, and she would never look back and wonder what might have been. She had done her best.

My description of labor may sound awful, but I was in control of my situation all the way through and had wonderful support with the doula. The doctor actually asked me and my doula what we thought several times and always went along with what I decided. The cesarean was my informed decision. It made all the difference in the world in my attitude about the surgery. The birth was a "failed VBAC" that wasn't a failure as far as I was concerned. One of the things that made me decide to have the cesarean was my baby's frantic kicking once the Pitocin was started late in labor. I could only go by my intuition, which made me worry he was in distress. Even with the general anesthesia he was brought to me as soon as possible and I was able to nurse him and really fall in love. It was just wonderful.

—Wisconsin

10

Appreciating Your Feelings

As a first-time mother I still find myself, more than half a year later, remembering my (our) birth experience. I think I am finally coming to an understanding of the many feelings I had then and accepting the miserable ones as well as the elation.

—A Mother Quoted in *Parents* Magazine

Few of us are prepared for childbirth's impact on our feelings. We open ourselves up—physically and emotionally—to a degree not thought possible. And if it's our first baby, ready or not, we're thrust into the new role of motherhood. We now see the world with different eyes, while coping with roller-coaster emotions. These feelings are normal.

You've looked forward to caring for your baby, but now that the baby's here, you worry. Maybe I really haven't prepared enough, you say to yourself. Bone-weary collapse seems just around the corner. As most of the 64,000 readers who responded to a *Parents* magazine survey in the 1980s said, the biggest surprise about parenthood is the fatigue. Fatigue alone can produce a kaleidoscope of feelings, most of them negative.

Women's intense feelings after childbirth are certainly not new. "As long ago as the 4th century B.C., the medical writer Hippocrates was theorizing about the biological basis of this strange sorrow and/or madness that could invade the mind of the new mother," reported therapist Maggie Scarf.

Some of the new mother's emotions bother both herself and those closest to her. She's just not herself, and no one knows why. She experiences mood swings, more than the usual amount of tears, irritability, and constant energy lows. These symptoms are usually labeled postpartum depression. On the other hand, when the new mother thrills at feeding and holding her baby, and when her tears are tears of joy, these emotions are labeled maternal. But the truth is, to some degree, all of these feelings are normal, not just the so-called positive ones. No one, including a new mother, is ecstatically happy all the time. Nor is her partner. A 1986 study showed that husbands have an emotionally unique time after the birth, too. They experience nervousness, worry, and anxiety, as well as enthusiasm and happiness.

Some combination of all of these feelings is normal, but the actual numbers of women who experience the continuum from having a bad day to the baby blues all the way to postpartum depression are unknown. Estimates in this country and Europe are that about 50 percent of women experience the bad day/baby blues, and 10 percent have true postpartum depression (loss of sexual and other interests, irritability, undue fatigue, inability to cope).

But when a woman does experience postpartum depression, are hormones the culprits? If they are part of the reason, they're certainly not all of it. Maybe it has something to do with being in the hospital. British research shows that postpartum blues are less likely in women who return home forty-eight hours after giving birth. To exonerate female hormones even more, in many other cultures and in homebirths in this country, women reportedly seldom experience postpartum depression.

At The Farm, a once-thriving agricultural community in Tennessee, head midwife Ina May Gaskin found that of the thousands of births that have taken place there, only .03 percent of those mothers experienced depression. However, a homebirth by itself is not a guarantee of avoiding depression. If the new mother is isolated, which she wasn't at The Farm, for instance, that loneliness and lack of support might result in depression.

Missing Pieces

A combination of birth experiences labeled the "missing pieces" can cause your emotional seesaw to continue on the downside longer than is comfortable, and you don't have to undergo all these experiences to feel a negative impact. Many women feel the effect with only a few. The missing pieces are unfulfilled expectations, unrealistic expectations about pain and self-control, invasion of your privacy, distractions, memory loss, unwanted interventions, and separation from your baby.

Unfulfilled Expectations

There are reasons why today's new mother may be especially perplexed and sometimes profoundly confused by her feelings. Women, especially younger women and those in the educated middle class, have come to expect the best.

You're harder to please. Simply having a live baby is not enough anymore. You want the best experience, too. Maggie Scarf points out, "You're told now you can do it all, have it all; and when you end up not having it all or not doing it all well, you feel guilty—and depressed."

Because there's more information available on birth now, the process is not so mysterious anymore. Nearly all of you go to childbirth-education classes. You know to eat well and avoid drugs. As far as you know, you're doing everything you can to have a good and safe birth. Why, then, doesn't childbirth always result in what you wanted? Because birth isn't that predictable and neat a package.

Then *Parents* magazine writer Leah Yarrow said that the letters the magazine received after its poll "suggest that women spend considerable time struggling to come to terms with the disparity between the expectations they had of their labors and births and their actual experiences." This is especially true with women who have unexpected cesareans.

The truth is that the act of giving birth plunges you into the hands of a force much bigger than your ability to control it or fully anticipate it.

Pain

Nobody knew or cared whether or not I could stand the pain. And *nobody* was willing to help me and my husband through those awful contractions. I kept telling myself over and over: They can't let me die—it would look bad for them and the hospital.

—Oklahoma

Many women are stunned by the pain they felt. No one said it would hurt so much, or if someone did, you didn't think it would happen to you. Pain in childbirth is not new, of course. When your mother or your aunts, perhaps, told you a horror story about birth, you knew those were pre-Lamaze times your relatives were talking about. After all, you had much more information available to you now than they had.

Many of us have been told that if we did it right—breathed and relaxed correctly—we'd feel a contraction, not pain. For some laboring women, that's true. For most others, it's not. In the *Parents* magazine survey, most of the mothers found childbirth to be painful, and one-third said childbirth was "the most painful experience" they had ever had. Only one-third of the mothers reported that "medication took all the pain away." Research in 1987 confirms the same low rating of satisfaction with pain relief from drug use. Not only does pain persist with drug use, but many a new mother feels that the medical profession—not she—produced the child.

British sociologist Ann Oakley says, "The deliberate misrepresentation of the pain of childbirth adds to the risk of postpartum depression, since it makes realistic anticipation impossible." She continues, "A woman who has been misled about 'painless childbirth' has been found to be more likely to panic and request drugs when those sensations turn out to hurt.... Furthermore, a man who withstood hours of severe pain, refusing anesthetic to benefit another, would be a hero, but a woman who experiences pain is made to feel inadequate." Her pain becomes a "mark of failure."

Loss of Control

> Prepared childbirth classes lead you to believe that you will be making your own decisions about how delivery will be handled. My own experience was quite the opposite. The staff treated me as a "body," not a person. They administered anesthesia for delivery without asking me if I wanted it, but simply because that was the usual routine.
>
> —Survey

"Loss of control in any form," says researcher R. Rubin, "may result in loss of self-esteem and bring on a feeling of shame and humiliation." There's much appropriate interest, of course, in controlling pain. And many—particularly nurses, doctors, and reportedly some childbirth educators—advocate controlling emotion, as in "A good laboring woman is a calm and quiet one." Maintaining control, however, for laboring women—based on what they say—often focuses on who was in charge of the birth.

We've heard stories from women who were totally satisfied with their unplanned cesarean births because they were consulted through every step in the decision-making process and felt supported by the people around them. On the other hand, we've received stories from women furious about events that might seem benign in comparison to a cesarean. However, these unwanted, not-in-the-birth-plan procedures, which ranged from pubic shaves and enemas to staying on the fetal monitor longer than agreed upon, generated intense negative feelings in these women.

Lack of Privacy

Niles Newton believes that people, being territorial animals, are more relaxed in the home. However, birth in our society usually takes place in a hospital. What is it that women don't get in hospitals that is part of their biological need? Privacy, for one thing. It's difficult to provide true privacy for any hospital patient. You are handled by strangers (the nurses on duty, a doctor on call, perhaps medical students, interns, residents, nursing students).

Thousands of hospitals are taking a step in the right direction by offering a more homelike appearance with wallpapered and curtained birthing rooms. But having your baby in one of these rooms is no guarantee that you'll feel at home. For that, you need not just attractive decor, but caring, attentive people who treat you with dignity and respect (and who keep your door closed).

Distractions

A woman in labor craves peaceful surroundings, yet many laboring women have described how disturbing overheard conversations and laughter from the hall can be (or being asked questions by the staff when you're in the middle of a contraction). Because of the physical and emotional intensity of giving birth, laboring women's senses soar. According to psychologist Elizabeth Loftus, in her book *Memory,* hearing memory is apparently stronger in humans than touch, sight, or smell memory. Forty and fifty years after the event, many a woman still remembers the conversations staff members had (as if she, the woman in labor, was merely an object) while she was in labor.

In the first days after the birth, women's sensitivity to comments and distractions is still intense.

One nurse was extremely overbearing and even threatening. She worked very hard for whatever reason to undermine my self-confidence. Where breastfeeding was concerned, she was almost downright mean. I ended up trying to avoid her at all costs, which wasn't easy, since she was the head of the nursery. This goes to show how one experience you have at your birthing time can overshadow your other memories, no matter how joyous they are.

—California

Memory Loss About Birth

It's normal to talk about giving birth. You'll want to replay the experience again and again. In fact, you need to—so much so, that if you can't remember everything, you're often troubled and anxious.

Dyanne D. Affonso, professor of nursing at the University of Arizona, coined the term *missing pieces* to describe postpartum feelings after interviewing 150 women in Hawaii and Arizona. She found that "more than three-fourths of the women interviewed indicated that they could not remember, or were distressed by vague ideas of, some period or periods during their labors or deliveries." Women described finding themselves thinking often about what they could not remember. Researcher Karen Stolte in 1986 found that in the decade since Affonso's work was first published, women still had missing pieces, but fewer reported them. One aspect remained the same, though: Women still want to talk about their births.

One of the reasons for the memory loss Affonso gives is the use of the fetal monitor, which "may result in a laboring woman not hearing what is said to her, or if she heard it, she may forget it later." A woman's anxiety about the use of this equipment creates a crisis in her mind. Upset and distressed, she literally cannot hear what's said to her

Women who receive little feedback from doctors or nurses about their progress—where they are in labor, how fast they're dilating, and the condition of the baby—also have a sense of not understanding or remembering what happened, whether their labors were long or short, states Affonso. During their hospital stay women who couldn't remember found themselves asking the same question over and over to one person, or even asking "the same question to different persons such as the nurse, doctor, husband, or even the cleaning lady."

Not only will drugs used during a vaginal birth have their effect on memory loss, but those used during cesareans, particularly those cesareans that are unexpected, often leave big gaps in memory. Having someone there to remind you makes a big difference. "My friend stayed with me during the cesarean," a mother told us, "and never left my side. She was not only constant comfort, she was my memory machine. She told me everything that happened, and then told me again. It was so reassuring."

Unwanted Interventions

Ann Oakley found that "having the blues during postpartum hospital stay was associated with epidural block, dissatisfaction with the second stage of labor and instrumental [forceps] delivery." She also found that "becoming depressed at some point in the five months following birth was also preceded by obstetric intervention and feelings of dissatisfaction about the birth per se." She associates this dissatisfaction with the mother's sense of loss of control in labor and the management of the birth itself.

Routine hospital procedures often trigger a sense of low self-esteem. Birth therapist Gayle Peterson points to draping, shaving of the pubic hair, enemas, and routine episiotomies as unrecognized attempts to hide the fact that birth is sexual. They also serve to make many women feel demeaned.

Separation from Your Baby

"When the mother is really the first human being to have contact with the baby and that contact is continuing within several hours," said a midwife, "she is the expert for her baby, and feels it, and develops a tremendous amount of confidence, even skills."

Most of you want to be with your baby after the birth—that's clear. But many women still aren't, particularly the nearly one in four who have cesareans.

Rooming-in mothers developed maternal feelings significantly sooner, according to some research, and felt more confident and competent in caring for their newborns than did mothers having limited contact with their babies. Further, it was shown that mothers who felt confident about themselves consequently gave more affection and evaluated their own children in more positive terms, thereby increasing the self-esteem of their children.

In spite of all the pluses rooming in offers, American hospitals don't provide as much rooming in as you might suppose. The *Parents* survey published in the early 1980s, when the concept of rooming in had been discussed for at least twenty years, showed that "a little more than half (56%) did have some form of rooming in, but only a small percent (6%) of all mothers had their babies with them all the time."

The Need for a Support System

The missing pieces of your birth can be prevented or diminished by family and friends because they can let you know how special you are, a necessary ingredient to help you avoid depression. You probably will have your mate with you during your labor and the birth, so you will have the presence of someone who cares for you. What more could you need or want? Another women, that's who. As wonderful as it is to have your mate with you, we believe most of you will benefit from an additional support person. (See the next chapter for more on this.)

From the beginning of time, the traditional companions for a laboring woman and the new mother have been, and continue to be, women. In a study of 186 cultures, pediatrician-anthropologist Betsy Lozoff was able to "find only two cultures in which a man actually did something to help deliver the baby."

Traditionally, women have helped other women give birth. Isolated families where new mothers have only their mate for support are not the best environment for women. It's too easy for the new mother's needs and emotions—and her partner's—to be overlooked. A strong support system is particularly helpful for women who are single or having their first baby, those who have had a cesarean or whose baby died, or those who have a poor relationship with their mates.

Troublesome Behaviors

Your behavioral style may get in the way of getting what you want. If it's important for you to please other people and always play the *peacemaker*, if you want to avoid criticism at all costs, speaking out about your childbirth preferences may not be easy for you. The price you pay for silence, however, is perhaps anger and/or depression—now or later.

You may speak out daily on your job or in your home, but react differently in your dealings with the authority of doctors and hospitals. "Oh, what will they think of me?" you wonder. As women, we often feel responsible for everyone's comfort and well-being, including that of the hospital staff. We should learn to count to ten before taking the blame or backing off from a request we've made. And if that doesn't work, count to twenty.

How do you know when you're in your *apologizing* (or "I won't make trouble") mode? You'll know if you've said some of the following statements to yourself:

- It's very important to me that I don't have an electronic fetal monitor; I'm probably not right, though. After all, the doctor must know more than I do about this.
- My doctor doesn't agree with me that I should stay out of bed and walk around during labor; I must be wrong, so I'll do what she wants me to do.
- I couldn't convince the nurses to bring me my baby—they probably know better than I do. And I hate to be obnoxious by insisting.

And then there's *compassion*. Many women try to "out-good" everyone else by always being fair and understanding (especially of men). There's nothing wrong with compassion and fairness; they are noble attributes, and necessary ones for good parenting. But they can stand in the way of getting what is best for you and your baby. For example, one mother spent a miserable night anxiously listening to the cries from the nursery, fearing her baby was crying for her. She was in tears and her breasts were full, yet she didn't want to disturb the nursing staff by asking for her baby. And a Delaware mother wrote to us, "The nurse started to cry and told me that she had had a bad day. I spent the rest of my labor worrying that I had somehow hurt her feelings and apologizing every time I moaned too loud."

Many people adopt a passive attitude for coping with difficult situations. Even though that's not always the best response in our daily life, in pregnancy it is a perfectly normal response. For you, as a laboring woman, the most important reason for avoiding hassles in the hospital, for avoiding disagreements of any kind, is your physical and emotional vulnerability. That's true no matter how assertive a person you are ordinarily. Enlist the help of your partner or doula (see next chapter) to fend for you.

Sometimes, it's true, you may feel that yielding is simply the most rational way to cope with some situations. And it certainly can be. We only encourage you first to understand your choice of options, and their individual importance to you; then choose your own actions.

Anger from a Past Birth

I would have liked to have been allowed to find my own best position for comfort in labor and delivery. I found it excruciating to lie flat on my back—yet it was insisted that I do so (because of fetal monitor). I tolerated labor well in a standing, bent-over position, but I was forced to lie in bed—which I hated. Also, to be moved from a bed to the delivery room was further agony— I really didn't want to be disturbed at such a crucial point. It was only through the help of my husband that I managed. Then they kept me from my baby. I still get angry when I think about it.

—Survey

So what do you do if you're still mad? You find ways to cope with that anger and, even better, use that energy in a positive direction.

1. *Give yourself permission to be angry.* Having a baby is one of a woman's most important life experiences. If your baby's birth wasn't what you wanted, you have a right to be angry. You can't go back and do that birth over, but you can understand what you're angry about.

2. *Write down all the things about your birth experience that made you unhappy.* This may help you answer, "At whom am I angry?" Maybe you're angry at everyone. The nurse, for ordering you to lie down when you felt more comfortable sitting up. Your mate, because he or she didn't speak up enough to protect you or left the room during one of your worst times. The hospital, because you weren't allowed to use the facility you wanted—someone else got there first. Your friends, because they didn't tell you what to expect. Your doctor—ah, your doctor. Most of us don't allow ourselves to be angry at our doctor. Whatever happened, someone besides her is usually responsible: the nurse, the hospital, your friend, or your mate. But the fact is, most of what happens to a woman in a hospital is the responsibility of the doctor.

And what about being angry at yourself? Are you berating yourself, "If I had only stood my ground, or refused the fetal monitor/epidural/cesarean"?

Make a list and identify what you're angry about, and at whom. Now look at the list again. Is it enough for you to place blame? If it satisfies you, okay. However, most of us find it doesn't relieve us of our anger. Besides, placing blame just isn't so simple. If you blame your doctor for your treatment, remember she's only doing what she was trained to do. You could blame the nurse—except you know she's only doing what the hospital expects of her. So whom are you going to blame? Your partner? You have to live with that person. Besides, your partner probably did the best he or she could. Like you, the experience was far different from his or her expectations. He or she may be angry as well. Yourself? You have to live with yourself, too. Now that you know you're disappointed, perhaps betrayed, angry, or enraged, what are you going to do about it?

Make a decision about what you'll do next. What are your choices? Some of them are listed below.

3. *Do nothing.* One option that we all choose sometime or another is to do nothing. You can leave that anger buried deep within you. We've been asked why we would recommend doing nothing. Is it as productive as other suggestions? Maybe not. But we believe every woman has her own timetable for working through her feelings. And some of you will need to put that anger on a shelf in the back of your head for a while before taking it down, dusting it off, and deciding what to do next.

4. *Take action.* Anger creates energy that you can funnel into changing your own behavior when it comes to health care. A New York mother, infuriated by what she felt was an unnecessary cesarean when she was ten centimeters dilated, and who also felt insulted by what her doctor said to her, refused to pay the doctor or the hospital. Both had advertised that people didn't have to pay if they weren't satisfied, and she didn't, though her Blue Cross coverage would have reimbursed the entire bill. A Wisconsin woman channeled her anger into doing all she could to have a VBAC the next time. And she did.

5. *Talk about it.* Whether your birth expectations were met or not, whether you reacted with anger or not, whether you have missing pieces from the birth or not, you have a need, common to all women, to talk about your baby's birth. We've been stunned by the depth of feeling—often rage—of many women who answered our questions.

Get a friend who will listen to you, someone who will comfort you when you cry. For if you are grieving, you are grieving over a real loss. Grief therapist Marcia Lattanzi says, "You don't recover from grief, you manage it." And the more important the loss, the more profound the experience will be.

Women who had children long ago can still produce vivid accounts of their own birth experiences. One mother, who gave birth to twin daughters thirty years ago, still wonders what the twin looked like who was born dead and then immediately taken away. Another wonders what her labor was really like with her oldest son, now in his twenties. She was drugged as soon as she arrived at the hospital and was left alone to labor. There was no one to ask about what had happened. But you're not likely to be left alone in labor today. In fact, we encourage you to have at least two people with you.

One cesarean mother who had been asleep at her daughter's birth told us that when her baby was one day old, she asked the nurse who had been with her during her labor, and who also accompanied her to the operating room, to tell her, in detail, just what happened. That mother taped the conversation she had with the nurse and treasures it because it fills in some of the missing pieces of her memory.

Talking it out is cathartic, but it's more than that. Women have a need to preoccupy themselves with all the details of pregnancy, birth, the hospital stay, and those first few weeks at home. They talk of the pain and the pleasure, all the while putting the pieces of the experience together. Having a baby, especially the first time, changes your life dramatically. You're suddenly an equal with your own mother, and a sister to every other woman who has borne children. You're affected profoundly, and you yearn to understand.

6. *Write letters.* Even if it's been several years since your child's birth, you can still write a letter to your doctor or the hospital, telling them what you liked about their care, and what you didn't like. Hospitals pay attention to these letters, and will pay special heed if you also send a carbon copy to the chairman of the hospital's board of trustees. This board is responsible for getting patient/consumer input. You'd be helping the board to do its job by giving them your opinions.

If your complaint is about your doctor, write a letter, being as clear and specific as you can, to your doctor, as well as the local medical society. Do this especially if you had anything done to you against your wishes. Ask the medical society for a copy of the letter they send to the doctor. Your public librarian can tell you what medical society covers the geographic area of your doctor's office (it may not be the same as where you live). If you don't receive satisfaction locally, you can appeal to the state level, the state attorney general's office, the state medical licensing agency, or the grievance committee of your state's medical society.

7. *Tell doctors and hospitals directly.* Obstetricians tell us that they didn't think women were dissatisfied with their care because their patients hardly ever expressed these complaints to them (with the exception of those who sue, usually for a birth injury). Doctors are not likely to change if they believe women are satisfied with their medical care. We know it's probably a lot easier for all of us to tell our friends what we think, and we know that confrontation makes many people ill at ease. However, it's still most effective to tell your complaints to your doctor. To complain, plan ahead what you want to say, practice in advance, remain logical and self-controlled, and take a friend with you.

8. *Become hospital changemakers yourselves.* That's what we did. Why and how we worked with our community hospital to make maternity care changes that women wanted is described in Appendix A.

9. *Do things differently in the future.* If you're angry about previous birth experiences, the most important step for you to take is to resolve to do things differently in the future. What happened then, happened, and it's over now. Do what you can and move on.

But you don't have to be angry to want to do things differently the next time. Take what you learned from your experience and, step by step, develop a new relationship with health professionals.

11

Your Childbirth Support Group

I had the same kind of labor with my two children, but my experience with them was totally different. As my labors start with intense contractions, close together, the first time I went to the hospital right away. The second time I stayed at home for the first nine hours of my labor. I ended up having a cesarean both times, but the woman who was with my husband and me the second time made all the difference. And I don't mean only in my happier experience with labor and birth, but afterwards, too. I got my strength back quicker this last time, and the scar healed faster.

—Massachusetts

In this chapter we'll discuss the role of four different supporters for you. The first is your mate. He is not necessarily the choice, however, for the more than one in four U.S. women today who are single when they give birth, nor are men the partners of the growing number of lesbians who give birth. The next supporter is the childbirth educator. The other two are innovative in hospital births in our culture—the doula and the monitrice. *Doula* is a word (popularized by anthropologist Dana Raphael and the leading researchers in this field, pediatricians John Kennell and Marshall Klaus) describing a woman who nurtures and cares for a mother in labor and birth, as well as for her and her baby later—a woman who "mothers" the mother. *Monitrice* is the 1960s Lamaze word for a labor coach, but in our use, the monitrice is more than a compassionate, helping woman. She is a nurse hired to give one-to-one care to you in the hospital.

Your Mate

"Pam and Gerry stared at each other during her labor continuously—each strengthening the other," said a doula. "He kissed her face often and she thanked him with both looks and words for understanding her need. When she finally got to the pushing stage she was most comfortable standing up. Gerry held her up for hours, letting Pam's body be as limp as possible. Immediately after both of their babies were born, the voices in the delivery room hushed as we watched Gerry and Pam. Each was lovingly cradling one of their twin daughters and gazing into the eyes of that infant."

When the Lamaze method of prepared childbirth was developed in France, a woman trained to be a labor coach stayed with the mother. When this childbirth education method crossed the Atlantic to the United States, the husband took over the role of that woman. We believe your mate's presence is crucial and not to be duplicated by any other person. He is most important to the mother as her lover and the father of her baby. During the last twenty-five years, more and more fathers-to-be, originally encouraged by obstetrician Robert Bradley, entered labor and delivery rooms. For most women, their mate is the most important support person for them. The husband's presence and participation is necessary for the woman to have a "peak" experience in childbirth, according to psychologist Deborah Tanzer. Tanzer's research found evidence that joy and ecstasy in childbirth are directly related to the mate's presence. This peak experience is also possible for cesarean mothers whose mates stay with them through the birth. Fathers are not only there now, but occasionally a father catches his own baby in a hospital setting.

It's clear that the more that's done to keep birth in the hands of the new parents, the better they each feel about themselves and each other. This intimacy, says psychiatrist Lucy R. Waletzky, can reduce the stress many new fathers feel. She states that the most common negative reaction of a new father is jealousy. Among Waletzky's suggestions to men for more enjoyment of their fathering, she includes: Attend prenatal birth classes; stay with your mate when she's in the hospital for the labor and birth; and then stay with your baby and your mate as much as you can after the birth.

Historically, a man has not been the person who gives the major support to the laboring woman. And not every father wants to be present for his child's birth or throughout labor. That's his choice. Having your mate there is not the only way to have a baby. Some mates feel guilty because they don't want to be there. If he's not interested, plan to have at least one doula with you. What's important is that you receive the physical and emotional support that you need.

When the mate is there, his role in childbirth has become more than that of a lover. Most of the time, he is also labor coach and doula. He helps the woman to cope successfully with contractions, and comforts her with word and touch. And furthermore, he attempts to keep track of the hospital options the couple wants as well. But if the mate's presence were enough, more women would be satisfied.

The Doula

"No childbirth class can totally prepare a couple for what happens in the hospital," a childbirth educator/doula said. "I don't just mean the labor. It's more than that. It's being in a strange place. It's expecting that you'll get what you want just because you talked to your doctor about it before. It's just not that simple. I'm the go-between for the couple and the staff. I try to clarify any confusion, especially when the staff suggests interventions the couple said they didn't want. But most of all I do what I can to create the best environment for the woman and her husband. I know it's one of the most important days in their lives."

In a hospital birth today, having a good and safe birth requires a doula not only as comforter, but as both buffer and advocate with doctors and nurses for the laboring woman and her husband. Ideally, a doula is someone who already knows and cares for the pregnant woman, though many women have been helped by compassionate strangers. Preferably, she's a mother herself, wants to help other women, and pays attention to the wishes of the laboring woman. She could be a friend or a childbirth educator who is part of a growing group of trained doulas (also known as professional labor assistants and birth companions).

Some women may want more than one doula. In fact, it is common to find several women in attendance in out-of-hospital birth centers or at homebirths. When you have your baby, you, too, may want several women there; but check with your hospital in advance (going to the hospital administrator if you need to), since many hospitals have a limit on how many people can be with you in the labor room. You may have to negotiate to have more.

Many studies now show that the compassionate presence of a doula results in a reduction in labor time, risk for cesarean, and use of epidurals. (See Chapter 1 for a detailed description of the benefits.) Although these results are clear, opinions about whether a doula needs special training are mixed.

On one side are those, such as researcher Marshall Klaus, who told us that the doulas used in their research "have twelve to eighteen hours of training." Many of the childbirth educators, who often are also nurses, and midwives who are hired as doulas often agree that the most competent doula has some training or special background knowledge. On the other side are people like us, who receive enthusiastic stories every year from readers about helpful women who had no training.

It's true that professionals will probably know more about the birth process than a woman without their training or experience, but that doesn't mean that the presence of a trusted friend or a compassionate relative will not be just as helpful.

Whether you choose to have a friend whom you don't pay or hire a doula, think through what arrangement you would be most comfortable with, and then proceed.

What follows is our description of what the doula does.

Nurtures the Mother

The doula rubs the mother's back, holds her hand, and, as much as possible, keeps in soothing body touch with her. Since the father is doing this, too, isn't that enough? "Husbands, especially with the first child, are going to be frightened and inexperienced," says John Kennell.

The doula also offers the "female" connection, a same-sex empathy much like the identification men have with other men in a time of crisis—like soldiers on a battlefield. The doula probably has had a baby herself, so she has the link of experience. She understands the physical, emotional, and spiritual processes of childbirth. Some mothers who have given birth with doulas present tell of receiving an energy from these women, often described as a healing strength. Giving birth draws women together, while not precluding the simultaneously special relationship the laboring woman has with her husband. Often doulas describe reliving their own birth experiences—a feminine link through the ages.

It seems right to be with other women. Another woman present at the birth often can help the mother discard inhibiting social concerns, such as worrying about making too much noise, or complaining too much, or not pleasing others. A doula can help the mother know that she—and she alone—is the center of this birth. Her needs and the needs of her baby are the only ones that matter.

Calms the Father

Though the father's unique role makes him the key to the mother's joy and rapture, he can also benefit from the doula's presence. Fathers, especially first-time dads, can be unsure of what's expected from them during the birth process. As labor becomes progressively more intense, the woman becomes consumed by her body's contractions, and all attempts at casual conversation are gone. Some fathers may worry that all is not well. Even experienced fathers need help sometimes. A California mother wrote, "My first two births went so smoothly, another person wasn't needed. This third birth, however, needed someone else to step in and reassure the staff *and* us." It is at this point, especially, that the doula can encourage and reassure the father—telling him that the things he's doing (talking softly to the mother, kissing her face, wiping her brow, whatever) are all comforting and crucial. Also, though the father is not physically giving birth, he's still investing enormous energy. The doula's helpful presence and her kind and encouraging words can help to reduce the father's anxiety.

Serves as a Buffer

Some nurses understand the laboring mother's need for encouraging glances and comments, but they can also be severely limited in how much time they have for each patient. Others, though well intentioned, deflate mothers and may delay the progress of the labor by comments like, "Gosh, your contractions aren't as strong as they should be," or "Get hold of yourself—quiet down," or "If you don't hurry up, they'll probably give you a c-section." The mother doesn't need any negative statements during labor. In contrast to this, the doula continually reminds mom of how well she's doing.

The doula can also calm the staff. During the course of one labor a doula reported that the nurse would look visibly upset when she'd come into the room and find out the electronic fetal monitor was malfunctioning because of the position of the belt on the mother's abdomen. Knowing that the mother now thought she had done something wrong or that her baby was in trouble, this doula intervened and cleared up an accelerating misunderstanding. "The machine's malfunctioning again, isn't it?" said the doula to the nurse. "The baby's just fine. It's the machine that has the problem." When the nurse readily agreed the mother visibly relaxed.

Just having another person present during the labor, in addition to the father, reduces the chance of negative comments from the staff, since we're all generally on our best behavior when there's an audience.

One mother reported that she wanted to get up and move around during labor, even though she had an IV hookup and fetal-monitor attachments. The doula's reminder to the nursing staff, along with her readiness to help the staff work out the problems of the patient moving while attached to machine cables, led to a satisfactory solution that allowed the mother to walk around. If someone hadn't taken the role of the diplomat, the go-between, it's unlikely that mother would have moved from her bed.

The doula's there to see that hospital routine does not overshadow the parents' needs. The presence of the father and the doula can form a protective bubble around the laboring woman.

Becomes an Advocate

Active labor is not the time for a pregnant woman to be assertive. She has more important things to do than to have to remind nurses and doctors of what birth options have been agreed to. The mother needs to focus her mind solely on her body sensations; she can hardly do otherwise. So it might fall onto her mate's shoulders to renegotiate options. But this is a dissipation of his energies as well. Having a doula there to handle these matters allows the father to concentrate solely on his mate and her needs during labor.

As labor progresses, you may feel yourself getting "bogged down" in middle labor (four to seven centimeters) or when approaching the pushing stage. Quite normally you'll wish you were somewhere else. Or you'd give anything if the birth could happen "right now." You may even reach the point where you don't care whether you have anesthesia or not, a cesarean birth or not. That's normal.

If labor seems to slow, a lot of people (especially nurses and doctors) get nervous unnecessarily. That's when the doula can step in and gently remind everyone that the baby is fine. She can also monitor to see that the mother's preferences—from no routine IVs to a sitting-up position for birth (which may require a special prop behind her in the bed or on the delivery room table)—are honored. When the doula calmly reminds those present of what the mother wants, she helps everyone—parents and staff alike.

This part of the doula's role may make the parents uneasy before they even get to the hospital. What if the doctors and nurses become angry with the mother because this person is interfering? And what if parents in the future won't get what they want because the doula is too demanding now?

It's not the doula's intent to tell the staff how to perform their jobs; it's her purpose to remind everyone of what the mother wants. Nurses and doctors, of course, want to do their jobs well. They, too, want a healthy, satisfied patient. Although parents may have an initial fear of reprisal, women who have played the part of the interface between staff and parents have not usually been criticized. Although there's always been some concern that the presence of a doula would aggravate the staff, John Kennell and Marshall Klaus have observed that the staff really appreciates doulas, particularly after they've seen one or two in action.

You may be convinced that you want a doula with you and your husband when you're in labor, but are reluctant to ask a friend to come with you. It seems like a lot to ask of someone. But women we've talked to who have played the role of the doula consider it a privilege, a rare opportunity.

Once you've selected a doula—whether friend or hired labor assistant—before you go into labor, review with her what's important to you for your birth. Describe what agreements you have with your doctor or the hospital. Be as specific as you can about what you want her to do. You may not be comfortable with a doula providing all the functions we describe in this chapter. Fine. Tell her what *you* want her to do for you. And if, as occasionally happens—perhaps with family members, more so than with friends— your doula gets upset and becomes a burden, not a blessing, in labor, ask her to leave. Or ask your mate to ask her to leave. (Of course, the same is true of unhelpful nurses; ask them to leave as well.)

Helps after the Birth

While you've been pregnant, you've probably gotten a lot of attention, especially if this is your first baby. After birth, who is there to turn to? Your baby's needs take from you; that's your infant's right. A mother needs mothering herself to love and care for her infant. A doula is priceless after the birth. We know from the surveys that such friends are important breastfeeding supporters, and they are essential for mothering after you go home, too. She may or may not be the same person who was your doula during your labor and birth. Find someone whose attitude mirrors that of the midwife who told us that her most important role with a woman is to help her through her transition to motherhood—to give her encouragement and confidence as she learns to be a mother.

Lucy Waletzky encourages the mother's mate, too, to find a support system after the baby's born. She says, "Perhaps it would help to have someone mother the father." Mothers have friends and family to call, plus volunteer organizations like La Leche League. Men can talk to their own fathers, their friends, or men they work with who have children.

No one cares for you as much as your family and friends. Inviting them to help you is a plus for them, too. It's an invitation to share in some precious moments in your life and the life of your baby and for some mothers, can be a form of insurance that the doula will care for your child. Klaus and Kennell report in *Parent-Infant Bonding* that Raven Lang, lay midwife, "noted that the observers of the labor and birth became more attached to the infant than other friends of the family who did not witness the birth."

What can you do if you live a thousand miles from your nearest relative and none of your friends have babies? Make new friends. Find someone else who has a new baby—she'll speak your language. What about your neighbors, a co-worker, someone from your childbirth education class or La Leche League? Create your own circle of supporters.

The Childbirth Educator

Childbirth education in the United States began in the forties, largely influenced by British obstetrician Grantly Dick-Read and his book, *Childbirth without Fear: The Principles and Practice of Natural Childbirth*. During the 1950s and 1960s Dick-Read was followed by Robert Bradley and his husband-coached childbirth; ASPO (American Society of Psychoprophylaxis in Obstetrics), a teacher-certification group responsible for the widespread use of the Lamaze method; and ICEA (International Childbirth Education Association), an umbrella organization of childbirth educators and consumers. Now, in the 1990s, there are many more classes. (See Appendix D.)

Childbirth educators offer instructions on relaxation and breathing during labor, physical exercises, and a description of the course of labor. A tour of a local hospital ob unit is included, and most instructors give information on analgesia and anesthesia, breastfeeding, and changes in sexuality. Classes are taught at the end of pregnancy for six to eight sessions as well as early on, with one or two classes in the first trimester.

In addition there are classes that specialize, such as those for women who are having cesareans, women planning VBACs, and women who want homebirths. The typical childbirth educator also keeps herself well informed about birth interventions, such as ultrasound, fetal monitors, and drugs.

Today, although American women in general expect childbirth to be painful and an event that requires drug use for pain relief, women who attend classes often anticipate that the childbirth educator will "fix" that. But attending classes is no guarantee for most women that they will have a painless, fast, and easy labor.

Millions of women are more informed today because of the work of childbirth educators; nevertheless, childbirth educators are often criticized for failing to deliver more. Repeatedly women say, "My birth experience didn't match what she said it would be." "She led me to believe that I would get what I wanted." Why didn't she teach me how to cope with the pain better?" Maybe the mother didn't hear what the childbirth educator said. Or maybe she never experienced as much exertion as labor requires. Or maybe she was expecting more than the educator could give.

Many childbirth educators say they walk a fine line between giving consumers information and getting along with doctors. Independent childbirth educators, those who are not in the direct employ of hospitals or doctors, receive the most praise and least criticism from our readers. Some couples choose a class because of a suggestion from a friend, but most couples choose a childbirth educator because of a referral from their doctor. So even some self-employed childbirth educators try not to go out of their way to anger local doctors by volunteering negative information about the routine use of birth interventions, for example.

In years past, Lamaze instructors taught women distraction and conditioned responses (like special breathing techniques) to use during labor. Bradley instructors, on the other hand, encouraged women to breathe normally and tune into their bodies. Childbirth educator Penny Simkin told us that many Lamaze instructors changed their classes because of the influence of British childbirth educator Sheila Kitzinger. Today, most Lamaze instructors encourage women to have a greater awareness of their bodies during labor. And like many Bradley instructors and others, they take an eclectic approach—they teach their students techniques from many sources, including yoga breathing and visualization.

Shop for a childbirth educator as you would for a physician, midwife, or hospital. Childbirth educators vary enormously in what they offer, in their beliefs, and in their experience. Take the issue of pain, the most important for most women. If you want to cope with pain drug free, you need to be taught *how* to do that, not just that it is safer for the baby if you do. Some instructors, midwives in particular, describe nondrug methods of coping with pain. Others spend a whole class and more describing analgesia and anesthesia—with the admonition, "Don't be a martyr."

Interview childbirth educators on the phone. Ask your friends. If possible, look at each teacher's class kit (the handouts couples get). How consumer oriented is the material?

Childbirth educators cannot guarantee that you'll have your version of a good experience. The person to ensure that is you, by virtue of information you gather, your choice of both birth attendant and location, and whether you have enough support during your labor and birth.

The Monitrice

"I do not consider myself a complainer—but believe me, when you need something, have a question, or are in pain, and ring for a nurse, you don't expect to wait for two hours before they answer your call," said a New York mother. "Many a time I had to call two or three times." Although the hospital you plan to use may be fully staffed with nurses, most of you will be having your baby at a hospital that's not. Eight out of ten American hospitals do not have enough nurses for routine care. And the shortage may be on the ob floor.

What can you do to avoid paying the consequences of a nursing shortage when you're in labor? Choose a nurse-midwife as your birth attendant if you're having a hospital birth. (Women who give birth at freestanding birth centers or at home always have at least one-to-one care.) Traditionally they stay with a woman throughout all of the labor, so there is no need to have a nurse with you, too. If hiring a nurse-midwife is not an option for you, hire a private-duty nurse, a monitrice, to be with you. This practice is uncommon for hospital births but not new.

Philip Sumner and his partners at Manchester Community Hospital in Manchester, Connecticut, had their own monitrice program for about ten years. Fourteen maternity nurses trained in the Lamaze method of prepared childbirth were on call on a rotating basis. They were hired privately by the patients, came to the hospital when the woman arrived in labor, and stayed with her through labor, birth, and recovery. The monitrice monitored the fetal heart rate with a fetoscope, continuously if necessary, so that electronic fetal monitoring was used for normal births only when the monitrice felt she would like the additional data it might provide. Other U.S. physicians have since used monitrices, too, particularly if insurance paid their fee.

Do you definitely need a private-duty nurse in addition to your mate and your doula? Will your care suffer if you don't? Yes and no. It won't if your birth attendant is a midwife. What if you're in a hospital that routinely uses electronic fetal monitors on all patients, and you want to be an exception to the rule? When you discuss this preference with your physician, your argument will be much more persuasive if you tell her that you're willing to hire a private-duty nurse who will monitor your baby's heart tones by fetoscope. Your willingness to hire a nurse also shows how important this preference is to you.

To find a monitrice, ask your childbirth educator first. Since most childbirth educators are also nurses, some of them are already being hired as monitrices, also known sometimes as labor assistants or labor coaches. If your educator doesn't provide this service, she might know a colleague who would. Other options are to ask your doctor if she knows of someone who provides this service, or call the hospital ob unit and ask if they have a list of nurses who do this.

When you find her, suggests Polly Perez, co-author of *Special Women: The Role of the Professional Labor Assistant*, ask her about her training and background, her experience as a monitrice, how she sees her role, her willingness to come to your home in early labor, and her ability to monitor your labor with a fetoscope. Ask, too, for the names of other women she's helped, so that you can get their opinions.

If you plan to have your baby in a hospital, you can't expect one-to-one care. You'll have to provide that yourself by hiring a monitrice. All women benefit by having their mate, doula, and monitrice present. But if you are expecting your first baby, these supporters are especially helpful to you. First-time mothers are likelier to have interventions of all kinds than women who have already had a baby. Labor and birth will be an entirely new and untried experience to you, and you will need all the help and reassurance you can get.

12

How to Have a Normal Vaginal Birth (and Avoid an Unnecessary Cesarean)

Why, I asked him, is medicine so resistant to new ideas? "It's not just medicine," (Sacks) said. "In any activity new ideas find it difficult to enter the world... because new ideas force people to think differently, to give up their ways of thinking in the past. In physics it's said that it takes twenty-five years for a new idea to get accepted. This is because It takes twenty-five years for the older generation to die off. They're so fixed in their thinking and attitudes."

—Oliver Sacks responding to a newspaper reporter

In her seventh month of pregnancy Kathy finalized her birth plan with Dr. Right. By then she had discovered there were a lot of things that seemed very important to her, such as checking into the hospital as late as possible, hiring her own nurse to be with her at all times (a monitrice), and having other women there with her (as well as her husband).

When Kathy told her doctor she wanted to stay home as long as possible in labor, and to call him when she felt like coming to the hospital, he agreed. But his sudden laughter showed that he felt she wouldn't last very long at home. Hiring the nurse was okay with him, too, since there was a shortage of ob nurses at the hospital. To avoid having a fetal monitor, he said, the private-duty nurse, or monitrice, would have to check the fetal heart tones. Getting him to agree to these things was easier than she had expected. However, *getting him to agree to the presence in labor of her mother-in-law, Maria, and her friend, Julie, was more difficult. He suggested the monitrice and her husband were enough. He couldn't understand why she wanted other women to be there, but finally he agreed to that point as well.*

When Kathy was negotiating with Dr. Right, she noticed that he paid more attention to what she said when she talked about what was safe for her baby. When she told him what she wanted, he listened, but not as carefully as when she said she wanted to avoid interventions unless absolutely necessary because they might not be safe for her baby.

Kathy listened and agreed when her doctor said that her birth-plan preferences might have to be overridden in an emergency situation. Kathy typed up two copies of her birth plan. Both she and Dr.Right initialed them. Then he took one copy for her hospital chart, and she kept the other with her.

Kathy had been a light smoker when she became pregnant. Cigarettes had not tasted good to her during the nausea of early pregnancy, so she quit smoking. She had been an occasional drinker but she found, as her pregnancy proceeded, that alcoholic drinks didn't seem to taste good anymore, either, so she quit this too.

Take Care of Yourself and Your Baby

Avoid Drugs and Alcohol

The unborn baby is the loser when a woman smokes or drinks during her pregnancy. Studies done in various medical centers have linked smoking with an increase in the risk of sudden infant death syndrome (SIDS), miscarriage, premature birth, premature separation of the placenta from the uterine wall (placental abruptions), placenta abnormality low in uterus (placental previa), premature rupture of membranes (PROM), fetal distress during labor, and low birth weight. Heavy smokers tend to gain less weight during pregnancy than nonsmokers, and this is one reason for their baby's lower birth weight. However, studies indicate that smoking directly affects the unborn baby, reducing the amount of oxygen that reaches the baby and causing growth retardation. National Center for Health Statistics personnel estimate 20 percent of pregnant women continue to smoke.

Pregnancy and alcohol don't mix either. Doctors have long known that a heavy daily use of alcohol is connected with a set of birth defects in the baby known as fetal alcohol syndrome. As researchers began to take a closer look at the effects of alcohol use in pregnancy, they discovered that they simply could not find a safe level of use. So strong is the evidence that the March of Dimes, the National Council on Alcoholism, and the U.S. Surgeon General recommend, "If you are pregnant, don't drink alcohol."

Two huge social problems in the United States are cocaine-addicted pregnant women and HIV-positive pregnant women. An estimated 160,000 babies were born addicted to cocaine in 1990. Medical costs for addicted babies to the point of hospital discharge total half a billion dollars annually, conclude Ciaran Phibbs *et al.* from the Columbia University School of Public Health. The researchers confirm that effective treatment programs for pregnant cocaine abusers would give immediate savings.

Human immunodeficiency virus (HIV) is another growing problem for pregnant women and birth attendants who care for them. HIV is a precursor to AIDS which leads to early death for most people infected with the virus. Although heterosexual transmission of the virus is now the fastest growing route of transmission in the United States, intravenous drug use is still the number one avenue through which the virus is transmitted in this country.

The highest rates of HIV-positive pregnant women are in the cities of New Jersey, New York, Massachusetts, Florida, and Puerto Rico, reported Jody Kaigh, an obstetrician speaking at the 1991 ASPO (American Society for Psychoprophylaxis in Obstetrics) Lamaze conference. In her review of the literature, Kaigh reported that babies born of HIV-infected women can be infected with the virus in utero, but should be considered *not infected*. Because infants have their mothers' HIV antibodies for up to fifteen months after birth, screening tests for infants are useless up to that age. Most infected infants develop AIDS symptoms by the age of one year, so infants well at age fifteen months should be considered uninfected, said Kaigh. After fifteen months of age, three-fourths of babies born to HIV-infected women will test negative for the virus and can be considered free of the disease.

If the HIV-positive pregnant woman has no AIDS symptoms, she has no increased risk of poor pregnancy outcome, said Kaigh. If disease symptoms are present, however, pregnancy can worsen AIDS symptoms for her. No internal fetal monitoring should be used during labor because of the risk of transmission of the HIV virus to the

baby through the scalp electrode. Babies should be considered uninfected by birth attendants and protected from exposure to the
mother's blood when possible. Whether the infant is delivered vaginally or by cesarean does not make a difference in HIV infection of
the infant, reported Kaigh, but because cesareans may *expose* the infant to more of the mother's blood, they are a greater risk.

The same guide for intervention in birth can be applied to any
drug use in pregnancy: Avoid use unless the benefits outweigh the
risks.

Eat Well and Practice Relaxation

*Earlier in her pregnancy Kathy had taken a relaxation class. As her
pregnancy progressed, she tried to practice relaxation half an hour
before bedtime. The evenings when she practiced were followed by a
better night's sleep than those evenings when she skipped practicing.
Now well into her eighth month, she noticed that sometimes her
stomach became firm to the touch and she became conscious of the
heaviness of her abdomen. After a few days she realized that these
sensations were the uterine contractions of late pregnancy. She was
thrilled at her discovery. She decided that whenever she experienced
these very mild contractions, she would practice her relaxation—as a
sort of conditioning to respond with relaxation whenever she felt a
contraction. Her days seemed very full because she needed to move
more slowly, and she tired very easily. Some days she could hardly
make it through her teaching job, often going directly to bed when she
got home from work.*

*Early in her pregnancy her doctor had referred her to his nurse to
discuss a good diet. Gaining weight rather than trying to hold the
line was emphasized. So Kathy was astonished to find that some
women in her childbirth education class had recently begun dieting
because they had "gained enough weight," according to them.*

Current research is very clear in showing that having a healthy
baby of normal birth weight is linked to the woman's prepregnancy
weight, to whether she has gained enough during pregnancy, and to
whether she has gained throughout pregnancy. Even women who
are twenty pounds or more over their normal weight when they become pregnant need to gain weight. "It is never appropriate for a
pregnant woman regardless of her size, to lose weight or avoid gaining," wrote Carol Pietz, a specialist in maternal/infant nutrition.

In a national study of weight gain and outcome of pregnancy, Selma Taffel, a statistician with the National Center for Health Statistics, reported that a significant number of women do not gain enough. A majority of women either are given no advice or are given a weight gain limit that is too low. Both these groups were likely to gain too little weight, putting their babies at higher risk of low birth weight or fetal death. Women gaining less than twenty-two pounds were at the highest risk. The more weight women gain, the better the birth weight of their babies and the better the outcome. The best fetal outcome came with a weight gain of twenty-six to thirty-five pounds, only slightly better than gaining more than thirty-five pounds. These figures are much higher than many doctors and women themselves are using. Madeleine Shearer reported that a survey showed 25 to 80 percent of women in childbirth education classes were dieting to hold the line at their seven-month weight gain.

The end of pregnancy is not only the time when the baby has a huge growth spurt, doubling her weight from four to eight pounds, but it is also a time of rapid growth of her brain cells. "Even mild degrees of maternal undernutrition in the last few weeks can interfere with the normal growth and development of the normal fetal brain," says John Dobbing, British research professor, quoted by Gail Brewer in *What Every Pregnant Woman Should Know: The Truth about Diets and Drugs in Pregnancy*. Written in consultation with Tom Brewer, an ob/gyn, this book advises women:

- Don't worry so much about weight gain; eat according to your appetite.
- Make good nutrition your primary concern.
- Don't restrict salt intake.
- Be very careful about drugs, especially diuretics, which are dangerous to women and their unborn babies.

The Brewers' advice resulted from Tom Brewer's research on toxemia, a metabolic disease of pregnancy. For years, doctors prescribed weight control and salt restriction, together with diuretics (water pills) to prevent toxemia. The Brewers explain, however, that these prescriptions contribute to low birth weight and brain-damaged babies, and may actually trigger toxemia by promoting malnutrition in the pregnant woman.

In normal pregnancy the woman's circulating blood volume expands by more than 40 percent to take care of the nutritional needs of the woman and her growing baby. The expanded blood volume is determined and maintained by adequate salt intake. If you have ever tasted your own blood, you know it is very salty. The crucial need for salt is the reason that salt should *not* be restricted in pregnant women, the Brewers say.

Given the American passion for being skinny, it's not easy for a woman pregnant for the first time to watch her body contours change, to see her waistline go, her stomach begin to protrude, and her body put on fat where she never had it before. So it's important for you to realize that you'll gain the right amount of weight for you if you eat when you are hungry, taking in nutritious foods and avoiding empty calories. Women underweight before pregnancy will need to make special efforts to eat enough to gain more than normal-weight women, up to forty pounds and more.

It's hard to cut out cakes, pies, cookies, candy, and fried foods, which have a lot of calories and few nutrients; but it's also important to get all the nutrients you and your baby need each day by concentrating on milk products, fruits, vegetables, whole-grain cereals, breads, fish, poultry, and lean meat. However, you need not be a meat eater to get the high-protein nutrition essential in a healthy pregnancy if you use soybean products freely and combine grains and vegetables to form the complete proteins your body needs. *Diet for a Small Planet* gives an excellent explanation of ways to combine foods to get complete proteins, without eating meat.

Exercise Regularly

Kathy had arranged to stop working by the eighth month of pregnancy. By then her baby's movements reminded her of its presence many times a day. She began to turn away from outside interests and to turn inward. She decided not to fight it, but to go with her feelings. At least once a day, but especially when she was changing clothes and could see her nude body, she would put her hands on her stomach and talk to her baby. The uterine contractions of late pregnancy—which some experience and some don't—came a little more often. Wherever she was, she used them as an opportunity to practice her relaxation, letting calmness flow through her body.

Kathy had tried to take a walk every day during her pregnancy. Now that she was no longer working, she had more time for walking. Every day she looked forward to getting out to walk a mile or two.

Pregnant women need regular exercise to stay fit. As Elizabeth Noble, author of *Essential Exercises for the Childbearing Year*, writes:

> Walking, swimming, and bicycling are enjoyable activities that not only provide excellent general exercise but bring you into the fresh air and sunshine. Done regularly, they combine many of the desirable features of prenatal exercise planning: to strengthen muscles, build up endurance, improve circulation and respiration, adapt to increasing weight and changing balance.

Women who have been inactive prior to becoming pregnant need to ease slowly into exercise. Strenuous exercise that leaves a pregnant woman gasping and exhausted, either right after exercising or later, is not good, for her or her baby. Easy does it. Exercise, done regularly, in a way that causes you to breathe deeper and faster, helps you to be physically fit and better able to cope with physical and mental stress.

Another benefit of regular exercise while pregnant may be an increased secretion of endorphins in labor. Endorphins, the "wellbeing" hormones we mentioned earlier, are linked to reduced pain and your pleasure in the birth process. Daniel B. Carr *et al.*, reporting in the *New England Journal of Medicine*, demonstrated an increased endorphin response in women who exercised regularly. Exercise increases the blood levels of endorphins, and conditioning enhances the effect. Women who exercise regularly have higher levels of endorphins when they are exercising than women who exercise irregularly. Although we know of no such research on pregnant women, it may be that by conditioning in pregnancy, a woman may increase her endorphin levels when she is in labor and her uterus is working strenuously.

Even if it's late in your pregnancy, you still have time to do one exercise more important to you for your health than any other. The pelvic floor (made up of the pubococcygeous or Kegel muscle) supports your expanding uterus, which holds your baby. Exercising your Kegel muscle makes your perineum stronger, yet more "stretchy," more resilient, in the pushing stage of labor. Relaxing the pelvic floor while pushing with the abdominal muscles eases your baby's way out and helps prevent tears and episiotomies.

You exercise this muscle by contracting or tightening and then releasing. To find the Kegel muscle, try stopping your flow of urine. The muscle that tightens at that moment is your Kegel muscle.

Elizabeth Noble describes the Kegel exercise:

Remember: Quality is more important than quantity. Slowly contract the muscles as you would in making a hard fist, not just closing your fingers but clenching to bring in every muscle fiber. About 5 in a series, holding each contraction for about 5 seconds.... Always end with a contraction.... Fifty a day, at least, during pregnancy and postpartum. Fifty a day, at least, *for the rest of your life.*

Seek Out the Company of Women

Kathy especially enjoyed her contacts with other pregnant women and nursing mothers in her childbirth preparation class and in La Leche League meetings. There was a common bond of excitement, anticipation, and fear that these women instantly understood. Women who already had their babies talked about how helpful friends had been before, during, and after birth. Kathy realized a few weeks before her baby was born that having other women with her during her birth was not just a preference, it was a really strong need. She was glad her husband's mother, Maria, who had four children, would be there because she was experienced in giving birth, was a loving, calm person, and was the grandmother-to-be. She was also a supportive friend to her daughter-in-law Kathy. She was especially glad that her friend Julie, who had a three-year-old son, had agreed to be there. Kathy wanted Julie to handle any questions or problems there might be with the hospital staff, so that Kathy and Tim could concentrate on the labor.

As we discussed in chapters 1 and 11, a laboring woman needs to have another woman or women with her. In many other cultures the grandmother-to-be, midwife, or another experienced-in-birth woman is always present with a laboring woman. Most of the time their reassuring message is unspoken but understood: "You will give birth; you can stand the pain; you can find your own way to labor; I have done it, and I am here to let you know you can do it too. Your body is made to give birth, and all will be well." Women learn about giving birth and breastfeeding from other women. They instinctively trust other women.

When Kathy's due date came and went, she was not too depressed because half the women in her childbirth class still had not delivered.

By the forty-second week of her pregnancy, however, she was tired of lugging around thirty-five extra pounds. She felt very discouraged to learn at her routine prenatal visit that the baby's head was not yet engaged in her pelvis. Her friend Julie had arranged to call her every day so that Kathy would know where she would be and could reach her. This time when she called, Kathy wept and said, "I'm so tired of being pregnant." Julie said all the right things. She even correctly anticipated Kathy's unspoken thought that maybe—just maybe— she'd accept induction just to get the pregnancy over. Kathy felt better after talking with Julie. She returned to her acceptance of the truism that the baby would come when it was ready, and not a moment sooner. But it felt good just to know that someone else could empathize with her impatience.

For those last five days all Kathy thought of was the baby. It seemed to her that her brain had turned to mush, and that she must be the most uninteresting conversation partner. All she wanted to talk about was the baby. Concentrating on anything else seemed impossible. One morning in the grocery store where she always shopped, she became very frustrated when she couldn't find half the things on her list. She just felt weird. When she got home from the grocery store, she had some gentle contractions, not any different from before, and automatically relaxed through each one. When she had four contractions in an hour, however, a feeling came to her that maybe this was the real thing. She called Tim and asked if he could take off work for the rest of the day. "Are you in labor?" he asked. "I don't know, but I need you," said Kathy.

Stay Home in Early Labor

Almost all women know when they are in true labor that will soon lead to the birth of their baby. The problem comes from thinking and worrying about being in labor when you are not. Everyone, women and their birth attendants, has "difficulty in accurately timing the onset of labor," says Gordon C. Gunn of the Department of Obstetrics and Gynecology at the University of California at Los Angeles and Torrance. "This problem is especially true in primigravidas where regular uterine contractions may not result in cervical dilation and where cervical effacement [thinning of the cervix] usually precedes the onset of true labor." True labor consists of regular uterine contractions resulting in a progressive opening of the cervix. Early labor, when the cervix gradually thins, can precede true labor by many hours or days. If you are near term and are having regular contractions, you may be in early labor. The contractions could go on for several days, perhaps alternating hours of regular contractions with periods of rest (when you should!).

Avoid an early rush to the hospital, counsel Susan and Peter Rosegg in *Natural Childbirth: The Bradley Way.* Delaying your hospital arrival until you are well established in labor just may prevent an unnecessary cesarean from a staff anxious over your typically longer, slower first labor. The Roseggs describe emotional signposts to look for. Excitement and nervousness, the first signpost, is when most women go to the hospital. The Roseggs counsel waiting until some hours into the second emotional signpost, during which the woman is concentrating and seriously working with her contractions. "The signpost you want to see is absolutely dedicated seriousness, aggravation at having to move, and wondering if, in fact, she even can. (She can, of course—she only thinks she's made of glass.)"

What's the rush to get to the hospital? If you are in the one percent of women who have a very rapid labor and birth (an hour or two), you may end up among the tiny number of women who have a baby in the car on the way. In her review of all available data, Doris Haire reported at a La Leche League International conference in Chicago that infants born in cars have the lowest infant mortality of any group. Everyone else may be anxious, but mothers and babies do fine. "Nature unaided will usually conduct a successful delivery," says family practitioner Gregory White, homebirth attendant to over 1,000 women during thirty years of practice, and author of *Emergency Childbirth.* "Childbirth is not nearly so dangerous as a wild ride in an automobile."

White says to stop the car for the birth. "The mother, sitting in a slumped down position in the back seat, can deliver the baby over the edge of the seat into the hands of the attendant; or she may lie across the seat. As soon as the baby has been born and is breathing freely, it may be placed between the mother's legs and the trip to the hospital continued; it is not necessary to deal with the cord or wait for the afterbirth."

Stay home until you feel sure you are in well-established labor and will deliver soon. If you are feeling very uncertain, consider having a vaginal examination to establish dilation. If it is during a weekday, you can go to your doctor's office. Call his office first, of course, to alert him you are coming. Set this up ahead of time with him, so you can be taken right in for a quick check, rather than facing a possible long wait. If it is outside office hours, go to the hospital emergency room for a dilation check. If you are not at least four to five centimeters dilated, you will not have checked into the hospital, and you can return home without upsetting hospital routine.

Turn Inward and Trust Your Instincts

For nine hours, from ten in the morning until seven in the evening, the contractions continued, never too close together, never really regular, but always there. As each one came, Kathy stopped what she was doing and allowed a wave of relaxation to pass over her body, at the same time breathing slowly and deeply. She wasn't interested in regular meals, but did become hungry during the day and had a small snack three or four times. Between six and seven o'clock in the evening the contractions were so light she was hardly aware of them. She felt very sleepy because she had missed her nap that day, so she decided to go to sleep. Because he felt he might be up later for the real thing, Tim got into bed with her, put his arms around her, and the two of them fell asleep.

Two hours later Kathy woke up because she felt she had to have a bowel movement. A half hour later she had another bowel movement, and a half hour later another one. The contractions had come back, about every twenty minutes now, and seemed stronger than she had ever felt before. Suddenly Tim laughed and said, "You know what, I think the baby's moving down and you have labor diarrhea." Kathy wasn't at all sure of anything at this point, except that she knew that she felt a little hungry again and wanted to take a shower. So first she snacked, and then she stood under a warm shower. She found that the water not only helped her relax during the contraction, but the sensuous feeling of the water on her skin seemed to help her tune into her body better. She decided she wanted Maria and Julie to come. After Tim called them, it seemed only minutes before they arrived. Kathy was surprised at how relieved she felt just to have them there.

Supported and cared for in a safe, quiet place, a woman can turn inward and listen to what her emotions tell her to do in labor and birth. Such a philosophy of care was used by obstetrician Michel Odent and the six midwives who practice with him in Pithiviers, France. "What we try to do at Pithiviers is to rehabilitate the instinctive brain, the emotional brain, the brain which is close to the body, in a world that generally just knows and takes into account the other brain, the rational brain," said Odent at a 1982 conference, "Birth,

Interaction and Attachment," moderated by Marshall Klaus and John Kennell. "Michel Odent has put together clinically much of what is known from recent research to be of value in human childbirth," said Klaus and Kennell.

Odent, author of *Birth Reborn*, directed the obstetric unit at Centre Hospitalier in Pithiviers for years. In a 1983 interview, he told us about his unit in a public hospital that gives all maternity care for the local population, without selection, including immigrants and women with complications (for example, previous cesarean delivery). Induction, amniotomy, oxytocin to speed labor, and medication or anesthesia (unless for cesareans) are not used. The episiotomy rate is 5.8 percent and the cesarean rate is 6.9 percent.

The emphasis at Pithiviers is on providing a milieu, a setting for the woman "to forget what is cultural and to reach a level of consciousness in which she listens to the instinctive, emotional brain, to find for herself positions for labor and birth," said Odent in the journal *Birth*.

The change in level of consciousness, the regression of a woman to the more primitive, feeling level of awareness results in a safer, smoother, faster, and less painful labor and birth in the thousands of women who have given birth at Pithiviers. The average primipara (first-time mother) labors five hours from two centimeters to ten centimeters dilation, less than half the average labor reported for American primiparas. Yet a short labor is not a goal of the birth attendants. When we asked Odent how long he's willing to wait for a birth, he said, "As long as it takes. We have no clocks anywhere in the birth rooms."

During pregnancy, couples can attend weekly group meetings (with the midwives), which emphasize the excitement, happiness, and normal nature of childbirth. Group singing is included to enhance familiarity with the midwives and to reduce women's inhibitions. Odent described five needs during labor affecting the woman's ability to tune into her emotional, instinctive brain.

1. *The human factor.* The midwife acts as a substitute for the laboring woman's mother, expressing love and support and giving skin-to-skin contact in preference to talking, which is kept simple and to a minimum.

2. *The setting.* The birth room, where the woman labors and gives birth, is like a living room with a large comfortable platform with soft cushions. To avoid the suggestion of the "right" place to labor or give birth, there is no bed. There is a wooden birthing chair.

3. *Reduced sensory stimulation.* Absence of noise, talking as little as possible, and reduced lighting even to the point of semidarkness help the laboring woman tune out the world and turn inward.

4. *Warm water in labor.* "The efficiency of water during the first stage is mysterious," says Odent. "We observe many times that a good bath in warm water with semidarkness is the best way to reach a high level of relaxation." Some women prefer to shower. Some immerse in the small pool in the unit. Women are encouraged to use the pool if their labor has stalled at five centimeters. "It is common that within an hour the woman is fully dilated," Odent told us. Sometimes the women have felt so comfortable they have stayed in the pool and given birth there, very quickly. "Our purpose is never to have a baby born under water," says Odent. "But it is important to know that it happens. The baby will not breathe until it contacts air—like a dolphin."

5. *Positions for labor and birth.* There is no confrontation at Pithiviers, no telling a woman what she must or must not do. Women search for the position of most comfort. Many women kneel, bending forward during a contraction. Odent has observed that this particular posture often helps a woman forget what is cultural, turn inward, and regress from logic to feeling. (It also helps the rotation of the baby's head in the pelvis, as in a posterior presentation of the baby.) But there are no "best" postures. Some few women deliver in the birthing chair, some lying on the platform. The most common position sought out for births is a "standing-squat": The woman's knees are bent as if she were seated, but spread apart. Her full weight is supported by someone standing behind her, holding her. "When the mother is at risk, or the baby is at risk, as in twin or breech deliveries, for example, the standing-squat position for delivery is imperative," says Odent.

After delivery, the mother, usually in a sitting position, is active (rather than prone and passive), and ready to hold and caress her baby. The naked mother and baby, comfortable in a birth room warmed for them, have easy touching access to each other. Cradled against the mother's breast in a natural nursing position, most newborns find the mother's nipple and begin nursing with no effort on the mother's part.

From his experience at Pithiviers, Odent believes the optimum level of consciousness in birth is reached in a safe, quiet and supportive environment, and is accompanied by optimum secretion of oxytocin by the mother, and, very likely, a secretion of endorphins that protect both mother and infant against pain. "It is easy to understand that any drug given to the woman in labor can disturb the system of endorphins," says Odent. "More generally speaking, one cannot study protection against pain without studying at the same time the capacity to have pleasure and a sense of well-being."

Having an Active Birth

Kathy found she was most comfortable if she changed positions often or slowly walked. With each contraction she would automatically relax and breathe deeply. In between contractions she felt nothing at all. Though she was concentrating on the present moment, she suddenly realized she was really getting very good at what she was doing. The long labor gave her a chance many, many times to use her relaxation with each contraction. About two o'clock in the morning she found that she was no longer comfortable relaxing and breathing through a contraction. She had to stop and lean against a chair, or the wall, or Tim, for the contraction to stay manageable.She felt somewhat irritable at one point when Tim laughed nervously in response to her abrupt command to stop walking. She said, "If you think it's so funny, why don't you try this for five minutes?" Then they both laughed, and Kathy said, "You know what? I want to go to the hospital."

Tim called the doctor's answering service to let them know they were coming in, and also called the nurse they had hired to be with Kathy. Maria, Julie, Kathy, and Tim all went in one car for the fifteen-minute drive. Kathy did not feel comfortable sitting in the car. When one contraction came during the trip, she asked Tim to pull over and stop because she couldn't relax as they bumped over the road. After she arrived at the hospital, Kathy realized that she was most comfortable if she just kept walking, so she walked in a little circle in the labor room. She undressed, making a trail of clothes behind her. The hospital admitting nurse examined Kathy and told her she was five centimeters dilated. She was disappointed, until her cheering section reminded her that "you're halfway there." The monitrice arrived half an hour after Kathy and began the procedure she would carry out every thirty minutes during labor. She listened for the baby's heart tones for thirty seconds immediately after a contraction. She pronounced the baby doing "just fine." She drew a little flower on Kathy's stomach in the place that was easiest to hear the baby's heart tones.

Kathy was finding the contractions more difficult to handle and felt there must be something she should do. Then she remembered what another friend had told her. "You don't have to do anything, just relax and let your uterus open up your cervix." She thought of this often and it helped her to let go and allow her body to work. She even tried visualizing the uterus and cervix working together with each contraction.

Contractions are the means by which a woman's body labors and gives birth. Ask any woman who has had a baby how many contractions she had during labor, and she'll likely guess in the hundreds if not higher. Actually a Swiss study shows the average first-time mother has 135 contractions and a multipara has an average 68 contractions. In her book *Preparation for Childbirth*, Donna Ewy explains contractions:

Probably one of the greatest fears a woman has concerning childbirth is how can a baby pass through such an obviously small opening without excruciating pain. The whole function of "labor" is to allow the contractions of the uterus to open the cervix (the lower part of the uterus) to about 4 inches, the diameter of the baby's head. After the cervix has opened the baby passes through the birth canal. The tissues of the vagina are extremely elastic, and once the cervix opens, the baby passes through with relative ease.

The great opening of the womb happens only once or a few times in your life," writes Janet Balaskas in *Active Birth*. "In a way, you need to lose control, to surrender to and trust in the birth process, which takes place without your conscious control.... This is the time to turn inwards, to abandon oneself to the unknown."

Balaskas tells how to give birth actively:

You will want to move around freely during the early part, or first stage, of labor, choosing comfortable upright positions such as standing, walking, sitting, kneeling, or squatting. In between contractions you will find ways to rest in these positions, comfortably supported by pillows.... Most women find that, as labor intensifies and advances to the last part of the first stage (7 to 10 centimeters dilation), kneeling, upright, or on all fours is the most comfortable position.... Some find it helpful to move the pelvis rhythmically during contractions, either rotating or rocking as they kneel.... The kneeling positions are especially helpful if you have "back labor" or if the baby is lying in a posterior position.... Rhythmic rotation or spontaneous movement of the pelvis can help the baby to turn to the more usual anterior position.

At the end, for the actual birth, you will use a natural expulsive position (probably supported) like squatting or kneeling.... Because it makes optimum use of gravity, the supported standing squat is the most efficient position for the rapid descent of the baby. You stand or walk between contractions, but as a contraction comes on, your knees bend and you feel the need to hold on to something. You can hold your partner around the neck (in the "hanging squat"), or your partner can support you from behind, while you let go of your weight and surrender to the force of the contraction. After the contraction passes you move freely until the next one, when you are supported again.

Recognizing that many women need to try out and become comfortable with upright positions during pregnancy, Balaskas offers simple yoga exercises to prepare the body easily to seek positions of comfort in labor and delivery. "The emphasis during pregnancy needs to be on developing trust and confidence in her own body," affirms Balaskas.

I got it my way! Though I was nearly completely dilated the baby was still high. The midwife helped me get into a squatting position on the bed. After fifteen minutes of pushing, I had the baby. "You told me if you'd just get upright, you'd be able to deliver," the midwife said to me after the birth. I used to be afraid of delivery. Now I know it was because I wasn't upright for the five previous births, but flat on my back.

—New York

Kathy continued her slow walking or sitting with Tim right beside her, his arm around her upper back, partially supporting her. When a contraction came, she leaned her full weight against him to relax. When the contraction was over, she complained of the pain and suggested that she must not be doing very well. Her childbirth education class had given her the impression that if she relaxed and breathed correctly, she wouldn't have any pain. Her monitrice explained that even though she was relaxing and breathing very well, the intensity of the contractions was stretching her cervix open. That's something some women simply feel to be more painful than do others. But Kathy was reassured that they would all help her get through it.

As they discussed the intensity of the experience, Kathy's mother-

in-law, Maria, said that, of her four births, three had been without medications or anesthesia. She had a mixture of experiences with those three, she said: With one labor and delivery there was no pain at all; with another, there was a kind of searing pain at the peak of contractions; the last birth, a five-hour labor, hurt most of the time. Sometimes she felt as if she just couldn't stand the pain anymore, but the people she had with her got her through. They were going to do that for Kathy too.

Maria mentioned one thing that had helped her was to yawn and stretch between contractions. It seemed to help get rid of extra tension. Kathy tried it, and it did seem to help her relax fully between contractions. As the morning rolled in, more suggestions were offered. If what was suggested felt right to her, she would try it. More often than not, everything she tried worked for a while. But then a pain would build again during a contraction, and she would feel overwhelmed. She tried several different positions seeking comfort, turning inward, moaning.

Tim could see she was getting very tired and very hot, and he suggested they take a shower together. Kathy was so involved with her contractions that she couldn't think of things to do and the idea of a shower right then sounded like a clever one. (Tim had brought his bathing suit to the hospital just in case Kathy wanted to shower during labor.) It was slow going because, although Kathy had a good three minutes between contractions, she walked slowly. Before she got from bed to shower, she had two more contractions. While she waited them out, she stood with her arms draped around Tim, who supported her weight.

The shower cooled, refreshed, and relaxed Kathy, and once more she felt she was going to make it. In fact, there were moments when Kathy could almost laugh at herself. As the labor went on, she felt not only her body but her mind was opening up. She felt free to express whatever it was she was feeling—early in labor, her pleasure and excitement that the baby was almost there, and now, later in labor, her pain and despair at ever getting through it. She felt that those around her gave her permission to do whatever it was she needed to do, and that was probably the best help of all.

When things frequently got tense, Julie's job seemed to be to remind everyone that the baby was just fine. The monitrice was continuing her regular monitoring, and the baby's heart rate was strong. Tim drew strength from his mother and from Julie, both of whom praised him for the way he was helping Kathy. Sometimes he was uncertain that he was being helpful, because of Kathy's irritability. But

Julie and Maria reassured him by saying things like, "Oh, I know that feels good to Kathy." They could see that Kathy was responding to his touch. Tim opened up too, as the labor went on, and felt free to kiss, touch, and hold Kathy, to express his love and support for her. Tim noticed that sometimes when they were kissing, Kathy's mouth was tense and she was feeling a lot of pain. He suggested she might be tightening up her bottom. They discovered that smooching a lot helped to keep her mouth and her bottom much more relaxed. There seemed to be a connection between the two.

About seven o'clock in the morning, after five hours in the hospital, and about twenty hours since labor had started, Kathy was flushed and sweaty. It didn't seem possible that the contractions could hurt more, but they did. She felt confused because now she felt she had no time to recover between contractions. The monitrice told Kathy she had all the signs of being in transition, and she was going to alert Kathy's doctor. When he arrived, he agreed Kathy was in transition, and there was no need for a vaginal check. He did suggest that they might move labor along now if they broke the bag of waters. Julie reminded him how strongly Kathy felt about not artificially breaking the bag of waters. He said yes, he had remembered that, and it was fine.

Kathy was in transition for two hours. It was the worst time for her. Her pain, discomfort, and confusion were at their height, and she needed the quiet assistance from those around her.

The intensity of pain experienced in childbirth is often unexpected by prepared women, who assume that if they just relax and breathe well enough, there will be no pain. It is difficult to predict ahead of time which women will have pain and how intense it will be. The childbirth literature suggests that about 10 percent of first labors and one-fourth of later labors are painless. So, clearly, most women do have pain in labor and delivery.

In our culture, pain is considered abnormal, either due to disease or injury, and a symptom to be avoided or medicated. Obstetricians see the relief of pain as an obligation. It goes against their training to see a woman suffering in labor, and many feel the woman is a martyr, a little crazy, or both, to refuse medication or anesthesia. Mothers who have had painful labors and deliveries without drugs, but with caring and supportive birth attendants, family, and friends there, usually see it differently. They describe the pain as a catalyst that pushed them deeper within themselves, almost a guide to lead them to discover a physical and mental capacity they had not previously known. This change of consciousness is described by Michel Odent. It does not involve a control of pain but a surrender to it that leads to the woman's own body producing pain-tolerating hormones, endorphins, which also cause the after-birth high. Many of these mothers remark on the tremendous euphoria immediately following birth. They have found that the exquisite pain of labor in a loving, supportive, peaceful environment is followed by the most exquisite pleasure after birth.

> *Kathy had not felt hungry all night and had only felt the need for drinking water and apple juice. However, during the transitions, she was aware that she was tremendously thirsty and, over a two-hour period, drank about six full glasses of water. About every hour, the monitrice reminded Kathy to get to the bathroom and try to urinate, "so a full bladder won't be in the way of the baby."*
>
> *The last two hours of labor were truly the hardest work that Kathy had ever done in her life. She frequently felt overwhelmed and at one point during a contraction started to pant the words, "Help, help, help, help." Julie picked up on the word and repeated it with her over and over, then put her hands on Kathy's shoulders, looked into her eyes, and said, "Now breathe with me, Kathy." And slowly Kathy got back into the rhythm of breathing and relaxing with the contraction. Julie's eyes never wavered from Kathy's during the contractions of those last hours, and to Kathy it was a lifeline.*

Author Donna Ewy includes many comforting techniques in her book *Guide to Family Centered Childbirth.* She summarizes them by saying, "Three key methods that will help you get her back in control are eye contact, firm voice, and a secure touch."

Peggy Vincent, a nurse, discusses the power of eye contact with a laboring woman in *Birth* journal:

One of the many useful ideas discussed in *Spiritual Midwifery* is the technique of "catching eyes" with the woman during those parts of her labor when she feels like she is disintegrating or losing her perspective. The transference of power and feeling between two people whose gaze is fixed on each other and who are breathing in rhythm during a very intense moment in their lives is so charged with energy that it makes one stand back in awe. The power is tremendous. The problem is that, as a culture, we are not comfortable with prolonged eye contact. It is something that people need to be taught. However, in my experience in the hospital, it has been worth the effort to try. When a woman suddenly looks lost or desperate, I say,

"Open your eyes and look at me, I'll breathe with you." If she'll do it, if she will allow herself to trust you enough to maintain eye contact, you can get her through almost any kind of a contraction just by the power of being there and experiencing it with her on a level that is difficult to appreciate unless you have been there yourself.

Tim was sitting next to Kathy, massaging her thighs where she seemed to be feeling a lot of tension, lightly stroking her face, kissing her between contractions, and telling her she was "almost there" and doing great. Gradually, over the space of about three contractions, Kathy started grunting at the end of each one. The monitrice felt she was probably fully dilated, did a vaginal check, and found that Kathy was indeed ten centimeters dilated.

The contractions seemed to change. There was much more time in between, and Kathy felt like pushing with each one. The monitrice notified Kathy's doctor, who was waiting in the doctor's lounge. He checked Kathy and confirmed that the baby's head was well engaged, that she was fully dilated, and that she could go ahead and push. Kathy felt as if she wanted to stand, knees bent, and lean against Tim. He stood behind her, supported her under her arms, and held her full weight during each contraction as she pushed whenever she felt like it. Marie remarked that it was a good thing that her son had been a football player, and the laughter broke some of the tension.

Kathy spent the next hour and a half pushing in different positions. She stood, hanging onto Tim. She squatted, supported and balanced by Tim and Julie. She lay on her side. Near the end, she sat on the bed with Tim behind her, supporting her, the top of the bed tilted up, pillows supporting Tim's back.

Historically, the most common position for birth in various cultures has been some form of the upright position. For first-time deliveries, which normally have a longer second stage, the upright position (standing, sitting, kneeling, or squatting) and changing positions shorten second-stage labor. Contractions are stronger and more regular and the woman seems to be able to relax more completely between contractions. Women seem able to push more effectively because of the assist from gravity in the upright position.

Late in pregnancy, try out several positions for birth, so you are familiar with how they feel.

- Lie on your side curled up. (Good if the birth is going very fast.)

- Kneel on the floor, then lean forward, on all fours, or with your upper body leaning on the couch. (Good for back pain and for rotating a baby in a posterior position.)
- Stand, bend, and spread your knees as if to sit in a chair, and have your partner hold you under your arms from behind, supporting your full weight.
- Sit on the toilet, upright, with back support, hands on your knees to simulate a birth chair. Better yet, try out the one your local hospital may have. The birth chair does limit free movement of the pelvis possible in the fully supported standing squat position. This limitation probably accounts for the increase in tears or episiotomy with the birth chair.
- Do a full squat. (The pelvic opening is increased 20 to 30 percent.)
- Sit with your back supported and your legs comfortably spread apart, knees flexed.
- To get a feel for the "uphill" lithotomy position we hope you can avoid: Lie on your back on the floor with your bottom close to the couch. Bend your legs so your calves rest on the seat of the couch.

In each position, practice your Kegel exercise, so you are familiar with the feeling of releasing your pelvic floor in a delivery position.

"Okay," said the doctor, "now here's what I want you to do. When a contraction begins, take two deep breaths, in and out. Take a third breath and slowly release it as you push for just as long as you want. You will be making some kind of a sound as you push. Relax your bottom while you are pushing. Whenever you need another breath, inhale slowly and then slowly release your breath as you push. When a contraction is over, take a deep breath and relax."

Julie, who was standing next to Kathy and who had her hand on Kathy's arm, felt her tense when the doctor was telling her what to do. "Hey, you don't have to remember those instructions, Kathy," said Julie, "because your doctor is going to talk you through each contraction until it's old hat for you. You don't have to worry about anything—you just have to keep your bottom relaxed." Julie could feel Kathy's arm relax. With each contraction the doctor gave his instructions. Soon Kathy picked up her own natural pushing rhythm. It felt good to make "uhhhhhh," grunting sounds, letting out her breath while she was pushing for about five or six seconds with each breath. Her doctor told her to bear down only when she felt the need to push, without trying to hold her breath or prolong a push. He told her that by pushing this way she was getting lots of oxygen to her baby. For several of the contractions the monitrice placed her hand on Kathy's perineum, the area around the vaginal opening. It helped in two ways. The monitrice could feel when Kathy's perineum was tense or when it was relaxed, and she could tell Kathy. It also helped Kathy because by having a firm hand on her perineum, she could visualize better where she needed to relax.

Kathy pushed whenever she felt the urge; then, suddenly, the bag of waters burst. Kathy felt a warm jet of water between her legs. She was astonished at how much water it seemed her body was putting out. Soon a few centimeters of her baby's head could be seen at the vaginal opening. The monitrice, who sensed that Kathy was tiring, took Kathy's hand and guided it down to touch her baby's head. "You see, Kathy, there is your baby's head; it's almost here." Touching the top of the baby's head with the baby still inside her thrilled Kathy. She felt renewed energy. Slowly the head stretched the perineum until it bulged so large it looked ready to burst. But the slow stretching was doing its job. It looked as if the doctor could avoid doing an episiotomy. Kathy felt better when she was pushing. When, suddenly, the doctor told her to stop pushing so he could ease the baby's head out, the sensation of stretching and pain was tremendous. As the head emerged, Kathy screamed in pain. She felt that she might rip up the front, but there was no tearing. There was another short wait before Kathy felt the next pushing contraction. When it came, Kathy's baby was born with one push. Immediately the doctor gave the baby to Kathy to hold. Her eight-pound, one-ounce baby boy was born just before ten in the morning, twenty-four hours after she started early labor the previous morning.

Kathy was laughing and crying at the same time and all sensations of pain were gone. She felt only enormous pleasure. About ten minutes later the doctor clamped the cord on the baby's side, but allowed the cord on the mother's side to bleed freely into a bowl. During her pregnancy Kathy had taken medical articles to him showing that when the cord was left unclamped on the mother's side, it shortens the third stage of labor (the delivery of the placenta), blood loss is greatly reduced, and the mother has less risk of any backup of fetal blood left in the cord. There was close to a half cup of blood in the bowl when Kathy felt a mild contraction, then felt the soft placenta fill her vagina. She pushed and expelled it easily.

Kathy loved the feeling of her wet, warm newborn lying against her breast, the two of them covered with a blanket. Tim put his hand *under the blanket on his son's back. Kathy's love for her husband and baby seemed to expand moment by moment until she felt her love radiating out to include the whole world. The words that kept passing through her mind were "miracle—it's a miracle."*

A Checklist for a Normal Vaginal Birth

Pregnancy

1. Choose a place of birth where there is the least intervention, or a hospital with very flexible routines.

2. Choose a midwife, a doctor with a midwife philosophy, or a doctor with whom you can negotiate for your preferences.

3. Decide what is important for your birth, write up a birth plan, and ask your doctor to sign it.

4. *Gain* weight, using nutritious foods and liquids.

5. Do not smoke or use alcohol.

6. Avoid any drug use unless the benefits outweigh the risks. Avoid aspirin, which has been found to cause bleeding in mothers and babies even when taken days before birth.

7. Learn deep relaxation, slow deep breathing, and other breathing techniques that you may use in labor.

8. Practice labor and birth positions.

Labor

1. If you have premature rupture of membranes, stay home and wait for labor (it may be days; see page 153), unless you have active genital herpes.

2. If you are near term (within three weeks of the due date), stay home in labor until you feel you must go to the hospital. Return home if you are not at least four to five centimeters dilated. (Particularly important for first labors, which tend to be longer.)

3. Eat and drink as you desire. Sleep when you can.

4. Urinate frequently.

5. Avoid efforts to intervene in a normal labor.

6. Hire a monitrice for labor support and to monitor your labor and your baby's heart rate, especially if that is the only way you can avoid a fetal monitor.

7. Walk, stay upright or in a side-lying position, unless your

labor is going very fast and you are more comfortable in another position. Try different positions to find the ones of most comfort to you. Change positions.

8. Alternate resting and walking for a long labor.

9. Have at least one woman you know and like with you—your doula—in addition to your mate.

10. Use warm water, a soaking bath, or a shower to help you relax and open up if your labor stalls at five centimeters or so.

Delivery

1. Use almost any position but the lithotomy position (on your back, legs in stirrups). Upright positions allow gravity to help—especially important for first-time mothers whose deliveries tend to take longer.

2. To give your baby a good oxygen supply and to allow time for the perineum to stretch slowly (and avoid an episiotomy) use exhale-pushing, also known as gentle or physiological pushing:

- Push only when you feel the need.
- Release your breath very slowly when you push.
- Push no more than five to six seconds at a time. Take another breath when you still feel the need to push.
- Take a deep breath when each contraction is over.

13

The Nurse: Your Help on the Inside

Before the baby was born, I read many books and talked with my friends. All the time I was focusing on the birth process itself. Then, there I was, in the hospital. I was dealing with hospital bureaucracy, and I'd never been in a hospital before. I was flabbergasted. I was on my back, and all my defenses were down. I found out that nurses can be either condescending or helpful. Nurses make *all* the difference. The nurses really count. They're the ones on the line. They're there all the time.

—New York

While you may have carefully scrutinized your physician and the options available at your hospital, you're not likely to have given much thought to the nurses, the people with whom you'll spend more than 95 percent of your in-hospital time. Perhaps no one has told you that how you're treated during your stay depends mostly on the nurses. So that you'll have more understanding of, and perhaps more control over your hospital stay, we'll describe what you can expect from nurses, why they do what they do, and how you can get what you want from them.

Nurses, 97 percent of whom are female, are the largest group of health professionals in the world. They all pass the same state exam after graduating from an approved degree program, which varies from associate degrees to doctorates. In 1990 the typical nurse earned from about $28,000 to $38,000 a year, though some positions, such as nurse anesthetist, pay more.

A nurse can always get a hospital job, in part because of a nationwide nursing shortage (or more accurately, an excess in demand) that is expected to continue at least until the year 2000. However, although jobs are plentiful, they're not necessarily easy. A hospital nurse takes on enormous responsibilities. And while working rotating shifts and holidays—times when hospital floors are traditionally understaffed—she may also be expected to assume housekeeping tasks. In addition, defensive medicine has increased the amount of time a nurse spends with charting and other paperwork, while the nursing shortage means this same nurse has more women to care for. A common complaint for many nurses is that they can't spend enough time with patients and give quality care, and this directly affects you.

What Mothers Want from Nurses

A nurse stayed with me the entire labor and delivery, holding my hand, answering my questions, giving support. She was a stranger to me, but very helpful and warm.

—Pennsylvania

I would like to comment on one nurse in particular. She tried in every way possible to make my stay as uncomfortable as she could—even after my daughter was born. She came into my room and gave me this long lecture on how bad and childish I had acted during my labor. And on the day I was discharged, she gave the information to me for postpartum care and then said to me, "Now this is your responsibility for eighteen years and don't forget it!"

—Washington

We've read hundreds of comments from mothers regarding the nursing staff and find that most comments fall somewhere between the two quotes above. The care most mothers receive is neither perfect nor perfectly horrible.

Labor and Birth

The theme throughout all the comments from mothers is that they want help, not hindrance; respect, not tolerance. They crave information about the labor and pain relief. Although nurses are still the hands-on practitioners of the health-care profession, in their

training, knowing about new medications and emergency procedures takes precedence over knowing how to help the normal laboring woman with breathing or relaxation techniques.

> My labor nurse only seemed to know how to offer me drugs
> when I was uncomfortable. I know she wanted to help me, but
> it wasn't the right kind of help. I wanted her to encourage me
> and show me what to do with my breathing.
>
> —Survey

But when mothers got that support, they were indeed grateful.

> Without the labor nurse at Community Hospital in Boulder I
> would have folded. My comfort was her main concern. That
> labor nurse was super!
>
> —Survey

Breastfeeding

Nurses are trained well to show you how to hold your baby and the
bottle, as well as when and how to burp your infant.

When mothers rate the hospital staff for breastfeeding help, however, they don't fare as well. Women say that nurses help more than
doctors, but nurses were not as uniformly helpful as were La Leche
League leaders, midwives, and childbirth educators. The higher the
breastfeeding rate in your town, however, the better the help from
the nurses and doctors there will likely be. Like the rest of us, they
do best what they do on a regular basis.

New mothers expect nurses to be as competent with their infant
feeding advice as they are with blood-pressure checks or the use of
drugs. Is this a reasonable expectation? Yes. The nursing mother is
in the majority.

However, the nurses who are on duty when you're in the hospital
may not have had access to current information in breastfeeding, or
they may have no personal experience with breastfeeding their own
children. Lawrence Gartner of the Pritzker School of Medicine at the
University of Chicago states, "I agree that both hospital practices and
the support available for the majority of mothers who are breastfeeding are quite inadequate. A lot of bad advice is handed out about
breastfeeding, even within good hospitals.... You do, in fact, have to
go through a formal retraining of groups of nurses, some of whom in

234 A GOOD BIRTH, A SAFE BIRTH

fact are resentful about the mother who wants to breastfeed."

Paula J. Adams Hillard, an obstetrician herself, wrote of her own childbirth experience, "The person who meant the most to me was a breastfeeding counselor; I now feel that every postpartum floor in the hospital should have someone available to encourage women to breastfeed their babies. Even though I had relatively few problems with breastfeeding, it meant a great deal to have my questions answered and to be able to read the excellent material I was provided."

The best breastfeeding counselor is a woman who has breastfed and who thinks breastfeeding, in general, can work for nearly any woman who wants to do so. She does not perceive breastfeeding as a problem, and does not think it is messy or inappropriate in our culture. This breastfeeding counselor realizes that no one knows the baby better than his own mother and, most importantly, makes no value judgment about the new mother's lifestyle, whether she's married or single, employed away from home or at home all day. She conveys the pleasure of breastfeeding and helps the mother feel good about her choice.

If you have a doula who fits this description of a breastfeeding counselor, you need look no further. Or perhaps your hospital is one of the many today that has its own lactation consultant on staff. (See Appendix D for information on lactation consultants.) Also, La Leche League counselors and many childbirth educators and midwives, nearly all of whom have breastfed their own children, help their clients with breastfeeding.

And Please! No Criticism

"One time when the nurse came into the room, I said to her: 'Isn't it incredible how patient Pam is with this labor? She has this machine hooked up to her, she is in a strange environment, and she's really tired,'" said a doula. "'You are not letting her eat or drink. And she puts up with all of it, is so patient, and she allows her body to labor.' The nurse said, 'Yes, she's doing so well. We are proud of her, but we wish she'd hurry up her piddly labor. We hate to have to do a cesarean just because she's so slow.'"

A negative comment like this strikes fear in many mothers. It certainly doesn't enhance a laboring mother's belief in herself. And she won't forget that comment either—not if she's like other women we've spoken with. Nor will her labor go faster because of the threat. It may only serve to convince mom that she's a failure. She can't even get a baby born on time.

But wait a minute! Whose time are we talking about? Why did the nurse say that? Perhaps because many nurses are incorrectly taught in school that normal labors should progress one centimeter an hour. Or perhaps, as we've been told by nurses, that particular nurse is just having a bad day. Frankly, we think birth is too important for caregivers to have bad days, difficult as that may be to control.

Being criticized about your "noisy" behavior during labor or being taken to task because your baby gained "only" half an ounce after a feeding is *never* helpful. If there's a better way for you to do something, there's also a helpful, encouraging way to tell you.

You wouldn't want your mate in the throes of lovemaking to whisper in your ear, "Darling, you're wonderful, but gee you're so slow" (or noisy, or quiet). Comparisons that suggest you're somehow not up to standard are just as inappropriate when you are giving birth or nursing a baby.

As a laboring woman and new mother, you'll thrive on praise and support. Insulate yourself with the affectionate bubble of family and friends. Have your husband and doula with you. Protect yourself from demeaning comments by nurses, unintentional as they may be. Although all of you will not be subjected to these remarks, many of you will. Anticipating them in advance may deflect their sting.

How Nurses See Their Role

Labor and Birth

Maternity floors can be a tranquil oasis in a hospital filled with the sick and dying. Birth, after all, is not an illness; it's a celebration. But there's the other side of the picture, too. "Most people don't recognize that the maternity floor is also an extremely stressful and high-tension area," said one ob nurse. Even though it may not happen often, a nurse never knows who the next emergency patient will be. Just like the doctors she works with, her eye is trained to look for problems.

The emphasis in nurses' training is on what to do when nature can't seem to manage by itself. Nurses are taught how to put an IV in your arm, and, at a doctor's direction, how to measure the appropriate amount of Pitocin to get your labor started or speeded, and when to give you drugs for pain relief.

For some nurses, childbirth is nothing new; they've seen

hundreds of births. And when they report to the nursing station that they have "five in early labor," you may be seen as just part of their job on that particular shift. It's very exhausting for nurses to get emotionally involved with each birth. Many nurses learn early to keep themselves at arm's length. In addition, patients are not a nurse's only responsibility. There's paperwork to be done, and, above all, she must do whatever the physicians tell her. The nurse's role is not an easy one. She has enormous responsibility, but often little authority.

Other nurses, though, still see each birth as sacred, not routine. Each birth for them is new and exciting. They get involved with the couple during labor and enthusiastically make personalized arrangements for the parents whenever possible. They don't talk loudly and laugh in the halls with other nurses. And they keep their voices hushed in a room with a laboring woman. They avoid examining her during a contraction, because they know that can be painful. And they tell her what to expect next in her labor. They believe the mother's needs are paramount.

Maybe you'll be fortunate enough to have one of these enthusiastic, helpful nurses. Are there very many? Not enough. Not because nurses don't want to give you the best of care—they do. But there may not be enough staff on the floor to permit your nurse to spend much time with you. Or her training or lack of experience with what you want gets in the way.

The View from the Nursery

Although hospital planners usually continue to include large nurseries in the blueprints for new ob units in the United States, the concept of nurseries—a place to keep babies away from their mothers—is under fire. We humans are the only species that routinely separates mothers and babies. Forty years ago, when nearly all mothers were totally unconscious by the time they gave birth in hospitals, it might have been logical to appoint someone else (the nursery nurse) to be the infant's caregiver. However, despite the fact that hospital nurseries may become the health-system dinosaur of the future, if you're pregnant now, you'll probably still have to cope with nurseries during your hospital stay.

Nurses who choose to work in the nursery lavish love on their small charges—which, as a parent, is exactly what you want them to do. However, sometimes this affection becomes misguided. Mothers have told us of nursery nurses who insist they know what's best for "their" babies and that moms don't.

Mothers' complaints range from nurses insisting on supplemental water or synthetic milk feedings for breastfed babies, to rigid feeding schedules—which suggests misinformation and attachment to routine. Nurses might want to keep to the routine, however, because it's easier for them, and they know you can do what you want when you get home. But why not do what you want while you're still in the hospital?

Of course, not all nursery nurses are unhelpful. But enough are that if you're forewarned, you're forearmed.

A Help, Not a Hindrance

Some of the nurses were really mean, but I was dependent on them. Had there been an emergency, I wanted them to be on my side. I was afraid that if I was a difficult patient, the nurses might take forty-five minutes to answer the bell—just when I needed them the most.

—Survey

The Role Intimidation Plays

You're flat on your back and feeling helpless. You know doctors and nurses don't like "troublesome" patients. (Translated, "troublesome" refers to patients who make requests outside the routine.) And, yes, hospitals are intimidating.

Your best guarantee of getting what you want, of not having to cope with unpleasant personnel, or having your stay be the best it can be, is to have your mate and/or doula with you all the time. All of us, including nurses, are on better behavior when there are witnesses present. A deliberately long delay in answering a bell is impossible if you have someone with you who can go out to the nurses' station and get a nurse in person.

Nothing terrible will happen simply because you are persistent. You have everything to gain by letting your wishes be known. You are dealing with people who want to be helpful. But understanding that it's possible for some nurses to be unpleasant, you can protect yourself with your family and friends. And if you should run across a truly nasty nurse, tell the head nurse or your doctor. One of them can arrange to have other nurses care for you.

Getting What You Want

Nurses want to give you good bedside care, but their employer is the hospital, not you. Be reasonable with your expectations, and don't plan on nurses automatically asking you what you want.

Communicate your preferences clearly, frequently, and repeatedly. If you don't, no one will read your mind—not doctors, not nurses. Be specific. Most misunderstandings occur when the nurse is confused about what you mean. You've had an opportunity to develop a relationship with your doctor over many months. You'll have only minutes, or maybe hours, with any one nurse.

There is a nursing hierarchy that's usually not obvious to patients because the nurses all wear uniforms; therefore, they all look alike. LPNs (licensed practical nurses) and nurses' aides are paid less and have fewer months or years of training than RNs (hospital-school nurses) and BSNs (college-trained nurses). The range of duties for LPNs and aides is more limited, and they are always under the supervision of an RN or BSN. In the 1990s, in addition to these established groups, new categories of nursing assistants are being formed to help relieve the shortage. A glance at the name tag of any nurse might very well tell you what category she is in and who's the boss. If you're not sure whom to talk to about a request you have, ask for the head nurse.

We've heard many comments from mothers who didn't get what they wanted in the hospital. But you can, if you're prepared to negotiate in advance with your doctor. When the nurse says to you, "We never do that here," or "It's against hospital policy," or "I've been working here for ten years, and I know Dr. X won't allow that"—or any other statement that doesn't get you what you want—tell her, "*Dr. X said I can* (walk around during labor, keep both my mate and friend with me, have my other children visit me, etc.)" or "*Dr. X said I don't have to accept* (an enema, drugs during labor, or sugar water for my baby, etc.)." Plan on someone saying it for you more than once, however. Shifts change, nurses sometimes rotate patients. If your mate and doula are there, you won't have to do the talking.

What if something you never anticipated happens and there was no prior negotiation with either your doctor or the hospital? Don't panic. Be clear and specific.

Example: With your first two births you were not "prepped" in the labor room. So it didn't occur to you to talk to your current doctor about that. But you're no sooner in your hospital room than the nurse comes in with her shaving kit. You could say, "I know you're just doing what you're supposed to do, but I don't get prepped during my labors. If you have any questions about that, please talk to Dr. X."

Now, if it's that simple, why would most mothers in that situation submit to the procedure? Because they are caught by surprise and, feeling so vulnerable, they perceive that the nurse really seems to be the one in charge. The mother feels helpless. If you are all alone, the struggle to disagree with the nurse might seem overwhelming. Don't be alone.

Reasonableness and persistence are the key. You don't have to submit to any procedure that you don't want. You are entitled to a full explanation of everything the staff wants to do to you. You are not obligated to participate in their routine.

The Most Troublesome Conflicts

Rooming In

Even though you may have arranged in advance with your baby's doctor to have your baby with you as much as you wanted, this option is often the most difficult to obtain smoothly.

Part of the problem is in the definition of "rooming in." For many mothers, either breastfeeding or bottlefeeding, it means keeping your baby with you as much as you want—up to twenty-four hours a day. But that's not the common hospital definition for rooming in. At one place, it means the babies come out during the day. At another place, it means the babies can be with the mothers all day and once at night (except, of course, during visiting hours). It's not often that hospitals intend for you to have your baby all the time.

If your experience is like that of many other mothers, you will have to remind at least one nurse on every shift that you've made different arrangements for your baby. When a nurse comes to take your baby to the nursery after the birth or after the feeding, you can explain to her that you've made arrangements for the baby always to stay with you, unless you decide differently. You'll probably have to tell every nurse you see that you're keeping your baby with you.

You may have to get a private room to arrange for rooming in, and you may have to forego visitors. Each hospital's rules differ in that regard, too.

Feeding Your Baby on Demand

Another common arrangement that mothers make that often doesn't go smoothly is "demand feeding." This means your baby mostly stays in the nursery, but comes to you when he wakes up. But sometimes this doesn't happen—nurses forget, or they get too busy.

When you want your baby and he's not available, the worst thing you can do is nothing. Hospitals are busy places, and it's easy for the staff to be occupied with other duties or simply to forget that you want your baby more than perhaps the other mothers.

What can you do? We know many mothers who walked down to the nursery and got their babies every two hours or so. If you're not up to walking there, have your mate or your doula go down to the nursery and get your baby for you. That's acceptable in nearly all hospitals. If it's not possible for you or anyone else to go to the nursery in person, just keep asking for your baby. Persist.

Breastfeeding

Though help for breastfeeding mothers is better than it was thirty years ago in hospitals, there are still many mothers who have experiences like the following:

> When I was in the hospital, the nursery nurses told me it was hospital policy that all babies, even my breastfed son, get two bottles of formula for a PKU test. They also told me that my baby, like all the others, gets sugar water between feedings because new mothers like me can't produce enough milk. When my breasts got engorged on the third day, the nurses showed me how to use a nipple shield so that the baby could suck more easily. Now that my baby is a week old, I'm wondering what's the matter with my milk. My baby doesn't seem satisfied and fusses at my breast even though I know he's hungry.
>
> —Colorado

Although the nurses who cared for this mother wanted to be helpful, their standard routine for breastfeeding mothers guarantees that many, if not most, new mothers will find that breastfeeding is not going well a week after the birth.

What went wrong? The number-one interference with successful breastfeeding in the hospital is not getting your baby as much as you want or need. Next on the "no-no" list are: synthetic milk in the nursery, sugar water or "Baby Coca-Cola" as some nurses label it (or even plain water), and nipple shields.

A test for PKU (phenylketonuria), a rare genetic disease, can be performed on a completely breastfed baby just as well when the mother's milk comes in. Many surveyed breastfeeding mothers didn't want their babies getting bottles of any kind in the hospital— but especially bottles of synthetic milk. Some babies become allergic to cow's milk (one of the most common allergens) with even the briefest contact with synthetic milk in their early days. Others get confused with trying to suck from two different nipples—the mother's and a rubber substitute.

And still other babies who drink anything from a bottle in the hospital may become too tired to nurse vigorously at the breast. There's another reason to avoid bottles in the hospital, too: The delicate balance between supply and demand of breast milk can only be maintained when the baby nurses frequently at the mother's breast. The more the baby nurses, the more milk the mother produces. This frequent feeding is also the key to managing newborn jaundice, which is discussed in the next chapter.

There are two kinds of shields associated with breastfeeding. One, the breast shield, is helpful. The other, the nipple shield, is not (with rare exception). The nipple shield, which is worn over the mother's nipple while the baby sucks, draws the nipple out so that the baby can grasp it. Theoretically, it might seem helpful; in practice, it's not. The breast shield is worn inside the mother's bra during the last months of pregnancy or in the early weeks after birth to draw out an inverted nipple. If you have true inverted nipples, buy breast shields (not nipple shields) and wear them before the baby is born.

Nurses often recommend the use of the nipple shield to relieve temporary engorgement when your breast feels hard. However, there are better solutions to that problem than wearing a nipple shield. Very frequent nursing will prevent or later alleviate engorgement. Or hand expression just before nursing relieves pressure and softens the nipple area so the baby can latch on.

With the inappropriate use of rubber nipples, a nipple shield, and supplements of either synthetic milk and/or water that the Colorado mother experienced, it's not unlikely that by day seven when she's home with her baby she's wondering what went wrong. Can this mother's problem be solved? Sure, with good help and support. After all, many mothers have successfully breastfed their babies after weeks of pumping or being separated from a sick infant. But without help, like many mothers in that situation, she will wean earlier than she wants and probably always believe her body couldn't produce enough milk.

What can you do to avoid synthetic milk for your baby in the hospital? Arrange in advance with your baby's doctor that your infant's chart indicates that he's not to get formula for any reason. Discuss with your doctor that you want your baby's PKU test given after your milk comes in.

Remind the nurses that your baby doesn't get synthetic milk. Many mothers tell us that nurses automatically bring bottles of sugar water periodically during the day. You don't have to give those bottles to your baby, especially if you've discussed that, too, with your baby's doctor. "No sugar water" can be put on the infant's chart, also. (Or pin a note to your baby's shirt or tape one to his bassinet if he goes back to the nursery—"No bottles, please.") (What about extra water if your baby has jaundice? See Chapter 14.)

A rule of thumb to use when you are in any hospital situation is: *Don't plan on getting everything you want without effort on your part.* That's especially true with breastfeeding. You, your mate, or your doula will have to remind nearly every nurse you see—on every shift—that your breastfed baby doesn't get bottles. Or that you want your baby now. That alone will improve the care that the nurses give you with rooming in, demand feeding, and breastfeeding.

Despite our criticism of some nurses, there are ob nurses who are not only extraordinarily helpful to mothers, but courageous as well. An increasing number of nurses refuse to give medications to mothers when they believe these drugs will be harmful. And many bend the rules as much as they can to accommodate patients' preferences. There are others who spend endless hours trying to change hospital policies from the inside to meet the needs of consumers.

Nurses make all the difference in your hospital stay. Work with them, so that you can have a good and safe birth, as well as a pleasant and helpful hospital stay for you and your baby.

14

Your Baby Doctor

We pediatricians know that 75 percent of our patients get better without us.... That knowledge keeps us humble.

—Charles Taylor

Just as other doctors do, the pediatrician-to-be spends most of her residency learning how to treat sickness, especially rare diseases in children. The emphasis in most pediatric training programs is certainly not on normal processes, although the bulk of any pediatrician's private practice is taken up with earaches, diaper rash, and anxious parents.

Special Influences on Pediatricians

A pediatrician's income depends on a regular influx of new patients. Even though an increasing number of her patients are adolescents, the largest share of a pediatrician's caseload is still younger children. Pediatricians care for more children in the birth-to-two-year range than do family doctors. As children get older, family doctors take a bigger share of the market. A pediatrician's income is doomed without newborns.

Not only are pediatricians competing against family practitioners and nonphysician specialists, pediatricians more than ever compete against each other because there is a reported surplus of them.

Dependence on Obstetricians

New parents usually base their choice of a baby doctor on either their friends' suggestions or their obstetrician's recommendation.

A pediatrician, who doesn't have the advantage of an already-established relationship with you or your family, depends on having a good word put in by obstetricians. Most are well aware that they can't "rock the boat" with obstetricians if they expect to get referrals.

For instance, most pediatricians know not to fuss at hospital meetings about the effects routine obstetrical interventions may have on babies. (Pediatricians are usually present at scheduled cesareans, but often do not consider it appropriate to suggest that the obstetrician wait until the mother's labor starts first—thereby reducing the chance of prematurity for the baby, a primary concern for pediatricians.) In the medical pecking order, obstetricians are near the top in income (because they're surgeons), and pediatricians are usually near the bottom (because they seldom use technology). Obstetricians don't have to listen to pediatricians.

When pregnant patients ask about a baby doctor, some obstetricians may refer them to the new pediatricians in town. That gives the new doctor a chance to build up her practice. But the newcomer will usually get the referrals only if she shares similar philosophies with the obstetricians and, in some cases, knows her place. Pediatricians are keenly aware of the need to get along with obstetricians. Economic reprisals are real. Peer pressure is intense among doctors, and the urgency to conform to whatever the local medical norms are is relentless.

Synthetic Milk Companies

Synthetic milk companies pursue pediatricians and family practitioners as earnestly as drug companies pursue all physicians. These manufacturers sponsor seminars and medical research, and help underwrite pediatric journals through advertising. Synthetic milk companies pay for some worthwhile projects that would never happen without their financial support. But medicine today has—at best—a tainted marriage with these companies. Much of a physician's information on synthetic milk comes directly from the manufacturers; there's seldom an objective, third-party source. Even many mothers get breastfeeding information from synthetic milk companies in free pamphlets.

Short-term breastfeeding is good for these companies. Synthetic milk sales have gone up as breastfeeding rates have increased, paradoxical as that might sound. The reason, according to one company representative, is that women who breastfeed are likelier to wean to synthetic milk during the first year of the baby's life, rather than to regular milk. (Most U.S. nursing babies are weaned to a bottle by the age of three months.)

If you plan to breastfeed at all, the influence of these companies can be insidious. Most mothers take home one of the ubiquitous new-mother hospital packs, which always contain some sample synthetic milk. A Canadian study shows that mothers who do take these packs home wean to a bottle and start solids in a matter of a few weeks—much earlier than mothers who don't take the free samples home.

And if you plan to bottlefeed your baby, the influence of the synthetic milk companies can be misleading. Naturally, each company promotes its own product as the best one, but typically, the chemical formulas vary little among the manufacturers. Infant formula is an enormously profitable, $700 million plus business annually. The supporters of breastfeeding, such as La Leche League, and even the American Academy of Pediatrics don't have the money to provide the information blitz that's standard in big-business marketing.

Obviously, there will always be baby bottles and parents who need them. But you as the parent, with adequate information, can make your own decision about what and when to feed the baby. The more you make your own decisions for your baby, the more self-confident you'll feel as a parent.

Finding Dr. Right

The Dr. Right who cares for your baby serves you best when she observes the child's health and development, and, equally important, reinforces your ability as a parent to make decisions about your own child. Taking your baby to a doctor who intimidates you will only delay your self-confidence, your own common sense, and your growing maturity as a parent. Your doctor's flexibility and willingness to listen to you are as important as her knowledge.

Review Chapter 5, in which we describe the steps for finding the right doctor for your pregnancy and birth. Here we'll describe those unique parts of the search process for finding Dr. Right for your baby. Just as in looking for your doctor, check with the nurses who work on hospital ob floors, childbirth educators, and La Leche League leaders. Nurses can tell you which doctors are most likely to have patients who room in with their babies or who are helpful and enthusiastic about breastfeeding. Nurses know which doctors are willing to arrange for your other children to visit even if it's not hospital policy, or which doctors will examine your baby in your room with you present instead of doing daily exams only in the nursery.

The Prenatal Interview

We suggest you interview doctors for your baby's care before your baby's birth—even though many parents don't. Take your partner or a friend with you; you are likely to "hear" better. If you currently have a family practitioner caring for you, you'll be able to ask her the appropriate questions about your baby's care as you see her through your pregnancy.

There are many mothers and fathers who meet their baby's doctor for the first time after she's already examined their baby in the hospital. Some mothers find they don't like this doctor once they meet her, but are extraordinarily reluctant to change doctors once they've gone that far. ("At this point," they say to themselves, "what difference does it really make?") Yes, of course, you can switch doctors at this point. But it's easier to interview them in advance of the birth and decide then.

Ten Questions for Baby Doctors

Some of these questions can be answered on the phone prior to your consultation visit. As with other question lists in this book, ask those questions that are most important to you first. You'll find information about other questions to ask on topics such as infant feeding, newborn eyedrops, and bilirubin lights following this section.

1. *How much are your hospital charges and fees for office visits?* In most places, pediatricians charge a similar fee. Family practitioners probably charge somewhat less. However, that varies from town to town.

2. *Does a pediatric nurse practitioner (PNP) work in your office?* A PNP is a nurse with additional masters-degree level training, the pediatric equivalent of the certified nurse-midwife in an obstetrician's office. A PNP can handle "well-child" checks and minor illnesses, and consults with the pediatrician as needed. Many parents like to work with PNPs, as they often spend more time with them, and their fees are lower than the doctor's.

3. *Do you charge for phone calls?* Most physicians do not charge for these calls, but some do. Typically, most parents of firstborn children call frequently.

4. *Do you return every call?* Some pediatricians make every callback. Others have trained personnel, usually nurses or nurse practitioners, return the calls. Some parents find that these trained personnel are very helpful. Occasionally, the person who handles your phone call may not have the same attitude about the issue in question that you or your doctor have.

For instance, in one city many breastfeeding mothers chose one doctor in particular because she not only had breastfed her own children, but was most helpful with any problems the mothers had with nursing. However, the people who answered some of her office phone calls were not as knowledgeable and supportive of breastfeeding as the doctor herself. In another instance, one mother chose her doctor because his philosophy of mothering was similar to hers. However, the nurse who took some of his calls had a different attitude. What the mother and doctor called "meeting the baby's needs" the office nurse labeled "spoiling."

If you find that the person who's handling your phone call is not on your wavelength, you can request that the doctor call you back instead.

5. *What is the scheduled length of your appointments?* The closer her appointments are (ten to fifteen minutes apart, rather than twenty or thirty, for instance), the more likely it is you'll do some waiting, as well as be rushed through your appointment when you do see her. Most doctors allow more time for complete physicals, and therefore charge more for them than they do for routine office visits.

6. *How often do you want to see the baby in the first year? Why?* Pediatricians more than family practitioners will schedule several "well-child" visits for your child. Pediatricians believe this to be a form of preventive care and an opportunity for parent education. Feel free to discuss in advance with your doctor the purpose of these "well-child" visits, so that you can decide in consultation with your doctor what's appropriate for *your* child's care. We all need encouragement as parents, but you decide if it's always worth an office-visit fee to find out how much your baby weighs and the fact that your doctor thinks your baby is doing well.

7. *Do you have a "sick-child" waiting room?* Some doctors try to avoid mixing the well children and the sick children in the same reception area. Young children are very susceptible to contagious diseases.

8. *If you share a practice, will I always see you?* Not likely, unless your doctor has no partners and never takes a day off. If you are scheduling an exam well in advance, it's easy to ask for a day that your doctor will be in the office. However, if you have a sick child and are calling up on short notice, you'll get whomever is in the office or on call. The same is true of night and weekend emergencies. As a matter of fact, your doctor and her partners may share their on-call times with other doctors. Just as with obstetricians, this means that you might have a doctor you've never seen before caring for your child in an emergency. If it's important to you, arrange to meet all the doctors who might cover for your baby's doctor in an emergency, or when you're in the hospital.

9. *Do you have evening or Saturday hours?* Although nine-to-five office hours are still the rule for many doctors' offices, a growing number of them are accommodating working moms and dads. And now there are off-hour pediatric centers that deliver immediate care at night and on the weekends in some cities.

10. *What is your philosophy about child rearing?* Suggested specific questions are: Do you think children should be fed on a schedule? Sleep in the same bed with their parents? Wean at a particular time? What is your usual recommendation for babies who cry when they're put to sleep at night? What is your philosophy about medication for children who have colds or other ailments?

You'll think of other questions over time as your baby grows up, but it's important to get some sense in advance of how much you and a baby doctor agree on child rearing. Otherwise, if you're disagreeing often, you'll probably change baby doctors later or you'll avoid discussing those conflictual issues, and you won't get the full benefit of a professional opinion.

In the last chapter we described three areas in which mothers and nurses sometimes clash: rooming in, feeding your baby—when your baby wants to eat regardless of the clock ("demand" feeding)—and breastfeeding.

You might have areas of conflict with your baby's doctor, too. True, you will spend most of your time in the hospital with nurses. But the doctor who cares for your baby has the power to make "good care" better and "bad care" worse. After you've asked the initial questions, discuss the following possible six areas of conflict that might come up during your hospital stay: breastfeeding, bonding, rooming in, newborn eyedrops, newborn jaundice, and circumcision.

Breastfeeding

Medical support for breastfeeding has come a long way. When our older children were born in the 1960s, the image of the breastfeeding mother was more bovine than madonna-like. (You can breastfeed, of course, my dear, but you'll lose your shape, perhaps your husband's affections, and eventually your milk.)

Now more doctors than ever favor breastmilk. But your baby doctor's help with nursing your infant is more than just her writing "breastfeeding" on your baby's hospital chart. Your pediatrician will not only check your baby every day, but she'll come in and talk with you, too. Much of her advice focuses on infant feeding.

For all the lip service given, many doctors' enthusiasm for breastfeeding still exceeds the amount of helpful advice they offer. Your doctor's "how to" knowledge might be lacking if:

- Accurate breastfeeding information was not part of her training, she has not breastfed a baby herself—particularly past the first few weeks—and does not now have a current interest in it.
- She has not learned what is helpful by observing her patients.
- The doctor is a man whose wife has not breastfed (or at least not past the first few weeks), and has not learned what's helpful and what's not by observing his patients.

Finding a "Helpful" Doctor

How do you know when your doctor's help is "helpful"? Inform yourself in advance. Read the excellent information available for consumers today. Many mothers have successfully breastfed without their doctor's support by learning from other nursing mothers. But why set up obstacles for yourself if you don't have to? Find a doctor who's not only enthusiastic about breastfeeding, but knowledgeable and supportive, too.

When you interview prospective doctors for your baby's care, go beyond asking them if they approve of breastfeeding. Ask if she'll be discussing breastfeeding with you every day that you're in the hospital. According to research in the *American Journal of Public Health*, mothers who receive well-informed counseling each day in the hospital have fewer breastfeeding problems later on than do the mothers who receive breastfeeding counseling only on the day they are discharged.

Ask what percentage of her patients are breastfed at birth. Then ask how many are still breastfeeding at three months or six months. If this number is almost nil (the number will be less than the number breastfeeding at birth), it suggests that she probably isn't very knowledgeable about breastfeeding problems, if only from lack of experience in managing them. Avoid doctors who say they are all for breastfeeding, yet have patients who are mostly bottlefed. Most likely, these physicians are all for nursing as long as you figure out how to do it without their help.

How does she handle breastfeeding problems? Ask if she thinks babies should always be weaned if the mother gets a breast infection or sore nipples, or the baby has diarrhea or what growth charts call "slow weight gain." These are all common problems that can be better managed without weaning the baby from the breast if you get the right information.

Working Away from Home

Millions of mothers have found ways to manage outside jobs and still nurse their babies. When you are having your baby doctor interviews, be sure to mention your intention to breastfeed and work away from home. You'll know soon enough what her attitude is. The doctor you choose may not know a lot of how-to's about this combination, but she certainly should be enthusiastic for you, and direct you to better sources of information, including other patients who have worked and nursed. Many moms who leave their babies feel guilty about the separation, whether bottlefeeding or breastfeeding. The last thing you need is a doctor telling you that you can't manage breastfeeding or that a good mother doesn't leave her child.

To find help if you plan to be a working and nursing mother, always talk with people whose emphasis is success—not failure—and look for the same in reading material. Read books about breastfeeding that have specific, practical hints on working and nursing. (Karen and Gale Pryor, for example, describe in detail the how-to's of morning-schedule arrangements in their 1991 book, *Nursing Your Baby*.)

Ask your childbirth educator for help. She will often know mothers who combine working and breastfeeding. Call La Leche League. (Although these women are the leaders in helping women to breastfeed, many of them have not worked and nursed.) If you find that the person you're talking with is not helpful, ask her for the name of a mother who has worked and nursed. These mothers are often quite enthusiastic and willing to share tips with other women. You can call a lactation consultant, too. (Look in Appendix D, or call the lactation consultant at the hospital or birth center where you gave birth.)

And don't wait until your baby is six weeks old, or six months old, and you're planning on going back to work in two weeks. Learn all you can well in advance—if at all possible. And, whether breastfeeding or bottlefeeding, surround yourself with people who are supportive of your decision to be a working mother.

Bonding

In the not-so-distant past, as new mothers, we were told that our infants couldn't see for days, couldn't smile for weeks. Now there's an explosion of information that describes almost endless sensory abilities of newborns. Much of the best-known research supporting the need for parents and infants to be together soon and often comes from Marshall Klaus and John Kennell.

Child abuse stimulated their early studies. They found that welcoming mothers into the nurseries and encouraging frequent contact between mother and newborns reduced the incidence of later battering. But as many now know, early, frequent contact benefits all babies, all parents, not just those at risk of child abuse.

Since many hospital personnel think there's a time limit to bonding, however, doctors and nurses may think they've satisfied you and your newborn's needs by giving you your hour. Kennell, Klaus, and others never meant to imply that the bonding process was one of glue, a magic sixty minutes at birth.

The idea that gazing into your baby's eyes while holding him lovingly for the first hour will create an attachment for life—at least through those first hard eighteen years—is misleading. That moment is an exhilarating experience for parents and should be encouraged for that reason alone. But attachment doesn't work like that. Love relationships are much more complicated. The issue really is getting acquainted with your baby, and she or he with you, as easily, as early, as continuously as possible. That takes time—lots of it. And hospitals don't always make that easy.

Talk with your baby doctor in advance about how much you want your infant with you immediately after he or she is born. Perhaps you'll want the staff to examine the baby while lying on your abdomen after the birth, instead of across the room on an examining table. And make arrangements, in case you have a cesarean, that your mate or a doula will stay with the baby in the nursery for the time period you would be unable to see and hold the baby yourself.

Rooming In

I want my baby with me at all times. If, however, there is some terrible reason that this could not happen, I would want my baby on request. The set schedule of seeing the baby is the worst possible idea!

—Survey

I was not pleased with the rooming in. My baby was taken to the nursery several different times for checkups, and I had to complain loudly in order to have her returned to me. It does not take three to four hours for a physical or for a heel stick!

—Survey

Don't assume doctors and nurses share your view of rooming in. If having your baby with you as much as you want—which is a primary preference of mothers—is important to you, too, then you'll have to negotiate with both your baby doctor and the hospital. Be specific. Describe what you want. Don't ask if you can have your baby with you as much as you want. You might get a clearer answer if you ask instead what hours of the day you cannot have your baby. Then, they may reply that you can have your baby whenever you want, except during visiting hours (three hours in the afternoon and another three hours in the evening); at night (nearly all mothers find out they don't want their babies at night, they might say; besides, it's not safe for the baby to be with you when you are asleep); and for an hour in the morning when the pediatricians come in to check the babies in the nursery.

From that answer, it's clear that they expect your baby to be someplace other than with you for two-thirds of any given day. If you know that you'll want your baby with you about eight hours a day, then this hospital has what you want. If, however, you want the option of having your baby with you more than that, you have several alternatives:

Talk to both your baby doctor and the hospital in advance. Ask if you can arrange for a private room. Often patients who get a private room can keep their babies with them during visiting hours. Since the hospital staff may then want you to forego having visitors yourself (except your mate), you may need to negotiate to have grandparents and/or a doula present, as well as the baby.

You can also tell them that although their experience at the hospital is that most mothers don't want their babies at night, you do. Many satisfied mothers can tell you that the more they roomed in with their babies, the more self-confident they were when they took the baby home. Rooming in doesn't necessarily increase your fatigue. Rather, it increases your knowledge of your baby and, therefore, your self-assurance. And if you're nursing, rooming in almost guarantees a good milk supply because you'll be feeding your baby whenever he's hungry.

Many pediatricians are happy to examine your baby in your room with you, but they are seldom asked to do so. If you cannot arrange to have your baby checked in your room, you can go to the nursery while your baby is examined there. Or, if you can't go yourself, your husband or doula can be with the baby in the nursery at all times.

If you cannot negotiate an acceptable compromise on rooming in, look for another hospital or a birth center. But what if you're part of an insurance plan that binds you to one hospital, and that hospital won't agree to your plan? If it's important to you, make an appointment with the hospital administrator and plead that your case be an exception. You'll get further than you would if you wanted to change the rules for everyone. (See Appendix A for more information.)

Let's say you've found a hospital that offers the rooming-in arrangement you want. Once you've arranged with your baby's doctor to write on your chart that you are rooming in, the doctor has not done everything she can for you.

If the arrangement doesn't work out the way you want (the nurses don't want to bring the baby at night, or you are receiving criticism from the staff because you want the baby with you all the time), *the next move is yours.* You can let your doctor know that you are not satisfied with the arrangement, and she can talk to the nursing staff. She is in charge of your hospital care; hers is the last word on the floor.

She can even remove a nurse from your care, but that's probably not necessary, or she can remind the staff of your special arrangements. Theoretically, every patient's care is unique, though in practice most patient care is routine. Only you, or someone acting in your behalf (your partner and/or your doula), can get personalized care for you.

Doing your part when you don't get what you want means speaking up, taking action. If you've arranged to have your baby whenever you want, but the nurses come to get your infant anyway, don't give your baby to the nurse. You have as much power as you choose to have. Tell the nurse if she has any questions about it to discuss it with your doctor (or the head nurse).

You'll spend only a few days in the hospital. But your doctor has to work with the nurses every day. For that reason, she won't be enthusiastic about complaining to the staff—especially if you haven't explained your preferences to the staff yourself. But she will speak up, and you'll make it easier for her if you've already done your part.

Newborn Eyedrops

One of the consequences of a pregnant mother's having a sexually transmitted disease (STD), such as chlamydia, gonorrhea, or syphilis, is that she may pass it on to her infant, who may develop newborn eye infections and other problems. (Newborn infections from maternal herpes or genital warts are handled differently.) That's why eyedrops of erythromycin, tetracycline, or silver nitrate have been put into all newborns' eyes within minutes after birth for years.

It used to be no one much objected to this procedure because everyone erroneously "knew" babies couldn't see anyway. But much more is known now about a newborn's capabilities. And many question a procedure designed to help a minority while inflicting an unnecessary interference of irritation and vision blurring on 100 percent of all babies.

"Infants with silver nitrate in their eyes do not follow an object or scan around the room," said pediatric researcher Perry Batterfield. "They also are fussier and rarely have their eyes open within the first three or four hours. Infants who have not had silver nitrate or other eye prophylaxis are quiet and alert after birth, able to scan the room and follow faces and objects. And their parents, especially fathers, are more affectionate and involved with their babies."

However, STDs are second only to the common cold now in the

number of infections, and many women have more than one STD at a time. What are your options?

- *Let's not assume all mothers have an STD.* You can sign a waiver asking for no treatment to the eyes of your newborn. You may feel more secure in doing that if you ask your health-care provider during your pregnancy to give you tests for a possible STD infection. Each STD is diagnosed with a different test, and none are 100 percent accurate, however, so you may want to get more than one, especially if your results are positive. False-positive (that is, you're told you have a disease when you don't) rates are as high as 20 to 30 percent for some STDs.
- *Postpone the treatment.* If there's no getting around your state law that your baby must have the eyedrops within the first twenty-four hours, then negotiate to delay the drops until later in the first day of the baby's life, when the infant is sleeping, rather than give them in the midst of a waking period, which the first hour often is.
- *Request a different antibiotic.* Though erythromycin is used more now than it once was, it's not used universally. This antibiotic ointment causes fewer eye infections than silver nitrate and is effective as a first line of defense against infant infections caused by chlamydia, which is far more common than gonorrhea. Researchers disagree over whether silver nitrate is equally effective. However, none of the eyedrops are used by themselves. If any infants show signs of STD infection, they are treated with other drugs, too.

With whom do you negotiate for an other-than-routine arrangement for these eyedrops? Since the authority for that decision may vary from place to place, talk to both your doctor and your baby's doctor.

Newborn Jaundice

My baby was two days old when she turned yellow on her face. I was still riding a wave of excitement over her arrival when the pediatrician came in to tell me there was a problem. It had to do with the jaundice which could in some way go to her brain and make her mentally retarded. I was terrified, and quickly agreed to the treatment with the lights in the nursery. I didn't understand whether or not she was in grave danger at the time, and the next 24 hours were difficult for me and my husband. I was given her for feedings every four hours and carefully looked to see if the jaundice was less noticeable, but she was as yellow as ever. She didn't nurse well as she received water in the nursery frequently to wash out the jaundice. The doctor came in that evening to tell me she needed further treatment. I left the hospital, as we couldn't afford to run up a hospital bill for me. I visited to nurse several times a day but it was difficult with another child at home, and I was very tired. Luckily she was better in 30 hours and came home.

—Mother Quoted in *Birth*

Obs are criticized from coast to coast, but pediatricians usually are patted on the back. Like obstetricians, though, they've made their mistakes, too, often because of inadequate testing of new procedures and products.

Visual impairment in premature babies, called retrolental fibroplasia (RFL), was epidemic in the 1940s and 1950s. According to William A. Silverman, in *Retrolental Fibroplasia: A Modern Parable*, fifty different causes were suggested before researchers found through randomized controlled trials that RLF was caused by hospital staff giving these premature babies what turned out to be too much oxygen. RLF was iatrogenic (doctor caused)—unintentional, but tragic. Research continues, however, as the proper dosage for oxygen has still not been established.

Silverman thinks RLF is more than a tragic mistake—it's a parable, a sign of our times. Careful testing is not always done. In his book, he lists twenty-six therapies used on babies; only 19 percent of the innovations led to sounder practice. The newest pediatric treatment on the list is "phototherapy for hyperbilirubinemia." Silverman placed a question mark by this treatment.

Jaundice is the most common reason why newborns are kept in the hospital, yet most of the time the condition is harmless. At least half of all full-term babies and eight out of ten preemies develop some form of this condition. Sometimes it runs in families. Newborns with prior siblings who had jaundice are three times more likely to have jaundice than other infants, 1988 research shows. This is true whether infants were breastfed or bottlefed.

Jaundice is a yellowing of the baby's skin and the whites of eyes. It's caused by excess bilirubin, a waste product formed by the body's creation of red blood cells. Most newborn jaundice is a normal reflection of the baby's adjustment to life outside his mother's body, and some researchers believe it serves a useful purpose.

The current medical concern about jaundice in the newborn is twofold. It's possible—though it actually happens rarely, and then only to infants who show signs of other illness—that if the level of bilirubin in the blood goes high enough, a condition called kernicterus develops, which can cause brain damage. The second concern, which is at the root of the proliferation of newborns being put under bilirubin lights, is that a certain level of jaundice (and pediatricians don't agree on what this level is) might cause neurological damage in the child.

Three Kinds of Jaundice

The most severe and rarest newborn jaundice is caused by Rh or ABO blood incompatibility. This jaundice is visible at birth or within the first twenty-four hours.

Another rare jaundice is caused by a substance in breastmilk that makes the baby moderately jaundiced for several weeks and is probably the result of mismanaged breastfeeding more than anything else. This jaundice doesn't develop until the baby is several days to a week old or more. At most, one in 200 babies might be affected. No brain damage has ever been reported from a case of breastmilk jaundice, although many mothers of affected children have been told to wean either temporarily or permanently.

The most common newborn jaundice is physiologic, or normal, jaundice. It first appears when the baby is two or three days old. It's the sometimes casual and cavalier treatment of this jaundice in otherwise healthy, full-term babies with phototherapy (bilirubin lights) that is unnecessarily exposing infants to phototherapy's side effects and increasing the number of babies being separated from their parents soon after birth. Our criticism is not aimed at the appropriate use of the bilirubin lights for the 10 percent of jaundiced babies who are premature or sick full-term infants.

Bilirubin Lights

Bilirubin lights, or phototherapy, combine bright blue (or green) and white fluorescent lights. When exposed to these strong lights, bilirubin in the baby's body decomposes. Though current treatment is phototherapy, tests reported in 1988 show that a drug that blocks the formation of bilirubin may be given to infants in the future. Certainly babies have benefited from phototherapy, but just as with most other birth and newborn interventions, the use of bilirubin lights was designed for a few and ends up being used on a large number of infants.

In many hospitals, babies, including the full-term healthy babies, are kept blindfolded and separated from their parents for most of the day for two or three days at a time while undergoing phototherapy. Although phototherapy has been used for more than twenty-five years, it is still not clear which babies should be put under the lights, how long they should be there, what wattage the lights should be, how effective the process is, and how extensive the side effects are—especially long term.

How can doctors and hospitals allow the management of normal newborn jaundice to be so unclear, you ask? Easy. Available research is not conclusive. Besides, each doctor believes her evaluation and method of treatment—whatever it is—is right. The hospital's job is not to police medical procedures; it is to keep the beds full, and the use of phototherapy contributes to this. Not only may the babies stay an extra two or three days, but often the mothers do, too. This adds thousands of insurance-paid dollars to the hospital revenue. Though hospitals do not coerce you or your doctor to use phototherapy, they are rewarded by your use of this therapy.

J. H. Drew *et al.* have shown that some of the very common short-term effects of the use of bilirubin lights are irritability and restlessness, intestinal irritation, lactose intolerance, feeding problems, riboflavin deficiency, water loss, diarrhea, short-term growth retardation, and skin rashes. W. T. Speck *et al.* stated that phototherapy "may alter intercellular DNA of human cells and may be a carcinogenic hazard." Cathy Hammerman *et al.*, reporting in *Pediatrics*, added to the list of cautions: "Since monochromatic blue light in particular has been associated with staff discomfort and vertigo, it is theoretically important not to deliver excessive doses of irradiance." Jerold Lucey reflected the opinion of many physicians when he stated in *Medical World News* that the long-term effects of phototherapy still are unknown. You as a parent might think all of these side effects, real and potential, are worth it if it prevents neurological damage. But therein lies the problem: phototherapy, as commonly used for full-term, healthy babies, is not likely to prevent anything.

Being blindfolded and deprived of touching, except for a few hours of feeding, for two or three days keeps infants from experiencing normal sensations. Oded Preis *et al.* reported that those babies who were not blindfolded, but whose eyes were protected from the lights by a screen, "had behavior patterns more like normal healthy newborn infants, as compared to those with conventional eye pad coverage, who tended to have more frequent periods of restlessness and irritability." To add to the baby's discomfort, he may have frequent heel sticks for blood sampling as well.

Touching is the most natural thing in the world. Hands hold, feed, and bathe the newborn. Arms rock him, and his mother's body gives comfort. Babies who are kept under the bilirubin lights, however, sometimes spend twenty hours out of every twenty-four just lying there, uncomforted by touch, sight, and the sounds of mother's voice and heartbeat.

Because babies lose fluid when they're under the lights, nurses are instructed to give them extra water. According to researcher Edward F. Bell *et al.*, some babies get so hot during phototherapy that they develop a fever. Giving water for dehydration is different, though, from the erroneous belief of most doctors and nurses that giving babies extra water helps "flush out" the bilirubin. Pediatric researcher and expert on neonatal jaundice Lawrence Gartner, and Kathleen Auerbach, both then at the University of Chicago, stated in 1986 that the feeding of water does not reduce the bilirubin levels. It does, however, interfere with breastfeeding. In some hospitals babies are not removed from the bilirubin lights at all, so that the breastfeeding mother is forced to temporarily (or permanently) wean. Unless a mother is highly motivated, it's often difficult for her to keep nursing.

Certainly no parent or physician wants to have a brain-damaged child, especially when it can be prevented. So doctors sometimes put a child under the bilirubin lights "just in case." But when to use the lights varies from hospital to hospital, doctor to doctor.

In the past, a significant number of infants demonstrated neurological damage when their bilirubin levels exceeded 30. (These were otherwise sick babies showing several signs of disease.) Many doctors, consequently, were taught that, in order for bilirubin levels to remain in a safe range, intervention should occur if the level exceeded 20.*

---

*The serum bilirubin level is measured in milligrams of bilirubin per 100 milliliters of blood. This ratio is then expressed as a percentage. A bilirubin level of 20 can also be expressed as "20 mg. percent."

The "danger" number has dropped drastically, so that today babies with levels as low as 9 are sometimes considered at risk. The worry is that if lower levels don't cause kernicterus, they may still negatively affect future intellectual performance. In fact, studies by several researchers, including Gerald Odell and Rosalyn A. Rubin, show *no* relationship between bilirubin levels up to 23 and IQ scores at five years. And a 1991 *Pediatrics* study of premature babies showed that bilirubin levels of 10 to 20 were no more associated with cerebral palsy or lowered IQ when these children were six years old than were lower bilirubin levels. Peter C. Scheidt, co-author, suggests that full-term infants are at even less risk for problems.

Despite these findings, in some U.S. hospitals full-term, healthy babies with bilirubin levels of 9 and 10—more often 12 and 13—are considered in danger. However, pediatricians who have been in practice for many years tend to pay less attention to the number, and more attention to the physical signs of the baby. For instance, is the baby lethargic or not sucking well? "If you start babies' phototherapy when the bilirubin level is at 10 to 13 (sometimes 15), which is where most people will start phototherapy," said Lawrence Gartner, "you will find the great majority of these babies, in fact, have already started on the decline of the bilirubin at the time that you started the phototherapy.... Ninety to ninety-five percent of those babies really didn't need phototherapy and were about to turn the corner anyway."

Researcher H. M. Lewis *et al.* found that jaundice may persist twenty-four to forty-eight hours longer if infants are not given phototherapy at these lower levels (13 and 14), but the level of jaundice itself won't increase; and in 1986, researcher R. Paludetto found that full-term jaundiced infants with bilirubin levels as high as 14.3 who were not treated with phototherapy were no different from other infants the same age who did not have jaundice. They all conclude that the risks of phototherapy outweigh the benefits at these levels.

Iatrogenic (Doctor-Caused) Reasons for Phototherapy

- *Fear of malpractice suits.* Surgeons are more likely to be sued than other doctors, so it's no surprise that ob/gyns have far more malpractice suits filed against them than do pediatricians and family practitioners. According to the American Academy of Pediatrics, lawsuits are mostly associated with the time immediately before and after birth. As there have been some cases involving newborn jaundice, the use of bilirubin lights will likely continue. With this in mind, a pediatrician told us, "If you're going to err, err on the side of intervention."

- *Drugs, especially Pitocin.* Studies show that the use of Pitocin, in particular, but perhaps also epidurals and other drugs (like sulfanamids, Valium, some tranquilizers, morphine, and vitamin K) increase jaundice in many newborns. According to P. C. Buchan, reporting in the *British Medical Journal*, there are indications that the higher the level of Pitocin in your body, and the longer it's been there, the higher the jaundice level will be in your baby. Some suggest this is caused by drugs temporarily overloading the infant's liver and its ability to process waste, while others think this may not be caused necessarily by Pitocin's chemical effect. If Pitocin is used at all, it can be an indication that the baby would have been born later and is premature, suggests P. Boylan. Researchers Chew and Swann include amniotomy, the breaking of the bag of waters (a routine procedure used with Pitocin), for the same reason.

- *Increased cesareans.* One of the most frequent complications of cesareans is jaundice in the baby. Now that nearly one in four births is a cesarean, there are more jaundiced babies. It's not clear why this is so. Perhaps jaundice is a common complication of cesareans because of maternal drugs. Also, delayed breastfeeding, a factor in jaundice, almost always occurs after a cesarean birth.

- *Use of vacuum extractor.* This is a metal or plastic cup that uses suction to "vacuum" the baby's head. Although it's believed to be less traumatic to the baby's head than forceps, babies who are born with the help of vacuum extractors are more likely to have jaundice and to be treated with phototherapy, according to 1986 European research.

- *Convenience —phototherapy is handy.* As one pediatrician said twenty-five years ago, "Now that every hospital is getting the bilirubin lights, for sure we pediatricians are going to diagnose more jaundice." And they have. Babies don't have to be sent to a high-risk center for phototherapy; it's as near as the nursery. In fact, in some hospitals even nurses can order blood tests for bilirubin counts without a physician's okay.

When a nurse tells a pediatrician that the bilirubin level is

10 or 12, the pediatrician may feel she has to do something about it. Not too long ago many of those babies wouldn't have had blood tests at all. Instead, the doctor would have made an evaluation of the baby by examining him. If the baby wasn't lethargic, if he nursed well and seemed normal, though jaundiced, the doctor would not have been likely to intervene.

Just as ultrasound equipment is used more when doctors have it in their offices, phototherapy use increases with availability. Prior to the bilirubin lights, babies were placed by a sunny window at home for a few hours, or the ultimate treatment for very sick infants was a blood exchange.

- *Fear of criticism.* If you're a doctor, using technology means you're up to date. Some pediatricians we spoke with told us they felt newborn jaundice was being overtreated. But even so, they sometimes put babies under the bilirubin lights just to avoid criticism from their peers. The pressure to use the available technology is great.

Avoiding Unnecessary Phototherapy

- *Avoid drugs.* Try not to go to the hospital too soon; wait until labor is well established. If Pitocin is suggested to you because your labor slows, consider the nonmedical techniques described in Chapter 8.
- *If you breastfeed, do it early and often.* An important key to preventing or controlling jaundice is to move the bilirubin out of the baby's body via meconium, the black bowel movement of a newborn. The most effective way to do that is to breastfeed early and often (every two hours or so), especially in the first three days without any supplements. Colostrum, which is produced by the mother's body until the "true" milk comes in, has a laxative effect and promotes the passage of meconium.

  Room in, if possible. If not, arrange for your baby to be brought to you as soon as he awakens. Protect yourself by finding a breastfeeding counselor, especially if this is your first baby. Go home early if you can, where feeding a baby frequently is easier, because there are no hospital routines to interfere. Nursing infrequently may actually increase your baby's jaundice, Lawrence Gartner says, by causing "starvation jaundice." Your baby needs you and your milk.

- *Ask your doctor why your baby needs phototherapy.* Let her know you know there is controversy about when to use phototherapy. Ask her to explain why a normal condition that affects most babies is not normal in your full-term, healthy baby. Ask her to describe the guidelines she uses and why. Ask her to tell you what symptoms your baby exhibits in addition to a certain bilirubin number. Ask her what the risks of treatment are. Blood tests for bilirubin are often inaccurate (a urine test may be more accurate). Several years ago in Indiana, sixty-seven labs measured bilirubin in blood samples that averaged a true value of 18. Lab results varied from 10.9 to 24. And if none of this satisfies you, you can always ask for a second opinion. Ask another doctor in your town. If you don't know whom to call for a second opinion, call La Leche League or NAPSAC (see Appendix D) and request names for referrals.

If Your Baby Needs Phototherapy

- *If possible, stay with your baby even if your infant needs to be under the lights.* Ask if the hospital has portable bilirubin lights that can be placed over both you and your baby (though you may find the lights just as uncomfortable as your baby does). Or request that the baby be wrapped in a special blanket, used for this purpose, so that you can continue to breastfeed. As a last resort, have the portable bilirubin light unit placed in your hospital room, so that you can at least be with your baby. You will quite naturally be concerned about your baby if the infant needs phototherapy— you will be reassured if you are able to see him.

  If your baby is treated with phototherapy, there is a valid concern about your baby having adequate liquids. Denver pediatrician Marianne Neifert suggests you can express your milk and give that to the baby for extra liquids in addition to nursing him frequently. (A breastfeeding counselor will be helpful in showing you how to express your milk.)

- *Discuss home phototherapy for your baby with your doctor.* Babies treated for jaundice in the hospital receive seven times as much phototherapy as babies treated at home, though the outcome of the babies was similar in British research. In 1985 the American Academy of Pediatrics stated, "Only equipment designed specifically for providing bilirubin reduction should be used for home phototherapy." (Portable bilirubin light units are available at rental agencies.)

Other doctors, like pediatrician and member of La Leche League's medical board Jay Gordon, have sent home hundreds of jaundiced babies with instructions for sun phototherapy with good results. Gordon suggests that you place your naked baby in a direct sunbath for five to ten minutes at a time two or three times a day. (Use common sense. "July and August in California would be too hot," he adds.) At other times keep the baby in front of the window in indirect light. Leave on all the lights in the house, since any light will help. Gordon has the parents bring the baby into his office at least once a day during home therapy and asks the parents to call him immediately if there's a change in the quality of breastfeeding—if the baby slows down or doesn't nurse as vigorously. If the parents are not comfortable with home phototherapy, or if the baby is not doing well and does need to be hospitalized, he suggests that the mother and baby go to a hospital where the mother can stay twenty-four hours a day, and breastfeeding never has to be stopped. It's been Gordon's experience that the vast majority of babies don't need to be hospitalized for phototherapy treatment.

- *Some physicians suggest giving your baby supplements of vitamin E.* Researcher Steven J. Gross, in his Duke University study, found that jaundiced premature babies had reduced bilirubin levels when they received fifty milligrams of vitamin E each day for the first three days of life. Premature babies are much more susceptible to the consequences of bilirubin than full-term healthy babies. (He did not study full-term infants.) Some lay midwives have told us that they recommend that mothers give their babies vitamin E once on the first day. Jay Gordon suggests to mothers that they pierce a capsule of vitamin E (200 or 300 units), spread it on their nipples, and let the baby nurse it off gradually.

Though the hospital staff may tell parents that their baby is in no danger because he's under the lights, most parents worry. Many are like the Illinois woman who wrote, "My pediatrician came in and said the baby has jaundice and has to stay. He handed me a printout, told me not to worry, and left. That was the beginning of about a week of tears and frustration." And many parents carry lingering doubts for years that there's something permanently wrong with their child.

If your doctor suggests phototherapy for your infant, let her know how important it is to you that your baby stay with you. Since treating newborn jaundice with bilirubin lights might be an every-day occurrence for her, she may not see the situation as the crisis you do. Discussing your baby's situation in detail may also relieve some of your doctor's anxiety about a malpractice suit.

You've got time to talk about this with your doctor if your baby has physiologic (normal) jaundice or even breastmilk jaundice. (We're not talking here about jaundice caused by blood incompatibility or a premature or sick full-term baby.) With physiologic jaundice, it's not a we-must-do-something-in-the-next-hour emergency, although being in a hospital often makes it seem so.

Circumcision

Circumcision is the removal of the foreskin of the penis. For some people, such as Jews and Muslims, it is a religious ritual. In the last three generations in the United States, however, the circumcision of newborn boys in the hospital has been cultural (like father, like son), and has been performed by obstetricians or pediatricians.

Most infant boys (60 percent) in this country are circumcised, though nearly all were in the 1960s, while the rate in England and Scandinavia is less than one percent. And as an indication of its dis-favor these days, circumcision is not paid for by many insurance companies. Medical and surgical complications from circumcision do occur, and the operation is painful for the infant.

In the 1940s circumcision became routine for two reasons, cleanli-ness and the prevention of cancer of the penis. Since then, research has shown that it is poor hygiene, not an intact foreskin, that causes rare infections, although uncircumcised males are nearly the only ones to contract penile cancer. Critics of circumcision, however, say that this particular cancer is very rare, and that's also true: In the past fifty-five years, there have been only 750 to 1,000 U.S. cases of penile cancer in a country where about 2 million boys are born each year.

It is not true, however, that circumcision reduces the risk for can-cer of the cervix in female partners, or that it improves sexual enjoy-ment for the male.

In what is perhaps a turnaround from their 1975 statement, the American Academy of Pediatrics (AAP) in 1989 said there may be a health advantage to circumcision after all, though it also made clear that "there is no absolute medical indication" for circumcision. In a study of 200,000 males in army hospitals, uncircumcised males were ten times more likely to have urinary tract infections, which are rare among men. However, critics, as well as the AAP itself, say there are problems with the study and consider the findings only tentative. And whether uncircumcised males are more or less likely to contract sexually transmitted diseases remains controversial.

When considering circumcision for your son, here are some suggestions:

- *Decide for yourself.* On one side are those in favor of this procedure for religious or cultural reasons. On the other side are those who believe it is a human rights issue that clearly outweighs religious or cultural beliefs.
- *If you decide not to have your son circumcised, don't sign the release that allows your physician to perform this operation.* This procedure is not required by law. The decision is up to you.
- *When you're wavering on this matter, ask someone to let you witness a circumcision.* Perhaps your childbirth educator could help arrange that, so that you won't have any surprises. A Kentucky mother of three sons witnessed the circumcision of her youngest a quarter of a century ago—and swore that no future son of hers would ever have this cut. She had permitted it because she didn't know what it was really like.
- *If you decide to have your son circumcised, arrange to be there, so that you and your mate can offer him comfort.* Some doctors recommend the use of a local anesthetic to block the pain. Others don't, because the administration of the drug is painful as well. No amount of medication, furthermore, really makes it okay for the baby. That's why it's so important for the parents to be there, too. In prior years, many people believed that babies couldn't feel the pain because of an undeveloped nervous system, despite infant screams. Many mothers didn't know how upset their sons became because the circumcision was performed in the nursery, and the mothers couldn't hear the cries.

A San Francisco pediatrician told us that "only a minority of people want the right to make decisions about their child. Many parents don't think they're capable. They forget to depend on themselves." But no one knows or cares about your child more than you do. Do your part, so that the care for your child is the best it can be.

Your baby doctor wants to do a good job for you and your child. She wants you to feel good as a parent, and she knows any baby has a better chance with self-confident parents. Choose a pediatrician who shares your philosophy, with whom you feel comfortable, and with whom you can build a partnership for your child's good health.

Epilogue

"I feel overwhelmed." "So much to think about!" "I think I'll leave everything up to the doctor." When you reach this point in the book you might feel a little panic.

We knew some of our information would be scary, and it wasn't until we were well along in writing that we realized how much information has been kept from pregnant women. Maternity care is the most important service we buy. If we are not informed, we don't know what good care is, much less how to get it.

"Okay, so you've informed me; but do I really have to do all those things you say to get what I want? It seems like so much trouble." Yes, it's work. But how many times in your life do you give birth? Isn't it worth the effort to get a good and safe birth?

By working for what you want you are contributing to better maternity care for all women. Thousands of women will read this book. Some will take one step. ("I will get a woman friend to be with my husband and me during my labor and birth.") Others will draw up a detailed birth plan and persist to get many options. Others will decide there are really one, two, or three things important to them, talk with their doctor, and get his agreement. Add up all these individual changes, and you have a widespread demand for better maternity care. Yet all you need to do is take one step for yourself.

"What happens if I do all that you suggest and my beautiful birth plan goes awry?" Your satisfaction with the birth will not be based on whether the birth goes according to the plan. Your satisfaction depends on your sense of accomplishment, your feeling of meeting the challenge of birth the best way you could. That sense of satisfaction depends on whether you are consulted and respected at every step of the birth or are treated as a container for the baby; whether you are in control of the decisions made about your care or decisions are dictated to you by the staff. If you have carefully chosen Dr. Right and a place of birth, and have set up a support system (your partner, one or more doulas, and a nurse for one-to-one care), your satisfaction with the birth is likely to be very high whatever happens. Why? Because the environment and supporters will ensure that even though the birth is different from what you planned, you can open yourself to whatever the experience brings. Dealing with the unexpected, with your supporters' help, you will find an inner strength, a capacity for courage and coping, you did not know was within you.

Appendix A

How to Be a Changemaker

So far, this book has focused on helping you get what you want for you and your baby. Appendix A is a guide to help you create improved maternity options in your hospital for all women. Of course, these same steps apply to changing other bureaucracies, too.

Our local hospital administrators never asked for our input. From day one, we offered our opinions totally unsolicited. In spite of our pariah status, we were very successful. When the local hospital announced plans for a new ob unit several years ago, we set out to persuade the hospital administrators to offer women the maternity options they want. All of our original goals were met. The hospital added to its blueprints what were then unusual and innovative additions in the late 1970s: an in-hospital birth center; facilities for labor and delivery in the same room in the traditional unit; mostly private postpartum rooms; and more.

If you're thinking, "What changes can I make? What makes me an effective changemaker?" remember, as a childbirth consumer, no one knows better. And you can't get fired. Doctors and nurses who want to make changes always face a threat of peer pressure, even dismissal. But as a consumer who is buying medical service, we're convinced that you, too, can be successful in making changes.

The strategies that worked for us didn't come to us neatly prepackaged. We learned a lot from trial and error. Other tactics were learned from watching hospital administrators, doctors, and board directors, or from talking with successful businesspeople. And though we first used this formula more than fifteen years ago, we know from reader responses that our formula is still effective.

If you believe that hospital administrators and doctors are all-powerful, all-knowing, all-doing—don't read on. But if you're not sure, take what is helpful to you from our formula for success. If we did it, so can you. We built our confidence and knowledge one step at a time. We didn't always know how we were going to accomplish the next step. We just knew we'd do it. You may not need to use each and every strategy, or you may discover new ones. Use what works.

We've divided the strategies into two sections that are equally important: what worked for us, and what strategies were used against us.

What Worked for Us

1. *Choose your partners well.* Look for optimists; avoid naysayers. As Henry Ford said, "If you think you can or you can't, you're always right."

Look for risk takers. Avoid those people who always say, "Yes but..." Beware potential partners who think they have to ask permission from those in authority; getting approval is unimportant and works against success. Some people will always disapprove of you, no matter what you do—especially when you're questioning the status quo.

Keep the action group very small, or energy dissipates when trying to achieve harmony. Rule by consensus is usually a guarantee you'll have only a discussion group. It's better to have a strong leader or two to implement the goals of the group. If you give your group a name, make it positive sounding—not negative. Be *for* something, not against.

2. *Do your homework.*

• *Set concrete, measurable goals and deadlines.* Don't just say, "Someday we want Hospital X to have more family-centered maternity care." Do say, "Within eighteen months (or twelve, or twenty-four) we want Hospital X to provide a birth room where families can stay together during the birth process, any mother can room in as much as she wishes, and siblings can visit both the mother and the new baby on the ob floor."

Having established your goal and deadline, then you can make your timetable. Sometimes events outside your control determine your deadline. We had to finish and publish the M.O.M. Survey within nine months because that's when the hospital was going to have the first set of blueprints for the new ob unit available, and we wanted the impact of the survey to come before the blueprints were literally set in concrete.

We established goals when we saw the M.O.M. Survey results. Because the results from all three surveys (Boulder,

Wenatchee, Baltimore) are the same, you are safe in assuming that these goals represent women in your area, too. Or do your own survey. Also, be sure to find out what other hospitals are offering.

- *Go to experts for help.* Once we decided our goal was to give the hospital input from consumers, we realized the best method was a survey. We consulted with a local university sociology professor, who counseled us on the appropriate way to do the survey and to train the telephone surveyors.

   When asking experts for help, remember that you don't always have to do what they suggest. Use your own common sense, too. One of the doctors we asked to review our survey results before they were published was aghast that not only did one in five women want a homebirth, but that we actually intended to print that information. Yes, we did want his input. But we didn't agree with him on deleting the data on homebirth preferences.

- *Know what's in it for the hospital to change.* Your success in changemaking will come as a result of a partnership with the hospital. When hospitals change their policies to offer the maternity care women prefer, hospitals benefit, too.

   —It gets the government off the hospital's back. Federal policymakers want hospital care to be more consumer oriented.

   —It will get women off the hospital's back, too (fewer complaints from consumers).

   —Most of all, these changes make money for the hospital. Administrators need healthy financial statements. Offering women what they want means more mothers use the facilities. And families who come to hospitals to have babies tend to return when they need hospitalization again.

   —If your town has more than one hospital with a maternity unit, you're in luck. Since the hospitals compete with each other for the same patients, they'll be especially interested when you tell them women will use the hospital that offers these options.

   —The hospital's prestige will increase. Hospitals like to make money and be progressive.

3. *Decide it's your battle.* You've done your homework. You've thought through your goals, established a timetable, selected your partners, found your experts, and come to understand what's in it

for the hospital to change. You're probably riding high from your initial enthusiasm and zeal, but somewhere along in the process you'll have to decide that it is indeed *your* battle—or that it's not.

Do you have the persistence to stay in for several years? Is this issue of maternity change paramount with you? If you feel you have only two or three months to devote to this project, you're not likely to accomplish your goals—unless your partners pick up the slack.

Persistence is the key. If you persist, you can find a way to succeed. But none of us can fight every battle that beckons. If you decide that this project *is* your battle, form a network of supporters. Feel free to call us.

4. *Go with what is, not what you wish were true.* It's counterproductive to insist otherwise. Let's say you've got your heart set on an out-of-hospital birth center. But your state's health department laws prevent such an establishment. You could work through the legislature to change the laws, but maybe you want more immediate results. So then you go to your local hospital and suggest they construct a birth center in the hospital down the hall from the traditional ob department. However, don't expect to find any building funds budgeted for your project.

When hospitals say they can't do what you want, ask what they *can* do. Remind them of the need for the facility. Back your requests up with some statistics. If the hospital is unwilling to make a long-term commitment, discuss a short-term pilot project. Compromise is inevitable. It's a necessary part of changemaking.

5. *Go to the top.* In most hospitals, including for-profit hospital corporations (privately held hospitals are an exception), the top is the board of directors. When we first published our survey, we were ignored. But we didn't allow that to go on for long (three weeks). You can't be ignored, either, if you go to the top.

To make sure that our hospital's board of directors knew about us, we sent a letter to the chairman. We also sent copies to the homes of all of the other members. The letter described briefly what women wanted, based on our survey, and what specific changes the hospital would need to make to provide those options. The list of changes the hospital would have to make was what we called our fat minimum. (That's more than we absolutely had to have, but allowed space for compromise.) The list of changes was also concrete and clear. Telling hospital administrators that women want "family-centered maternity care" is too vague. But telling them women want their other children to visit them in their hospital rooms is specific.

You'll increase your chance of getting what you want by offering

solutions, not just problems. That thoroughness separates you from those who "just want to complain."

Although hospital boards of directors are supposed to represent the community, they seldom hear directly from the public. These boards are predominantly male and are often composed of bankers, businesspeople, and university administrators. You cannot expect them to know much about childbirth if you don't educate them.

6. *Work on all levels, cover all flanks* We kept contact with other consumers, childbirth educators, hospital administrators, doctors, nurses, the board of directors, even a government agency (the Health Systems Agencies) that would eventually review the hospital plan to renovate and expand the maternity unit. We encouraged and helped organize public meetings with panel discussions on maternity options.

We didn't keep secrets. We sent copies of our letters to all, to let everyone know what we were doing. You cannot be ignored if you're obviously and persistently visible—by phone, mail, or in person.

7. *Use the power of groups.* Well-known Canadian obstetrician Murray Enkin once said that "one couple is weird, two are a committee, and one thousand are a movement." Swell your ranks, broaden your support by forming alliances with others. In union there is strength.

At about the same time we began our M.O.M. project, a new group, the Boulder Perinatal Council, began to meet at the hospital. This group was established as an information exchange, not as an action group. But because it did exist, we asked for and received support from many of the member agencies for our project.

The hospital increasingly recognized this group as the official consumer voice. Having this group accelerated our progress. If you're not already part of such a group, contact other organizations with perinatal interests and form your own. The local director for the March of Dimes Birth Defects Foundation, Becky Messina, was the key organizer for the Boulder Perinatal Council.

But don't just look for support from other health organizations. The hospital received support letters for changing maternity options—at our urging—from women's political groups, the YWCA, and other organizations that don't focus exclusively on health.

8. *Look for insiders.* When Woodward and Bernstein exposed the Watergate scandal in the 1970s, one of their sources was an unidentified White House insider labeled "Deep Throat." Do you know of a doctor or nurse who's on the staff who may be a closet supporter of your goals? He or she is likely to be a doctor who is more

progressive than the others, or a nurse who wants the hospital to make its policies more consumer oriented. Do you know a member of the board of directors who will let you know what discussion, if any, is made of your project at board meetings? Will this board member put the topic of maternity options on the board-meeting agenda? Do you have a relative, neighbor, friend, or member of your social group who has inside knowledge? For example, among our bridges was Roberta's husband, Bob, who, as a doctor, was a member of the hospital's staff and privy to many medical meetings.

These bridges can keep you apprised of the temperature inside the institution. Remember, you don't need their agreement with your project, just some interest.

9. *Use outside connections.* Outsiders can be influential. Sometimes there is nothing like a name. If they don't influence the hospital policymakers themselves directly, these outsiders can certainly make you—the changemaker—feel better.

In the early months after we published the survey, we got a lot of negative feedback. We heard complaints about our survey methods or criticism that we were butting into other people's business. Then along came a letter from internationally known pediatric researcher Marshall Klaus (we had sent him a copy of our survey results), telling us: "You've done an excellent survey." It certainly reassured us that we were on the right track.

At about the same time we asked fifteen or twenty medical professionals, both state and nationally known figures, for letters of support for our M.O.M. project in our attempt to get more funding for additional projects. We didn't get the funding, but we got the letters. Those letters increased our confidence. Don't overlook politicians and other public officials. They are potential sources of strong support.

10. *Seek publicity.* Get attention. No matter how much the other side wants to ignore you, getting publicity forces them to recognize you. It keeps the pressure on and prevents the hospital from sweeping your project under the rug. In a magazine interview, John Kenneth Galbraith commented that women at Harvard made inroads in getting equal treatment only when they presented a "mood of menace." This mood, he said, "must be strong enough so that it can induce a certain measure of alarm. That alarm is mostly achieved by uninhibited public criticism, which is something the people resisting women don't want to hear." We gave a copy of our survey to a newspaper reporter and invited an interview. The resulting article was the first of nearly one hundred nationwide about the

M.O.M. survey and maternity care in Boulder.

You, too, can make maternity care in your town a public issue. Following are steps that worked for us:

- *Keep journalists informed about your project.* The most likely person to contact at a newspaper is the one who covers what used to be called the women's page news. The best contact person at radio and TV stations is the public-affairs director. At cable TV companies, it's the local access director. Reporters are always looking for news, but that doesn't mean that they'll necessarily be interested in supporting your pet project. It's up to you to find the appropriate person and let her or him know that maternity care in your community is not just a local, isolated issue, but a national issue. Meet the reporter in person. Give that person background information to read. A media release, hand delivered, is helpful for newspapers, radio, or TV. It should describe what women want locally and what changes the hospital would have to make.

  Most reporters do not have the luxury of a lot of time to research issues. By giving them background material, whether it's newspaper clippings or surveys like ours, you're expanding their available information. But that doesn't mean they necessarily will write the story the way you want, or that they'll do a story at all.

  If a reporter does write anything on your project, thank that person afterward. Reporters seldom get anything but negative feedback. Get others to write or phone, too. Although women reporters may have a lot of empathy for your project, especially if they're mothers themselves, we found there are male reporters who are very interested in this issue also.

- *Encourage letters to the editor.* The letters to the editor mirror current concerns of the community. They are an ideal place for you and your allies to go public. But it's often tough to get people to actually write the letters and send them in. Make it as easy for them as possible, though, because these published letters can create a bandwagon effect.

  It can be very discouraging to send in a letter to the newspaper and then discover it's not printed. It's a fact of life, however, that newspapers don't publish all the letters they receive. Call or go in and talk with the publisher (that's going to the top) and/or the person responsible for that section of the newspaper. Tell that person of your project and ask if he or she will run all letters that come in on that issue. That person might agree. If so, you're that much ahead.

Give potential letter writers ideas for letters (or even rough drafts). Know the rules for letters to the editor. Do they have to be typed double-spaced? Do they have to include an address? Does it help if the letters are hand delivered? (It often does, especially if you bring a baby with you.) Give your letter writers all the information you can.

- *Consider petitions.* Getting petition signatures is a form of publicity, as well as a means to rally public support. It's a concrete way to acquaint the population with your specific requests. Petitions that have specific—not vague—wording with dozens (better yet hundreds) of signatures not only make a strong statement to a hospital, they may also spark the interest of the media.

11. *Act like an equal at meetings.* Eighty percent of the message you convey is in your body language, even when you're speaking. You may be uneasy, but you want to appear calm.

- *Dress like you mean business.* No jeans or casual clothes when you're in suit territory. That's going with what is. You want them to listen to you, not judge you unlistenable because of what you're wearing. You'll feel more successful and powerful if you look as though you belong there. Even if you feel anxious and insecure, you can become what you pretend to be by dressing for the part. You might think about wearing a so-called color of authority, such as dark blue.

  Yes, you can dress like you mean business with a baby in tow. As a matter of fact, having a baby along can be to your advantage. It's a definite visual reminder of the issue at hand, and we found that administrators and doctors were disarmed with a baby present. That's a disadvantage for them that can work for you. Roberta's infant daughter, Amanda, accompanied us for about a year. Roberta was sometimes distracted caring for Amanda, but Diana took up the slack. Besides, distractions gave us time to think.

  Be on time for meetings. You don't want to apologize for being late. You don't want to apologize for anything.
- *Be prepared.* Know exactly what you want to accomplish. If

you've done your homework, you'll feel more competent, tactful, and dignified. When we had meetings with hospital administrators, we knew what our fat minimum was before we went into the meeting. We expressed it to ourselves this way: "Today we'll find out their timetable for approval of the blueprints." Or, "Today we'll find out what the next step is in changing the policy on allowing siblings to visit their moms."

If you decide your goal in advance for any particular meeting, it's easier for you to say, as the time draws near for the end of the meeting, "We've covered many items in our discussion today, but I promised the others I wouldn't leave until I found out X."

- *Keep your cool.* You can often set the tone of any meeting by your own behavior. Avoid showing anger during the meeting. Ventilate your anger before the meeting or afterward— not during; save that for your "autopsy" meeting. (That's when you discuss later what you did right, where you went wrong, and how you can fix it the next time.)

  Don't burn your bridges with these people. An enemy today may be a helper tomorrow. The people you will be meeting with are just doing their jobs. If they don't want to give you what you want, if they disagree with your whole premise, it's nothing personal. It's just business.

  They may get angry and holler at you. (That's "saber rattling," a common technique for intimidating people.) Or they may think that once you're there, they'll tell you what's what. (That's known as the "king holding court.") But you can't be intimidated or made to feel inferior if you decide you won't be.

- *Keep your expectations reasonable.* Part of being prepared is knowing what's reasonable to expect. We knew when we arranged a meeting with one influential pediatrician that we could expect that for most of one hour he would tell us all the things wrong with our project. And he did. He certainly met our expectations. However, we did squeeze in an explanation of our project from our point of view.

  As it turned out, this particular doctor was helpful later in making some of the very changes we had suggested. No, it's not always going to work out that way. But it's important to remember that the people you are trying to persuade are looking at the issues from a different perspective. Don't take your marbles and go home just because they disagree with you. There are always areas of disagreement.

- *Don't go alone to any meeting.* Pad your delegation. If possible, have more people on your side than they have on theirs. Presidents of big companies travel with an entourage. You can do the same. You'll automatically be perceived as more important. Have all members prepared—if only to remain silent observers.

- *Know their deadlines* (and use them to your advantage). Before the hospital here could begin construction on its new maternity unit, it had to get an okay from the state. Consequently, we knew the hospital's deadline was the final state hearing. Because we were invited to testify at that hearing, it was important to the hospital administrators that we be in agreement with them on the plans. When we next met with them, they had to make concessions to us.

- *Be on the offensive in meetings.* Bring up your own issues, your own agenda. For instance, if you want to talk about special arrangements for cesarean mothers, say so. Don't expect them to say, "Now, what's on your mind?" They'll be busy bringing up their own issues instead.

- *Be a good saleswoman,* not an apologizer. Present your project in the best light. If you're convinced that women want maternity options your hospital doesn't now offer, be enthusiastic. Be unafraid to represent all women. All women do want individualized care. A hospital that offers women alternatives meets the needs of all women.

- *Use the "broken record" technique* if it helps you get where you're going. Sometimes it's clear that the administrators don't want you to give them the facts. Their minds are made up, and they don't want to be confused with the facts. Then use the broken record technique. When they tell you that they can't change the hospital policy to allow partners in the cesarean operating room, just keep repeating the same phrase, "It's very important to cesarean mothers that their partners be present at the birth." They may tell you that the anesthesiologists refuse or that the obstetricians refuse. You just keep repeating your original sentence. It's not your problem that the administrator might have some difficulty in making this policy change. That's his problem. He's paid to solve problems.

12. *Develop staying power.* Changemaking is a process, not a single

event. To be successful, you must let them know that the issue will not go away. Send regular reports to people at every level. Schedule meetings. Tell the other side you look forward to continued review of this project with them.

Part of staying power is follow-up. One West Coast hospital gathered a full day's worth of speakers to discuss what hospital-maternity-care options women wanted. However, for all the talk that day, no changes were made. A follow-up would have indicated a meeting with administrators to discuss *which* options would be added and *when*.

How long do you have to last? Your timetable may be different from ours, but two years passed from our first conversation about doing a survey until the hospital policies and blueprints contained all the major preferences of women.

No, you don't have to work on this project all the time, every day. But you must keep abreast of the issues. Take care of yourselves as well, and keep in touch with your network of supporters. Don't lose heart. There will be pitfalls. You'll be criticized. That's okay. Develop a watchdog committee to monitor the hospital after changes are made, or the hospital will predictably lapse back to former policies. After all, they have time on their side. Above all, persevere.

What Was Used Against Us

Bureaucracies don't like outsiders trying to rock the boat. That's understandable. If you were in their shoes, you wouldn't like it either. So what the hospital will do in response is what just about anyone in a position of power will try. You may find that not all of these steps are used against you, but if some are, you'll be forewarned and forearmed, so that they won't deflect you from your goals.

Hospital administrators, doctors, nurses, and board directors aren't bent on frustrating you, so don't take it personally. They're just doing the job they're hired to do. And they do it very well. Here's what they'll do—how they sock it to you:

1. *They'll ignore you.* An effective technique, guaranteed to weed out the faint of heart. You'll write a letter and get no response. Your phone calls won't be returned. You'll present a proposal, and they'll smile and say, "Thank you, the committee will consider it." Months will go by before you find out from a friend who's on the staff that it never came before the committee. Or it was voted down in the last

two and a half minutes of the November meeting. We circulated 125 copies of our survey to every doctor, health-care agency, hospital administrator, and nurse having anything to do with birth or babies in our community and asked each for a response. Out of 125 copies circulated, we got zero responses. Frankly, being ignored makes you feel like a balloon that just got stuck with a pin. We thought we had finished the job by circulating the survey, but we were wrong. Oh, you faint of heart. It was just the beginning.

You do the obvious then. Refuse to be ignored. Contact people. We decided who the opinion leaders were (one obstetrician, one pediatrician, one hospital administrator) and arranged to meet with them individually. When it seemed the information still wasn't going places, we went to the top. We wrote a letter to the chairman of the board summarizing in one page what women wanted. We asked other agencies to send a similar letter, using ours as a model. Many did, which forced the hospital to realize we were determined to be visible. So, keep plugging away. Make phone calls. Write letters. Solicit support from others. Do not accept silence as the final response. Never go away.

2. *You'll be told, "Don't call us, we'll call you."* When we first began our survey, we kept the original hospital administrator we worked with informed of what was happening—not to ask permission, remember, just to keep him informed. We had not been invited to do this project, but we were always open to talking about it. As a matter of fact, in the first conversation, he told us we didn't need to go to "all that trouble." "You and some of the girls could come in, and we could all just sit down and chat about it," he said. We thanked him kindly for his suggestion and went on with the survey.

Later, when we discussed the questionnaire with him, he complained about some of the questions asked. He said we had no business asking women questions about procedures that only doctors should decide.

Incidentally, in other cities when groups begin to make noises about wanting changes at the hospital, more than one group has been called in for a meeting, usually 7:30 A.M.—good for doctors, not so good for mothers with young children—and has been told, "Don't call us, we'll call you" (meaning "when it's too late for your input to matter" or "never").

Remember, when you accept their timetable, you have totally given away yours.

3. *They'll find flaws.* When our survey was hot off the press, and we had found a way to get them to talk to us about it, we were told

we had gone about it all wrong. "You only interviewed mountain hippies," one doctor said. Another told us the survey was heavily biased. Disappointed, we could have accepted their verdict. We could have nitpicked details, whined a little, and said, "Well, we did the best we could." But the issue (always remember your goal) was not defending *how* we did the survey. The issue was what options do women want. We said, "You may not have confidence in our methods, but are you saying that you don't think this is what women want?" Now what could they say? No one else had ever asked women what they wanted, so how could our detractors know? Doctors told us that their patients didn't tell them that they wanted these options. But women often don't tell their doctors what they like or don't like.

When your "fatal flaws" are pointed out, remember that's a sign of success. You're getting somewhere. It's usually the next step after being ignored. If you've done your homework well, and your project is well thought out, you're not likely to have a genuine "fatal flaw." Stick to the real business at hand: your goals.

4. *They'll placate you, even excite you, with their interpretation of what you want.* They'll use words like "homelike" and you'll think it's music to your ears. What's homelike to many hospital personnel (who live in a world of rules and regulations and gray-green paint) may be just a splash of color, a rug on the floor, a comfortable chair, and, the ultimate ruse, a cheerful bedspread. Is that what you really wanted when you said you wanted a "homelike birth"?

Specify exactly what changes you want a hospital to make. Follow up with a letter. Be specific and definite. State: "Most postpartum rooms need to be private, so that women may more easily have their babies with them," *not* "Women want more contact with their babies." State: "Based on survey results, two of the four planned delivery rooms should have the flexibility of labor and delivery in the same bed," *not* "Women want an alternative birth situation." Vagueness allows the hospital administrators to interpret as they wish.

5. *They'll appeal to your logic.* They'll say, "The doctors won't use a birth center, no sense in putting one in." "You may want to do that, but it's not safe." "It's not financially possible." "It's just not reasonable; be logical." In a world where books or rules and regulations are inches thick and numerous enough to line a wall, it's easy to pull a book out, open it to almost any page, and find a reason why you can't do something. Keep repeating what you want. Stick to your goals. Don't let their version of logic sidetrack you.

6. *They'll refuse you access to the facts, and then tell you your information isn't good enough.* When we questioned an administrator about government procedure, he said, "Well, it's so complicated, you wouldn't understand." The initial refusal to disclose facts is often just that—the first response. Keep asking. If you're still refused, try something else. Ask, "If you can't help me, who can?" You are signaling to them that you can't be put off. (We finally contacted the government agency ourselves for the information.)

We were refused the use of patient names from hospital records for our survey. We found another source (all the while keeping the administration informed). Naturally, they told us our results would not be valid. Remember, they'll find flaws.

7. *They'll keep you an outsider.* They won't let you into the system. They don't have to let you serve on the hospital obstetrics committee, for example. Typically, it's composed of eight men and one woman—and it's in the business of providing health care for women. So go with what is. Make sure that you contact individual members of this committee and tell them what women say they want. Do not always rely on hospital-appointed go-betweens to keep committee members informed.

8. *They'll appoint someone to listen to you, raise your hopes, and they'll make sure that person is powerless.* They'll send the head nurse of the maternity floor or the director of public relations. Yes, you finally get someone to listen to you, and though this person will write reports or whatever, there will still be no change.

A group in Oregon was told to take their requests to the head nurse. They did. Months passed; nothing happened. Finally they asked the nurse, "What's going to happen?" "Nothing," was the reply. The head nurse this group spoke to had no power to change anything.

Don't quit talking to nurses, though. Nurses are on the front line. They're key to getting the maternity care women want. They can either help wonderfully or sabotage changes thoroughly every day they're at work on the floor. But don't stop with nurses. Make an appointment with the hospital administrator. Always start at the top. If you're denied access, try again. Use another tactic. Call a member of the board of directors, explain who you are, what you want to do. Once you have the board's ear, the administrator will probably be available, too.

9. *They'll act as if they're playing along.* Ah, this is so effective. This is not usually immediately obvious. One changemaking group had drawn up its own list of needed maternity options. Then came one

of those 7.30-in-the-morning meetings with doctors. Told "Thanks for coming, meeting with us, and giving us input. We'll take care of it," the women went home excited about their "partnership" meeting. Nine months later, there were no changes in sight.

Another example is one of our own. Our group was told that our input on the kind of bed used in the birth center would be welcomed. However, only a short time later we discovered that the budget for the hospital—which is established six to twelve months in advance—already had another kind of bed planned for and ordered. And it sure wasn't the one we wanted. We goofed! When making requests for certain kinds of equipment, ask what the status of the budget is. How much money is allocated for equipment, when could it be bought, what is the timetable for purchase?

10. *They'll get frustrated and start retaliating.* Name-calling and sabotage are the two most popular ways to retaliate. Be ready to grow a thick skin for name-calling. You need to respond swiftly to sabotage. Nurses can be skilled at sabotage and it doesn't always have to be intentional. In one hospital, the nursing staff reluctantly followed a new policy that allowed siblings to visit their moms on the maternity floor. But in complying with the new policy, they sabotaged an old one that permitted mom to keep her baby during visiting hours if she had no visitors herself. Here's where you changemakers need to stay on top of things. This contradiction was pointed out right away to the director of nursing, who showed the staff a way to include both policies.

Another obvious retaliation is plain old lying, missed deadlines, or statements like, "Gee, didn't I tell you about that?"

11. *They'll try to make you feel guilty.* This can easily come from an ally. As a matter of fact, men have never intentionally or unintentionally used this strategy with us. It's always been other women.

An up-to-then-supportive board member accused us of "ruining the whole project and making mothers suffer yet another summer in that sweatbox of a hospital" because our testimony at a preliminary government agency hearing might have delayed the project.

Another time a fellow worker in the Perinatal Council told us that we were causing trouble for people like her who worked regularly with the hospital. She didn't feel as welcome there as she used to and suggested it was all our fault.

Your first response might be an anxious, "Who me?" Accept that momentary twinge of anxiety and realize that this tactic is used on all persons who try to change the system. Remember, it gets easier with practice to accept the grievance for what it is: one person's opinion.

You may not have all these tactics used against you. But when any one of them is used, pat yourself and your fellow changemakers on the back. You are right on schedule.

What's in it for you to be a changemaker? You'll feel a sense of accomplishment and develop your creative powers to a new level. You'll permanently share mutual respect with the other side, and you'll be able to get what you want in other areas in the future.

And the ultimate success? If you've done your job well, the other side will take credit for it when the project is completed.

Nobel peace laureate Betty Williams told us, "It is within the power of any individual to fight for what is right and to change the course of events." She was talking about achieving peace. But the fight for humane maternity care is just as important—perhaps the beginning of all other issues. And change doesn't happen just because the cause is right. Families are the backbone of every culture. Why not become a changemaker yourself and give families the best of starts by getting maternity care that women want for good and safe births.

Appendix B

Reader Questionnaire

Readers are invited to complete this questionnaire or use it for their own local surveys. You may wish to photocopy this or simply answer on a fresh sheet with reference to the question number.

1. Rate your satisfaction with your most recent birth experience. (Circle one.)

Completely satisfied   Mostly satisfied   Satisfied

Unsatisfied   Mostly unsatisfied   Completely unsatisfied

2. What would you have changed about your prenatal care, your labor, your birth, or your hospital postpartum stay?

3. Where was your baby born? (Circle one.)

Traditional hospital unit   Birth room   Out-of-hospital birth center

Home   Other (Describe.)

4. Who was your primary birth attendant? (Circle one.)

Obstetrician   Family practitioner   Nurse-midwife

Direct-entry midwife   Other (Describe.)

5. Who is the caregiver for your baby? (Circle one.)

Pediatrician   Family practitioner

Pediatric nurse-practitioner   Other (Describe.)

6. What interventions were used in your birth?

7. What complications did you have?

8. What complications did your baby have? (For example, was your baby treated for newborn jaundice? If so, how? Please include the baby's bilirubin level used to decide treatment, if you know it.)

9. If your baby had to stay in the hospital or be rehospitalized, please explain.

10. Did you have a doula or monitrice present during your labor? (Please circle which one.) How was this person helpful?

Doula   Monitrice

11. Did you attend childbirth preparation classes? _____ Yes _____ No

If you did, were they helpful? _____ Yes _____ No

If you did, what kind of class was it? (Lamaze, Bradley, etc.)

Who sponsored the class? (Circle one.)

My doctor   My hospital   The childbirth teacher   Don't know

Other (Describe.)

Do you wish you had been given any additional information? If so, what?

12. Circle which of the following were helpful to you with breast-feeding.

Lactation consultant   Friends   Hospital nurses

La Leche League   Childbirth educator   Family   Obstetrician

Pediatrician   Family practitioner   Books/publications   Midwife

Pediatric nurse-practitioner   Other (Describe.)

Circle which of the following were *not* helpful to you with breast-feeding.

Lactation consultant   Friends   Hospital nurses   La Leche League

Childbirth educator   Family   Obstetrician   Pediatrician

Family practitioner   Books/publications   Midwife

Pediatric nurse-practitioner   Other (Describe.)

13. Did you attend La Leche League meetings or have personal or phone contact with an LLL leader? (Circle which one.)

Meetings   Phone

Do you wish you had been given any additional information? _____ Yes _____ No   If so, what?

14. What information in this book helped you the most?

15. What information in this book was not helpful?

16. What information was missing in this book?

17. Anything else you'd like to tell us? (Birth stories are welcome.)

18. Please give your name, address, and phone number in case we decide to ask for additional information. (Omit if you prefer.) Send to: Diana Korte and Roberta Scaer; c/o Harvard Common Press, 535 Albany Street, Boston, MA 02118.

Appendix C

The Three Surveys

The three surveys of American women, asking what options they wanted in their hospital maternity care, were conducted in Boulder, Colorado, in 1976; in Wenatchee, Washington, in 1978; and in Baltimore, Maryland, in 1979. The first, the Boulder survey, was the impetus and model for the others.

The M.O.M. Survey; Boulder, Colorado

Boulder is an attractive college town of 100,000 in the foothills of the Rocky Mountains, thirty miles northwest of Denver. Many residents are highly educated, white-collar workers. The city is home to high-tech government research programs and private business. Most of the citizens think of Boulder as a progressive place. For example, 84 percent of new mothers breastfeed their babies (many of them in public).

The survey started with our concern that women weren't being asked for input into plans for the local hospital's new maternity wing. We didn't know what a radical idea that was; it seemed logical to us. And so the M.O.M. (Maternity Options for Mothers) Survey was developed, with a network of women friends and health professionals.

We are longtime leaders in the worldwide breastfeeding organization, La Leche League. We knew from our many years of working with mothers that many women were frustrated about the care given to them when their babies were born. So we knew there were things that hospitals could and should be doing differently. We were also mothers ourselves, so we had some ideas on how things could have been different for us.

We got together a proposal and the assistance of forty-two volunteers, and applied to the Northern Colorado Chapter of the March of Dimes for a grant to cover the costs of computer-assisted analysis of data and publication of survey results. With the grant approved, over a period of four weeks, we were able to contact and survey 694 women from a master list of 906 names. Three groups of women were surveyed: nearly 100 percent of the Boulder Area La Leche League Women (240 women), a sample of women attending child-birth classes (205 women), and a random sample taken from news-paper birth announcements over a one-year period (210 women). All three groups totaled 694 women surveyed by means of a tele-phone interview. Only 24 women refused to participate. The survey took about fifteen minutes, but some women stayed on the line an-other half hour or more. Once started, they wanted to talk more about their birth experiences.

The women were asked to indicate their preferences ("strongly agree, agree, disagree, strongly disagree") on thirty-eight maternity care options. We were greeted with great enthusiasm from the moms, and a willingness to cooperate. One of our surveyors said, "This is an experience many women feel strongly about, but have no convenient way to get their opinions to the proper people." When the results of the survey were published early in 1977, it was a first—not only for Boulder, but for the nation, and for the American health-care system. Never had health consumers been so approached.

The Mothers' Survey;
Wenatchee, Washington

Wenatchee is another attractive city, with a population of nearly 20,000. It is located in the rolling hills of apple-growing country in eastern Washington State. Wenatchee residents are mostly blue-collar workers with high-school educations.

The Mothers' Survey in Wenatchee was the result of the "radical-ization" of one woman. Here's her story:

"I was angry!" says Shannon Pope of Wenatchee, in reply to why she was the first person to duplicate the M.O.M. Survey. "When I was pregnant with my first child, I knew just what I wanted, and I kept telling my ob what I wanted at each visit, as he was rushing out the door. I knew the risks of anesthesia to the baby, and I wanted a natural childbirth. When I got to the hospital in labor, I found out that my doctor wasn't on call. I had to argue all over again for every-thing I wanted. I thought everything went well, until I got my bill and discovered I had been charged for a pudendal block. I had been given this without being asked. I hadn't wanted it and didn't need it. The doctor had exposed my unborn baby to anesthesia completely against my wishes. I was still upset months later when I came across and article in *McCall's* about the M.O.M. Survey and knew I had to do something."

Shannon went directly to the top and made an appointment with the hospital administrator. He suggested that the M.O.M. Survey represented women only in Boulder and asked her to do a similar survey and present the information to the doctors. After getting a copy of the M.O.M. Survey and consulting with Roberta Scaer by phone, Shannon did the second maternity-options survey. Central Washington Hospital of Wenatchee contributed money and staff time for the study. In a random sample of 173 women who were mailed questionnaires, 68 replied. As in Boulder, they expressed definite opinions about what they wanted in maternity care.

Committee on Maternal Alternatives; Baltimore, Maryland

Baltimore, with 1.6 million people, is one of the oldest cities in America. It is a port city famed for its Chesapeake Bay seafood, its rich immigrant culture traditions, its professional sporting teams, and its famed Johns Hopkins Hospital. In the fall of 1978, just as the Wenatchee survey was being completed on the other side of the country, Bobbie Seabolt and her committee were hard at work putting the finishing touches on the third and most extensive questionnaire of women's preferences in maternity care ever done. Bobbi, too, had read of the M.O.M. Survey in *McCall's*. She wrote us for a copy of the survey results and the M.O.M. questionnaire and passed it around her group of volunteers (who called themselves the Committee on Maternal Alternatives, or COMA). Bobbi, like Shannon Pope, consulted with Roberta Scaer before doing the survey. Her group received some funds from the Baltimore Childbirth Education Association and the March of Dimes, but, as in Boulder, it was a huge volunteer effort that enabled them to get the job done. A total of 6,000 questionnaires was distributed by the Nu-Dy-Per Baby Service to all women using their diaper service in the greater Baltimore area. Responses came in from 1,345 women, who told of their preferences in their birthing experience. In addition, they replied to a whole new section asking what kinds of medical interventions were used in their births, and what their opinions of those interventions were. A complete report, first published in the fall of 1979 by the Committee on Maternal Alternatives, is available for $19 from Bobbi Seabolt, 1822 Notre Dame Avenue, Lutherville, MD 21093.

Appendix D

Your List of Helpers

These organizations are mostly national, occasionally regional, and a few are located in Canada, England, and Australia, where we have readers. Many fine local childbirth teachers and groups are not listed (the national organizations that are included can give you referrals). That's because many local listings would be out of date by the time you read them.

However, you can call the reference room of your local library or contact your town's United Way office for leads to groups and contacts in your city. You can also call these places if you find that one of the following listings is now out of date, too. Every listing in this appendix has been confirmed by mail or phone at least once, and often the wording used is what the organization gave us. *The listing of any person or organization in this directory, however, is not an endorsement by us.*

When requesting information from these organizations (with the exception of the mail-order companies), please send a stamped, self-addressed, business-size envelope.

Index

Birth Centers

National Association of Childbearing Centers
Kate Bauer, Executive Director
3123 Gottchall Road
Perkiomenville, PA 18074
(215) 234-8068

Provides referrals to consumers for more than 140 birth centers, publications including newsletter.
Send $1 for postage and handling. No SASE required.

Birth Defects

March of Dimes Birth Defects Foundation
National Headquarters
1275 Mamaroneck Avenue
White Plains, NY 10605
(914) 428-7100

Provides materials on healthy childbearing, birth defects, and their prevention, with information sheets on individual birth defects, such as club foot, Tay-Sachs, and sickle-cell anemia.

Breastfeeding/Lactation Consultants

La Leche League International, Inc.
P.O. Box 4079
1400 North Meacham Road
Schaumburg, IL 60168-4079
(847) 519-7730 or (800) LA-LECHE

Provides mother-to-mother breastfeeding information worldwide to one million women annually. Publications, including information sheets, newsletters, and books for both consumers and health-care professionals, and catalog of publications. Also tapes and braille for the visually impaired regarding pregnancy, childbirth, and breastfeeding. Send for name of nearest LLL counselor.

International Lactation Consultant Association
200 North Michigan Avenue
Suite 300
Chicago, IL 60601
(312) 541-1710

Provides professional organization for lactation consultants and other health professionals interested in breastfeeding. Quarterly publication, *Journal of Human Lactation*, annual conferences, and consumer referrals.

Cesarean Birth

C/Sec, Inc. (Cesareans/Support, Education and Concern)
Norma Shulman
22 Forest Road
Framingham, MA 01701
(508) 877-8266

Provides support and information on cesarean childbirth, cesarean prevention, and vaginal birth after cesarean (VBAC).

Conscious Childbearing
Lynn Baptisti Richards
3455 Moki Drive
Sedona, AZ 86336

Provides workshops, and counseling for avoiding cesareans and having a VBAC in hospital or at home; also provides referral list of professionals who support VBACs. Write for a free pamphlet.

International Cesarean Awareness Network (ICAN)
Esther Zorn, President
P.O. Box 152, University Station
Syracuse, NY 13210
(315) 424-1942

Provides information on cesarean prevention and VBAC (vaginal birth after cesarean); more than seventy chapters nationwide; book catalog, quarterly newsletter.

Public Citizen's Health Research Group
2000 P Street, NW, Room 605
Washington, DC 20036
(202) 833-3000

Sells publications, including the report, *Unnecessary Cesarean Sections: Halting A National Epidemic*. $10 for individuals/nonprofits; $20 for businesses/hospitals.

VBAC (Vaginal Birth After Cesarean)
Nancy Wainer Cohen
10 Great Plain Terrace
Needham, MA 02192
(617) 449-2490

Provides VBAC information, workshops, and counseling.

Childbirth Education

Academy of Certified Birth Educators and Labor Support Professionals
Sally Riley, Judith Wika, Linda Herrick
2001 East Prairie Circle, Suite I
Olathe, KS 66062
(913) 782-5116 or (800) 444-8223

Provides certification course for childbirth educators, including curriculum development, relaxation, labor and support techniques, teaching skills, and teen pregnancy.

American Academy of Husband-Coached Childbirth
Jay and Marjie Hathaway, Directors
P.O. Box 5224
Sherman Oaks, CA 91413
(800) 42-BIRTH (in California);
(800) 423-2397 (national);
(818) 788-6662

Certifies and trains instructors in Bradley method of childbirth education. Publications and videos.

American Society for Psychoprophylaxis in Obstetrics (ASPO/Lamaze)
1200 19th Street, NW, Suite 300
Washington, DC 20036
(202) 857-1128

Certifies and trains instructors in Lamaze method and provides information for consumers, including referrals to instructors, books about childbirth and family-centered maternity care, and magazines, including *Lamaze Parents Magazine* and *Genesis*. Videos about parenting are available through ASPO instructors.

Birth Works, Inc.
P.O. Box 2045
Medford, NJ 08055
(609) 953-9380 or (888) 862-4784

Combines traditional childbirth education classes with prevention of unnecessary cesareans.

Childbirth Without Pain Education Association
20134 Snowden
Detroit, MI 48235

Offers classes to expectant parents and certifies and trains instructors in the Lamaze method of painless childbirth. Publications and films.

Gamper International, Inc. (formerly Midwest Parentcraft Center)
627 Beaver Road
Glenview, IL 60025

Teaches Gamper method of childbirth education. Numerous groups in the greater Chicago area. Publications, quarterly newsletter, *Heir Raising News*, $15/year.

International Childbirth Education Association (ICEA)
P.O. Box 20048
Minneapolis, MN 55420

Gathers together parents and professionals interested in family-centered maternity care. Classes for both parents and childbirth educators; national and regional meetings; local chapters; publications, including the *International Journal of Childbirth Education*; and films.

**Read Natural Childbirth
 Foundation, Inc.**
Margaret B. Farley
P.O. Box 956
San Rafael, CA 94915
(415) 456-8462

Provides a program to prepare expectant parents for a more satisfying pregnancy, labor, and postpartum birth experience.

Childbirth Organizations (General)

**American Foundation for Maternal
 and Child Health**
Doris Haire, President
439 East 51st Street
New York, NY 10022
(212) 759-5510

Promotes unmedicated childbirth by sponsoring research seminars, publishing literature, and exerting pressures on national and state legislators and agencies.

**National Association of Parents
 and Professionals for Safe
 Alternatives (NAPSAC)**
David and Lee Stewart, Directors
P.O. Box 646
Marble Hill, MO 63764-9726
(573) 238-2010

Promotes education about all childbirth alternatives. Newsletter, books, and other publications, including birth directory. Active in legislative reform and political action.

Circumcision

Childbirth Education Foundation
P.O. Box 5
Richboro, PA 18954

Provides information about avoiding circumcision, including a variety of publications, as well as pamphlets about other childbirth issues.

National Organization of Circumcision Information Resource Centers (NO-CIRC)
Marilyn Milos
P.O. Box 2512
San Anselmo, CA 94979-2512
(415) 488-9883

Provides information about avoiding circumcision. Publications, including newsletter and pamphlet, *Circumcision Why?*

Peaceful Beginnings
Rosemary Romberg
13020 Homestead Court
Anchorage, AK 99516
(907) 345-4813

Provides information about avoiding circumcision, and offers other pregnancy-related publications.

Doulas (Birth Assistants and Mother-Helpers)

National Association of
Postpartum Care Services
P.O. Box 1012
Edmonds, WA 98020
(800) 453-6852

Provides referrals to consumers for more than eighty individuals or companies who provide mother-to-mother help after the baby is born. Publications, including quarterly newsletter, and national conventions for providers of these services.

The following two organizations provide birth-assistant training through workshops and publications:

Association of Labor Assistants
and Childbirth Educators
P.O. Box 382724
Cambridge, MA 02238
(617) 441-2500

Doulas of North America
1100 23rd Avenue East
Seattle, WA 98112
(206) 324-5440

Homebirth

American College of Home
Obstetrics
P.O. Box 25
River Forest, IL 60305

Provides information for physicians who cooperate with couples choosing a homebirth.

Association for Childbirth at
Home, International
116 South Louise
Glendale, CA 91250
(213) 667-0839

Provides information and support for homebirth, including publications. They also have in-house birth center at this location.

Birth Day
P.O. Box 388
Cambridge, MA 02138
(617) 259-0362

Provides alternative childbirth classes, referrals, and certified teacher training programs.

The Birthing Circle
303 E. Main Street
Burkittsville, MD 21718
Robyn O'Brien-Molloy
(301) 696-9602
Diane Younkins (301) 662-0176
Rose Gerstner (304) 876-6392

Provides referrals to expectant parents for all birth alternatives.

Informed Homebirth/Informed Birth and Parenting
Rahima Baldwin, Ute Beck
P.O. Box 3675
Ann Arbor, MI 48106
(313) 662-6857

Trains and certifies homebirth teachers and attendants; offers classes for couples planning home-births. Publications, including news-letter, books; also cassettes.

Midwifery

American College of Nurse-Midwives (ACNM)
818 Connecticut Avenue, NW
Suite 900
Washington, DC 20006
(202) 728-9860

Provides certification of nurse-midwives; referrals for consumers; publications, including brochures, fact sheets, and pregnancy calculator (a gestational wheel that esti-mates due date).

Apprentice Academics
Carla Hartley
3805 Mosswood
Conroe, TX 77302-1176
(409) 273-5175

Provides midwifery education, teaching aids, midwifery gifts, cre-ative childbirth education seminars, quarterly newsletter.

Association of Ontario Midwives
P.O. Box 85
Postal Station C
Toronto, Ontario
CANADA MBJ 3M7

Provides consumer referrals for midwives in this area.

Association of Radical Midwives
Ishbel Kargar
62 Greetby Hill, Ormskirk, Lancs
L39 2DT ENGLAND
0695-72776

Provides study and support for midwives and mothers, and infor-mation on choices in childbirth.

"Midwifery and the Law,"
published by *Mothering* magazine

Provides current legal status and midwifery contacts in each state. (See *Mothering* magazine listing under "Mothering Organizations and Publications" for address.)

Midwives Alllance of North
America (MANA)
P.O. Box 1121
Bristol, VA 24203-2111
(615) 764-5561

Provides support for all midwives and makes referrals to midwives in your home state.

Seattle Midwifery School
JoAnne Myer-Ciecko
2524 Sixteenth Avenue South, #300
Seattle, WA 98144
(206) 322-8834

Certifies direct-entry midwives and offers continuing education, labor support course, obstetrics and gynecology nurse-practitioner course, and other lectures and workshops.

Miscarriage, Stillbirth, and Newborn Deaths

AMEND
Maureen J. Connelly
4324 Berrywick Terrace
Saint Louis, MO 63128
(314) 487-7528

Provides one-to-one contact with parents who lose a baby through miscarriage or stillbirth, or shortly after delivery.

Bereavement **magazine**
Andrea Gambill, Editor
350 Gradle Drive
Carmel, IN 46032
(317) 846-9429

Full-service magazine that comprehensively covers grief issues, including miscarriage, stillbirth, and neonatal death. There are features for widows, bereaved parents, children, and other bereaved individuals. $22/9 issues.

HOPING
Judy Boomer and Sandy Cruz
3288 Moanalua Road
Kaiser Hospital
Honolulu, HI 96819
(808) 834-5333, ext. 9903

Provides a perinatal loss support group for parents, lending library, newsletter, parent-to-parent phone support, and group meetings.

Intensive Caring Unlimited
Carol Randolph, President
910 Bent Lane
Philadelphia, PA 19118
(609) 848-1945

Provides information and support for those women who have a high-risk pregnancy; who have experienced a miscarriage, stillbirth, or death of a child; who have a hospitalized child and/or want to breast-feed a hospitalized child; or who have a child with a birth defect or who is developmentally delayed.

The Compassionate Friends, Inc.
Therese Goodrich
P.O. Box 3696
Oak Brook, IL 60522-3696
(312) 990-0010

Provides support to parents who have experienced the death of a child. Hundreds of local chapters. Publications, book list, newsletter.

Perinatal Loss
2443 N.E. Twentieth Avenue
Portland, OR 97212

Publishes booklet of suggestions for grieving parents.

Pregnancy and Infant Loss Center (PILC)
1415 E. Wayzata Boulevard, Suite 22
Wayzata, MN 55391
(612) 473-9372

Provides referrals to support groups nationwide; publications, including literature on pregnancy and infant loss, quarterly newsletter, *Loving Arms*; lending library; educational programs for parents and care providers; consultation for professional care providers.

PRIDE (Parents Resolving Infant Death Experiences)
Kate Luscombe
Jersey Shore Medical Center
1945 Route 33
Neptune, NJ 07754
(201) 776-4349

Provides self-help and support groups for parents who have lost an infant for any reason or who have experienced pregnancy loss.

Reach Out to the Parents of an Unknown Child, Inc.
Kathy Geldart, President
555 North County Road
Saint James, NY 11780
(516) 584-5525 or (516) 862-6743

Provides support for families experiencing the death of a child due to miscarriage, stillbirth, or early infant death. Quarterly newsletter, perinatal bereavement cards, and more.

SHARE National Office
Sister Jane Marie Lamb
Saint Elizabeth's Hospital
211 South Third Street
Belleville, IL 62222
(618) 234-2415

Provides mutual help for parents of miscarriage, stillbirth, or newborn death; local groups; publications, including bimonthly newsletter, manual for farewell rituals, and book on starting your own group.

Shattered Dreams
Cathy McDiarmid
21 Potsdam Road, #61
Downsview, Ontario
CANADA M3N 1N3
(416) 663-7143

Quarterly newsletter offering support, information, sharing, and hope for the future to parents experiencing miscarriage.

**The Southern California
Pregnancy and Infant Loss
Center**
c/o Marie Teague
5505 E. Carson Street, Suite 215
Lakewood, CA 90713
(213) 425-4889

Provides support, resources, information, and education on miscarriage, stillbirth, and infant death. Makes referrals to "Hoping and Sharing," as well as other parent support groups. Offers a monthly newsletter, lending library, and subsequent pregnancy support.

Mothering Organizations and Publications

The Doula
P.O. Box 71
Santa Cruz, CA 95063-0071
(408) 423-5056

Provides women and their families with support, inspiration, and resources to foster and emotionally satisfying pregnancy, birth, and mothering experience.

Healthy Mothers, Healthy Babies
Lori Cooper, Executive Director
409 12th Street, SW
Washington, DC 20024-2188
(202) 863-2458

Provides coalition that coordinates national activities of member and state groups to promote quality health care and education for mothers and children. Publications in English and Spanish.

Mothering **magazine**
Peggy O'Mara, Editor
P.O. Box 1690
Santa Fe, NM 87504
(505) 984-8116 or (800) 984-8116

Quarterly magazine that celebrates parenting, advocates the needs and rights of the child, and provides information on which parents can base informed choices. $18.95/year in U.S.

Mothers at Home
Deanne Dixon, President
P.O. Box 2208
Merrifield, VA 22116
(703) 352-2292

Provides educational support and advocacy for mothers who are at home. Monthly magazine, *Welcome Home*.

Mothers' Home Business Network
Georganne Fiumara
P.O. Box 423
East Meadow, NY 11554
(516) 997-7394

Provides information for mothers who want to work at home. Publications, including newsletter, *Kids and Career—New Ideas and Options for Mothers*, $6/year. Sample issue $1.

National Association of Mothers' Centers
129 Jackson Street
Hempstead, NY 11550
(800) 645-3828; (516) 486-6614 in New York State

Provides a community program where women meet to explore the experience of becoming and being mothers. Contact them for location of sixty local groups, or how to start a center in your area.

New Ways to Work
149 Ninth Street
San Francisco, CA 94103
(415) 552-1000

Provides clearinghouse for work-time alternatives, such as job sharing, permanent part-time, flextime, etc. Publications, including newsletter.

Pacific Postpartum Support Society
Christine Bender
#104, 1416 Commercial Drive
Vancouver, British Columbia
CANADA V55 431
(604) 255-7999

Provides treatment program for mothers suffering postpartum depression and educational materials on PPD, including the handbook, *Post Partum Depression and Anxiety: A Self-Help Guide for Mothers*, for $7.95, plus $1 postage.

Woman's Workshop
Christine Donovan and Deborah Dawson
P.O. Box 843
Coronado, CA 92118

Newsletter to help at-home mothers explore outside interests and plan for life after motherhood. $16/4 issues.

WOTO—Women on Their Own
Maxine Karelitz
P.O. Box O, Department W
Malaga, NJ 08328
(609) 728-4071

Provides advocacy, networking, loans, workshops, newsletter for women raising children on their own (divorced, separated, widowed, single).

Other Publications, Videos, Cassettes, and Supplies

Birth and Life Bookstore
141 Commercial Street NE
Salem, OR 97301
(800) 443-9942

Sells full range of mail-order birth, child-care, and health books.

Birth **journal**
Blackwell Scientific Publications
Three Cambridge Center, Suite 208
Cambridge, MA 02142
(617) 225-0401

Quarterly journal about birth issues for nurses, consumers, midwives, childbirth educators, and physicians. $20/year, single issues $5.

The Birth Gazette
Ina May Gaskin
42, The Farm
Summertown, TN 38483
(615) 964-2519

Quarterly magazine for midwives, physicians, childbirth educators, parents, breastfeeding counselors, and health planners and legislators.

Childbirth Graphics
P.O. Box 21207
Waco, TX 76702-1207
(817) 776-6461 x287

Catalog sales for childbirth education materials. Books, posters, pamphlets, cassettes, and videos.

Educational Graphic Aids
7762 Brentwood Court
Arvada, CO 80005
(303) 424-9221

Sells mail-order books, publications, films, slides, and videocassettes.

Maternity Center Association/ Publications
281 Park Avenue South, 5th Floor
New York, NY 10010
(212) 777-5000

Provides free catalog of publications available. MCA sells books; pamphlets; charts; slides; videotapes for prospective parents and health-care professionals, parent educators, and others interested in improving maternal, infant, and family health.

Michael Anderson
402 San Francisco Boulevard
San Anselmo, CA 94960
(415) 454-8099

Sells video (or 16 mm film), *Midwife*.

Midwifery Today
Box 2672
Eugene, OR 97402
(541) 344-7438

Quarterly for and by birth practitioners, childbirth educators, midwives, mothers, doctors, and nurses. Includes twenty regular features. $50/year.

Minot Childbirth Information Project
Jody Mclaughlin
Box 3154
Minot, ND 58702
(701) 852-2822

Provides information on pregnancy, birth, and infant care, especially nutrition, vertical/active birth, cesarean prevention, and breastfeeding.

M.O.M. magazine (Mothers and Others for Midwives)
Jeriann Fairman
P.O. Box 1068
Sugarloaf, CA 92386
(714) 585-4175

Quarterly magazine, as well as alternative birth referrals. $14/year.

Naturpath Medical and Birthing Supplies
1410 N.W. 13th Street, Suite 2
Gainesville, FL 32601
(904) 374-9655
(800) 542-4784

Nicholas J. Kaufman Productions
14 Clyde Street
Newtonville, MA 02160
(617) 964-4466

Sells video, *Once a Cesarean: Vaginal Birth after Cesarean*. This shows a VBAC with supportive people.

People's Productions
2115 Pearl Street
Boulder, CO 80302
(303) 449-6086

Sells video, *Special Delivery*. This presents options of hospital birth, freestanding birth center, and homebirth.

Perinatal Loss
Kay Mulligan, Managing Editor
5275 F Street
Sacramento, CA 95819
(916) 733-1750

Publishes nonaffiliated, nonprofit newsletter designed for those dedicated to improving the health care of the pregnant woman, fetus, and newborn. $17.50/year.

"Two Attune"
Box 12-A
Harborside, ME 04642

Provides information for do-it-yourself, wife/husband homebirth, newsletter. $10/4 issues.

WishGarden Herbs
Catherine Hunziker
Box 1304
Boulder, CO 80306
(303) 665-9508

Provides quality herbal preparations for childbearing and general health; free catalog; regular field trips offered to Rocky Mountains and Southwestern desert.

Premature Birth

Children in Hospitals, Inc.
31 Wilshire Park
Needham, MA 02192

Provides information about the need for ample contact between children and parents when either is hospitalized. Encourages hospitals to adopt flexible visiting and living-in policies. Publications, including *The Consumer Directory of Massachusetts Hospital Policies.*

Research Service

The Health Resource
Janice R. Guthrie
209 Katherine Drive
Conway, AR 72032
(501) 329-5272

Provides customized, thorough information on your medical problem, including reasons for and side effects from cesareans, with reports averaging 20 to 150 pages. Request copy of complimentary newsletter.

SIDS (Sudden Infant Death Syndrome)

**Counseling and Research Center
for Sudden Infant Death**
Kris Polzer
9000 W. Wisconsin Avenue
P.O. Box 1997
Milwaukee, WI 53226
(414) 266-2SID (2734)

Provides counseling support for families that have experienced a sudden unexpected infant death. Publications.

Illowa Guild for Infant Survival
Melanie Pangbuin
P.O. Box 3586
Davenport, IA 52808
(319) 322-4870

Raises funds for research toward the prevention of SIDS. Offers support to the families of SIDS victims, educates the public, and supports families using in-home monitors.

National Sudden Infant Death Syndrome Clearinghouse
8201 Greensboro Drive, Suite 600
McLean, VA 22102
(703) 821-8955

Provides publications about SIDS, apnea, apnea monitoring, grief/bereavement, current research. Makes referrals to national and local parent support organizations.

National Sudden Infant Death Syndrome Foundation
Mitchell Stoller
8200 Professional Place
Suite 104
Landover, MD 20785
(301) 459-3388

Provides peer counseling for SIDS families; education for SIDS families, general public, related professionals; promotion of research of SIDS and related issues.

Twins, Triplets, and Quads

Center for Study of Multiple Births
Linda Neglia
333 E. Superior Street, Suite 476
Chicago, IL 60611
(312) 266-9093

Provides information for parents of twins, triplets, and quadruplets. Publications, including mail-order books.

Double Talk
Mary Hurlburt
P.O. Box 412
Amelia, OH 45102
(513) 231-8946

Provides resource center for parents of twins, triplets, or more. Newsletter.

National Organization of Mothers of Twins Clubs, Inc.
Lois Gallmeyer, Executive Secretary
12404 Princess Jeanne NE
Albuquerque, NM 87112-0955

Offers opportunity for mothers of multiples to share information, concerns, and advice. Information sheets, quarterly newsletter, chapter development kit.

Parents of Multiple Births Association of Canada, Inc.
Sherly McInnes
P.O. Box 2200
Lethbridge, Alberta
CANADA T1J 4K9
(403) 328-9165

Provides referral to local clubs, newsletter, mail-order literature service, and research.

The Triplet Connection
Janet Bleyl, President
8900 Thornton Road, #25
P.O. Box 99571
Stockton, CA 95209
(209) 474-0885

Provides information to families expecting triplets, or more, as well as encouragement, information, resources, and networking for parents of other multiples. Newsletter.

Twinline, Services for Multiple Birth Families
Patricia M. Malmstrom, Executive Director
P.O. Box 10066
Berkeley, CA 94709
(415) 644-0861

Provides services, publications, resource referral, and advocacy for families with twins, triplets, quadruplets, and quintuplets. Hotline: (415) 644-0863, M–F, 10 A.M. – 4 P.M. PST.

Twins **magazine**
Barbara C. Unell, Editor
P.O. Box 12045
Overland Park, KS 66212
(913) 722-1090

Bimonthly, national magazine offers a wide variety of viewpoints on twins, triplets, and more with research-based child development and family-living guidance written by health-care authorities, as well as multiples and parents themselves. $21/year.

Water Birth

Global Maternal/Child Health Association
P.O. Box 1400
Wilsonville, OR 97070
(503) 682-3600 or (800) 641-2229

Rents and sells portable birth pools and provides free referrals to women seeking a water-birth practitioner.

Point of View Productions
2477 Folsom Street
San Francisco, CA 94110
(415) 821-0435

Rents and sells video, *Water Baby: Experiences of Water Birth*, which was filmed in a birth center with Dr. Michel Odent.

Appendix E

Mother-Friendly Childbirth

The following ten steps are from The Mother-Friendly Childbirth Initiative of the Coalition for Improving Maternity Services (CIMS). The Coalition represents tens of thousands of maternity care professionals, including midwives, nurses, childbirth educators, breastfeeding counselors, labor-support providers, physicians, and others.

A mother-friendly hospital, birth center, or home birth service:
1. Offers all birthing mothers:
   • Unrestricted access to the birth companions of her choice, including fathers, partners, children, family members, and friends;
   • Unrestricted access to continuous emotional and physical support from a skilled woman—for example, a doula, or labor-support professional;
   • Access to professional midwifery care.
2. Provides accurate descriptive and statistical information to the public about its practices and procedures for birth care, including measures of interventions and outcomes.
3. Provides culturally competent care—that is, care that is sensitive and responsive to the specific beliefs, values, and customs of the mother's ethnicity and religion.
4. Provides the birthing woman with the freedom to walk, move about, and assume the positions of her choice during labor and birth (unless restriction is specifically required to correct a complication), and discourages the use of the lithotomy (flat on back with legs elevated) position.
5. Has clearly defined policies and procedures for:
   • collaborating and consulting throughout the perinatal period with other maternity services, including communicating with the original caregiver when transfer from one birth site to another is necessary;
   • linking the mother and baby to appropriate community resources, including prenatal and post-discharge follow-up and breastfeeding support.

6. Does not routinely employ practices and procedures that are unsupported by scientific evidence, including but not limited to the following:

- shaving; • enemas;
- IVs (intravenous drip); • withholding nourishment;
- early rupture of membranes; • electronic fetal monitoring;

Other interventions are limited as follows:

- Has an oxytocin use rate of 10% or less for induction and augmentation;
- Has an episiotomy rate of 20% or less, with a goal of 5% or less;
- Has a total cesarean rate of 10% or less in community hospitals, and 15% or less in tertiary care (high-risk) hospitals;
- Has a VBAC (vaginal birth after cesarean) rate of 60% or more with a goal of 75% or more.

7. Educates staff in non-drug methods of pain relief, and does not promote the use of analgesic or anesthetic drugs not specifically required to correct a complication.

8. Encourages all mothers and families, including those with sick or premature newborns or infants with congenital problems, to touch, hold, breastfeed, and care for their babies to the extent compatible with their conditions.

9. Discourages non-religious circumcision of the newborn.

10. Strives to achieve the WHO-UNICEF "Ten Steps of the Baby-Friendly Hospital Initiative" to promote successful breastfeeding:

1. Have a written breastfeeding policy communicated to all health care staff; 2. Train all health care staff in skills necessary to implement this policy; 3. Inform all pregnant women about the benefits and management of breastfeeding; 4. Help mothers initiate breastfeeding within an hour of birth; 5. Show mothers how to breastfeed and how to maintain lactation even if they should be separated from their infants; 6. Give newborn infants no food or drink other than breast milk unless medically indicated; 7. Practice rooming in: allow mothers and infants to remain together 24 hours a day; 8. Encourage breastfeeding on demand; 9. Give no artificial teat or pacifiers (also called dummies or soothers) to breastfeeding infants; 10. Foster the establishment of breastfeeding support groups and refer mothers to them on discharge from hospitals or clinics.

Copyright © 1996 by the Coalition for Improving Maternity Services (CIMS). Permission granted to reproduce without charge in whole or in part with complete attribution. For a full copy of the initiative, visit the CIMS site on the World Wide Web, http://www.healthy.net/cims, or write CIMS, c/o ASPO/Lamaze, 1200 19th Street NW, Suite 300, Washington, DC 20036, enclosing $3.00 payable to ASPO/Lamaze.

Appendix F

Bibliographic References
(By Chapter)

Introduction

Areskog, B. *et al.* "Experience of Delivery in Women with and without Antenatal Fear of Childbirth," *Gynecological and Obstetrical Investigations* 16:1, 1983

Enkin, Murray, M.D., *et al. A Guide to Effective Care in Pregnancy and Childbirth*, Oxford, England: Oxford University Press, 1990

Freudenheim, Milt. "Health Insurers Rebound as Rates Increase," *The New York Times*, March 6, 1989

Garcia, Jo *et al.* "Mothers' Views of Continuous Electronic Fetal Heart Monitoring and Intermittent Auscultation in a Randomized Controlled Trial," *Birth,* Summer 1985

Hartford, Robert B. "The Ease of the Elusive Infant Mortality Rate," *Population Today*, May 1984

Kramon, Glenn. "Employees Paying Ever-Bigger Share of Medical Costs," *The New York Times*, November 22, 1988

Lumley, Judith. "Assessing Satisfaction with Childbirth," *Birth* 12:3, Fall 1985

Malone, Theresa. "American and Dutch Women Differ on Expectation of Pain During Childbirth," *The American College of Obstetricians and Gynecologists New Release*, May 24, 1988

Melzack, Ronald. "The Myth of Painless Childbirth," *Pain* 19, 1984

National Center for Health Statistics. "Advance Report of New Data from the 1989 Birth Certificate," *Monthly Vital Statistics Report* 40(12), April 15, 1992

Newton, Niles. "Laboring Undisturbed," *Newton on Birth and Women*, Seattle: Birth & Life Bookstore, 1990

Rhundle, Rhonda L. "Insurers Step Up Efforts to Reduce Use of Free-Choice Health Plans," *The Wall Street Journal*, May 11, 1988

Rooks, Judith P. *et al.* "Outcomes of Care in Birth Centers. The National Birth Center Study," *New England Journal of Medicine* 321:26, December 28, 1989

Sargent, Carolyn, and Nancy Stark. "Surgical Birth: Interpretations of

Cesarean Delivery Among Private Hospital Patients and Nursing Staff," *Social Science and Medicine* 25:12, 1987

Senden, I.P.M. *et al.* "Labor Pain: A Comparison of Parturients in a Dutch and an American Teaching Hospital," *Obstetrics and Gynecology* 71, April 1988

Stoner, Eileen. Phone interview, July 1989

Taffel, Selma M. *et al.* "U.S. Cesarean Section Rates 1990: An Update," *Birth* 19:1, March 1992

Thomson, Molly, and James Hanley. "Factors Predisposing to Difficult Labor in Primiparas," *American Journal of Obstetrics and Gynecology* 158:5, May 1988

Treffers, Pieter E. *et al.* "Letter from Amsterdam. Home Births and Minimal Medical Interventions," *Journal of the American Medical Association* 264:17, November 7, 1990

Ventura, Stephanie. Phone interview, June 1991

———. "Advance Report of Final Natality Statistics, 1989," *National Center for Health Statistics Monthly Vital Statistics Report* 40:8, Supplement, December 12, 1991

Wolfe, Sidney, M.D. "Unnecessary Cesarean Sections: Halting a National Epidemic," *Health Letter*, June 1992

1   What Women Want

Adams, Virginia. "Pain and Pleasure in Childbirth," *Psychology Today*, March 1983

Anderson, Gene Cranston, Ph.D. "Current Knowledge About Skin-to-Skin (Kangaroo) Care for Preterm Infants," *Journal of Perinatology* 11:3

———. "Infants and Mothers as Mutual Caregivers," La Leche League International conference, Miami, July 25, 1991

———. "Risk in Mother-Infant Separation Postbirth," *Journal of Nursing Scholarship* 21:4, Winter 1989

Anderson, Sandra F., R.N., M.S., and Leta J. Brown, R.N., C.C.E. "A Scientific Survey of Siblings at Birth," *Compulsory Hospitalization or Freedom of Choice in Childbirth?* Vol. 3, David Stewart, Ph.D., and Lee Stewart, C.C.E., eds., Marble Hill, MO: NAPSAC Reproductions, 1979

Bower, B. "Emotional Aid Delivers Labor-Saving Results," *Science News*, May 4, 1991

COMA (The Committee on Maternal Alternatives). *How Women Want to Have Their Babies*, Baltimore, MD: self-published, 1980

Eisenstein, Mayer, M.D. "Homebirth and the Physician," *Safe Alternative in Childbirth*, David Stewart, Ph.D., and Lee Stewart, C.C.E., eds., Chapel Hill, NC: NAPSAC, 1976

Green, Josephine M., BA, Ph.D., Vanessa A. Coupland, BA, and Jenny V.

Kitzinger, BA. "Expectations, Experience, and Psychological Outcomes of Childbirth: A Prospective Study of 825 Women," *Birth* 17:1, March 1990

Hathaway, Marjie and Jay, AAHCC, and Kids. *Children at Birth*, Sherman Oaks, CA: Academy Publications, 1978

Hodnett, Ellen D., and Richard W. Osborn. "A Randomized Trial of the Effects of Monitrice Support during Labor: Mothers' Views Two to Four Weeks Postpartum, *Birth* 16(4), December 1989

Hotelling, Barbara A. "The Childbirth Educator as Doula," *ICEA*, February 1988

Humenick, Sharron S., R.N., Ph.D., and Larry A. Bugen, Ph.D. "Mastery: The Key to Childbirth Satisfaction?" *Birth* 8:2, Summer 1991

Kennell, John, M.D. "Are We in the Midst of a Revolution?" *American Journal of Diseases of Children* 134, March 1980

_____, *et al.* "Continuous Emotional Support During Labor in a US Hospital," *Journal of the American Medical Association* 265:17, May 1, 1991

Kerwin, Mary Ann, J.D. "Reflect on Our Past, Rejoice in Our Present, Reaffirm Our Future," keynote address, La Leche League International conference, Miami, July 25, 1991

Kitzinger, Sheila. *Some Women's Experiences of Epidurals*, London: The National Childbirth Trust, 1987

Klaus, Marshall, M.D., *et al.* "Maternal Attachment," *New England Journal of Medicine* 286:9, March 2, 1992

_____, and John H. Kennell, M.D. *Parent-Infant Bonding*, St. Louis: C.V. Mosby, 1982

_____, and Martha Oschrin Robertson, eds. *Birth Interaction and Attachment*, Johnson and Johnson, 1982

La Leche League. *The Womanly Art of Breast-feeding*, Franklin Park, IL: La Leche League International, 1991

Montagu, Ashley, Ph.D. *Touching*, New York and London: Columbia University Press, 1971

Newton, Niles, Ph.D. "Trebly Sensuous Woman," *Psychology Today*, July 1971

_____, and Michael Newton, M.D. "Psychologic Aspects of Lactation," *New England Journal of Medicine* 277:22, 1967

_____. "Oxytocin, the Hormone of Love," La Leche League International conference, Miami, July 25, 1991

_____. *Newton on Birth and Women*, Seattle: Birth & Life Bookstore, 1990

O'Mara, Peggy. "A Time for Women," *Mothering*, Fall 1991

Palmer, Gabrielle. "The Politics of Infant Feeding," *Mothering*, Summer 1991

Phillips, Celeste R. Nagel, R.N., B.S.N., M.S. "Neonatal Heat Loss in Heated Cribs vs. Mothers' Arms," *Journal of Obstetrical, Gynecological, and Neonatal Nursing* 3:6, Nov.–Dec. 1974

Pitt, Jane, M.D. Phone interview, November 14, 1979

Pittenger, James E., and Jane G. Pittenger. "The Perinatal Period: Breeding
    Ground for Marital and Parental Maladjustment," *Keeping Abreast
    Journal* 1, 1977
Placek, Paul J., Ph.D., National Center for Health Statistics. Phone inter-
    view, November 25, 1991
Pryor, Karen, and Gale Pryor. *Nursing Your Baby*, New York: Pocket Books,
    1991
Reader questionnaire responses, 1984–1991
Sander, Louis W., M.D., *et al.* "Early Mother-Infant Interaction and 24-Hour
    Patterns of Activity and Sleep," *Journal of the American Academy of
    Child Psychiatry* 9, 1970
Shearer, Beth. "Forced Cesareans: The Case of the Disappearing Mother,"
    International Journal of Childbirth Education, February 1989
Simkin, Penny, P.T. "Women's Long-term Memories of Their Birth
    Experiences," ICEA conference, Denver, August 17, 1991
Sugarman, Muriel, M.D. "Review of Maternal-Infant Attachment
    Literature," presented at ICEA Eastern-Southeastern Regional
    Conference, 1977
Tanzer, Deborah, Ph.D. "Natural Childbirth: Pain or Peak Experience?"
    Psychology Today, October 1968

2 *The Pleasure Principle*

Bing, Elisabeth, and Libby Colman. *Making Love During Pregnancy*, New
    York: Bantam, 1977
Birch, Elizabeth R. "The Experience of Touch Received During Labor,"
    Journal of Nurse Midwifery 31:6, November/December 1986
Brewin, C., and C. Bradley. "Perceived Control and the Experience of
    Childbirth," *British Journal of Clinical Psychology* 21:4, November
    1982
Chute, Owen E. "Expectation and Experience in Alternative and
    Conventional Birth," *Journal of Obstetrical, Gynecological, and
    Neonatal Nursing*, January/February 1985
Hall, Elizabeth. "Mining New Gold for Old Research," *Psychology Today*,
    February 1986
Hodnett, Ellen D., and Daryl A. Simmons-Tropea. "The Labour Agentry
    Scale: Psychometric Properties on an Instrument Measuring
    Control during Childbirth," *Research in Nursing and Health* 10,
    1987
Masters, William, M.D., and Virginia Johnson. *Human Sexual Response*,
    Boston: Little, Brown, 1966
————, and Virginia Johnson-Masters. Interview, July 1979
Moore, Demi. "Transcript #1335," *Oprah*, ABC-TV, October 25, 1991
Newton, Niles, Ph.D. "Interrelationships between Sexual Responsiveness,
    Birth and Breastfeeding," *Contemporary Sexual Behavior, Critical*

Issues for the 1970s, J. Zubin and John Money, eds., Baltimore, MD: Johns Hopkins University Press, 1973

———. *Newton on Birth and Women,* Seattle: Birth & Life Bookstore, 1990

———. "Psychologic Factors in Birth and Breastfeeding," La Leche League International Northwest Area Conference, Seattle, September 28, 1979

———, with Michael Newton *et al. Newton on Breastfeeding,* Seattle: Birth & Life Bookstore, 1987

O'Connell, M.L. "Locus of Control Specific to Pregnancy," *Journal of Obstetric and Gynecological Nursing* 12:3, May/June 1983

Sherfey, Mary Jane, M.D. *The Nature and Evolution of Female Sexuality,* New York: Random House, Vintage Books, 1973

Tanzer, Deborah, Ph.D. "Natural Childbirth: Pain or Peak Experience?" *Psychology Today,* October 1968

Zweig, S. *et al.* "Patient Satisfaction with Obstetric Care," *Journal of Family Practice* 23:2, August 1986

3 If You Don't Know Your Options, You Don't Have Any

Bajo, Kathleen, director, Ross Marketing Associates. Interview, December 1988

Barber, Rebecca A., C.N.M. "Renaissance in Birthing: The American Nurse-Midwife," *Journal of the Colorado Institute of Transpersonal Psychology,* Summer 1984

Bennetts, Anita B., C.N.M., Ph.D., and Ruth Watson Lubic, C.N.M., Ed.D. "The Free-Standing Birth Centre," *Lancet* 1:8268, February 13, 1982

Berman, Salee, C.N.M., and Victor Berman, M.D. *The Birth Center,* New York: Prentice Hall, 1986

Berman,Vic, M.D. Letter with NACHIS statistics, December 3, 1981, and update on first 1,000 births, September 25, 1982

"Birthing: Home's as Good as the Hospital" (Missouri Department of Health Study), *Hippocrates,* January/February 1988

Branca, Paul, M.D. "Forum of Health Policy Issues of the Freestanding Birth Center; If It Is Safe, What Makes It Safe?" *NACC News* 2:1, Spring 1984

Burnett, Claude A. III, M.D., M.P.H., *et al.* "Home Delivery and Neonatal Mortality in North Carolina," *Journal of the American Medical Association* 244:24, December 19, 1980

Campbell, Rona. Homebirth conference, London, October 1987

———, and Alison Macfarlane. "Place of Delivery: A Review," *British Journal of Obstetrics and Gynaecology* 93, July 1986

———, and Alison Macfarlane. *Where to Be Born,* Oxford, England: National Perinatal Epidemiology Unit, Radcliffe Infirmary, 1987

Clark, Linda, C.N.M., in group practice with Richard B. Stewart, M.D.

Phone interview, October 6, 1982

Cranch, Gene, C.N.M., Ph.D., Maternity Center Association, New York City. Phone interview, January 1982

Denver Birth Center. Open house, November 1977

Ernst, Eunice K. M., C.N.M., M.P.H. "Outcomes of 20,000 Women Who Sought Freestanding Birth Center Care: A National Collaborative Study," Eighth Birth Conference, San Francisco, March 1989

Ernst, K.M., C.N.M., M.P.H., director, National Association of Childbearing Centers. Phone interview, November 18, 1991

Eshelman, Michael, M.D. Personal interview, January 1980

Feldman, Elizabeth, M.D., and Marsha Hurst, Ph.D. "Outcome and Procedures in Low Risk Birth: A Comparison of Hospital and Birth Center Settings," Birth 14:1, March 1987

Feldman, Silvia, Ph.D. Choices in Childbirth, New York: Bantam, 1980

Ferguson, Patty, administrative assistant, Denver Birth Center. Interview, December 1988

Gaskin, Ina May. "The Farm: A Living Example of the Five Standards," The Five Standards for Safe Childbearing, David Stewart, Ph.D., ed., Marble Hill, MO: NAPSAC International, 1981

———. Homebirth conference, London, October 1987

———. "International Conferences," Birth Gazette 4:2, Winter 1988

Goodlin, Robert C. "Low Risk Obstetric Care for Low Risk Mothers," Lancet 1:8176, May 10, 1980

Harness, Barbara, director, Section for Maternal and Child Health, American Hospital Association. Interview, December 1988

Hinds, M. Ward, M.D., M.P.H., et al. "Neonatal Outcome in Planned v. Unplanned Out-of-Hospital Births in Kentucky," Journal of the American Medical Association 253:11, March 15, 1985

Honton, Margaret, ed. "Contemporary Obstetric Design," Perspectives in Perinatal and Pediatric Design, Columbus, OH: Ross Planning Associates, Ross Laboratories, 1988

Hosford, Betty, R.N., C.N.M., and Ruth Watson Lubic, C.N.M., Ed.D. "Childbearing and Maternity Centers—Alternatives to Homebirth and Hospital," Safe Alternatives in Childbirth, David Stewart, Ph.D., and Lee Stewart, C.C.E., eds., Chapel Hill, NC: NAPSAC, 1976

Huey, Kenneth, C.E.O., Longmont United Hospital. Interview, May 1989

Ivory, Loretta, C.N.M., director, Denver Birth Center. Personal interviews, November 1981, March 1989

Kitzinger, Sheila. "Why Home Birth," Homebirth conference, London, October 1987

Korte, Diana. "Infant Mortality: Lessons from Japan," Mothering, Winter 1992

Levy, Barry S., M.P.H., et al. "Reducing Neonatal Mortality Rate With Nurse-Midwives," American Journal of Obstetrics and Gynecology 109:1, January 1, 1971

Lubic, Ruth Watson, C.N.M., Ed.D. "Midwifery: An Extended Role in

Nursing Practice," Maternity Center Association, undated
———, and Eunice K.M. Ernst, C.N.M. "The Childbearing Center: An
   Alternative to Conventional Care," *Nursing Outlook* 26:12,
   December 1978
Lumley, Judith, M.A., M.B., B.S., Ph.D., and Brian A. Davey, B.S., M.S.,
   Ph.D. "Do Hospitals with Family-centered Maternity Care Policies
   Have Lower Intervention Rates?" *Birth* 14:3, September 1987
Mehl, Lewis E., M.D., Ph.D. "Home Delivery Research Today: A Review,"
   annual meeting of the American Foundation for Maternal and
   Infant Health, New York City, November 15, 1976
Minor, Al, Statistics Division, Health Insurance Association of America.
   Phone interview, November 15, 1991
Moran, Marilyn. *Birth and the Dialogue of Love*, Leawood, KS: New Nativity
   Press, 1981
"More Women Using New Birth-Site Options," *Hospitals*, October 20, 1991
Nathan, Joann, Section for Maternal and Child Health, American Hospital
   Association. Phone interview, November 13, 1991
"New Study Highlights Need for Improvements in Managing Maternity
   Costs," BGS Marketing Resources, July 10, 1991
Odent, Michel, M.D. *Birth Reborn*, New York: Pantheon Books, 1984
Otis, Caroline Hall. "Midwives Still Hassled by Medical Establishment.
   Practitioners Battle for Recognition and Autonomy," *Utne Reader*,
   November/December 1990, first reported in *The Birth Gazette*,
   Spring 1991
Ozerkis, Robin, C.N.M., Natural Childbirth Institute. Interview, March
   1989
Palmarini, Terra, midwife, coauthor of *Pregnant Feelings*. Interview, March
   1989
Perez, Polly, R.N., B.S.N. "Hospital Birth Centers versus Single Room
   Labor-Delivery Units," Eighth Birth Conference, San Francisco,
   March 1989
Poppema, Suzanne, M.D. Interview, January 1980
Porter, Gail. "Research Needs Described for Evaluating Birth Settings,"
   summary of *Research Issues in the Assessment of Birth Settings*, com-
   munication dated January 5, 1983
Rooks, Judith P., C.N.M., M.S., M.P.H., *et al.* "Outcomes of Care in Birth
   Centers," *New England Journal of Medicine* 321:26, December 28,
   1989
Schlinger, Hilary, midwife. Personal communication, July 1984
Scupholme, Anne, C.N.M., and A. Susan Kamons, Ph.D. "Are Outcomes
   Compromised When Mothers Are Assigned to Birth Centers for
   Care?" *Journal of Nurse-Midwifery* 32:4, July/August 1987
Sheehy, Gail. *Passages*, New York: E.P. Dutton, 1976
Stewart, David, Ph.D. "The Philosophy of Proponents of Home Birth,"
   District IV Conference, The Nurses Association and Junior Fellow
   Division of ACOG, November 9, 1977

_____ . "Skillful Midwifery: The Highest and Safest Standard," *The Five Standards for Safe Childbearing*, David Stewart, Ph.D., ed., Marble Hill, MO: NAPSAC International, 1981

_____ , and Lee Stewart, C.C.E. Phone interviews, September 23, 1982, December 5, 1988, November 15, 1991

Stewart, Richard B., M.D., F.A.C.O.G., in group practice with four midwives. Phone interview, October 8, 1982

_____ , and Linda Clark, C.N.M., M.N. "Nurse-Midwifery Practice in an In-Hospital Birthing Center: 2050 Births," *Journal of Nurse-Midwifery* 27:3, May/June 1982

_____ , Asher Galloway, M.D., and Linda Goodman, C.N.M. "An In-Hospital Birthing Room: One Year's Experience," *Compulsory Hospitalization or Freedom of Choice in Childbirth?* Vol. 1, David Stewart, Ph.D., and Lee Stewart, C.C.E., eds., Marble Hill, MO: NAPSAC Reproductions, 1979

Strickhouser, Margaret, C.N.M., Decator/Douglasville Nurse Midwifery Service. Phone interview, April 1989

Sullivan, Deborah A., Ph.D., and Ruth Beeman, R.N., C.N.M., M.P.H. "Four Years' Experience with Home Birth by Licensed Midwives in Arizona," *American Journal of Public Health* 73:6, June 1983

Sumner, Philip E., M.D., F.A.C.O.G., and Celeste R. Phillips, R.N., M.S. *Birthing Rooms Concept and Reality*, St. Louis, Toronto, and London: C.V. Mosby, 1981

Tew, Marjorie. "Place of Birth and Perinatal Mortality," *Journal of the Royal College of General Practitioners* 35, August 1985

_____ . "Do Obstetric Intranatal Interventions Make Birth Safer?" *British Journal of Obstetrics and Gynaecology* 93, July 1986

_____ . Homebirth conference, London, October 1987

_____ . "Home Birth and Midwifery Safer Than We Thought," *NAPSAC News*, Summer 1990

_____ . *Safer Childbirth?* New York: Chapman and Hall, 1990

Tyson, Holliday, S.C.M., M.H.Sc. "Outcomes of 1001 Midwife-Attended Home Births in Toronto, 1983–1988," *Birth* 18:1, March 1991

Wagner, Marsden, M.D. Homebirth conference, London, October 1987

Ward, Charlotte, and Fred Ward. *The Home Birth Book*, Garden City, NY: Doubleday, Dolphin Books, 1977

Wilf, Ruth, C.N.M., Ph.D. "Alternatives: Booth Maternity Center in Philadelphia," Booth Maternity Center, March 1977

_____ . "Fulfilling the Needs of Families in a Hospital Setting: Can It Be Done?" *21st Century Obstetrics Now!* Vol. 1, David Stewart, Ph.D., and Lee Stewart, C.C.E., eds., Chapel Hill, NC: NAPSAC, 1977

_____ . Interview, March 1989

Wilner, Susan, M.S., M.P.H., *et al.* "Comparison of the Quality of Maternity Care Between a Health Maintenance Organization and Fee-for-Service Practices," *New England Journal of Medicine* 304:13, March 26, 1981

World Health Organization. "Appropriate Technology for Birth," *Lancet,*
    August 24, 1985

4   *Understanding Doctors*

American College of Nurse-Midwives. Phone interview, November 1991
Anonymous family practitioner. Interview, 1988
Anonymous obstetrician-gynecologist. Interview, 1983
Bogdanich, Walt *et al.* "Hospitals That Need Patients Pay Bounties for
    Doctors' Referrals," *The Wall Street Journal,* February 27, 1989
Boone, Richard W., J.D., Michael D. Roth, J.D., and John W. Scanlon, M.D.
    "What Every Perinatologist Should Know about Medicolegal
    Problems," *Contemporary Ob/Gyn* 18, October 1981
Braun, Jennifer, Midwives Alliance of North America spokesperson. Phone
    interview, December 1991
Brown, Stephen W., Ph.D. "How Physicians See Themselves," *Medical
    Marketing & Media* 17:2, February 1982
Califano, Joseph A., Jr. "Billions Blown on Health," *The New York Times,*
    April 12, 1989
Center for Health Policy Research. "Projected Active U.S. Physician
    Population, 1986–2010," *American Medical Association Demographic
    Model of the Physician Population,* 1988
Cousins, Norman. "Internship: Preparation or Hazing?" *Journal of the
    American Medical Association* 245:4, January 23–30, 1981
Davis-Floyd, Robbie E. "Obstetric Training as a Rite of Passage," *Medical
    Anthropology Quarterly* 1:3, September 1987
Eichna, Ludwig W., M.D. "Medical-School Education, 1975–1979," *New
    England Journal of Medicine* 303:31, September 25, 1980
Eshelman, Michael, M.D. Interview, January 1980
French, Howard W. "In Overhaul of Hospital Rules, New York Slashes
    Interns' Hours," *The New York Times,* July 3, 1989
Freudenheim, Milt. "Doctors' Concerns: Fixing Prices and Price Fixing,"
    The New York Times, December 18, 1988
Glandon, Gerald L., and Roberta J. Shapiro, eds., Department of Economic
    Research. "Profile of Medical Practice—1981," Center for Health
    Research and Development, American Medical Association
"GMENAC Predicts Physician Surplus," *Health Resources Administration,*
    Department of Health and Human Services, November 1980
Jonas, Harry S. *et al.* "Undergraduate Medical Education," *Journal of the
    American Medical Association* 262:8, August 25, 1989
Kirchner, Merian. "Doctor Surplus—What 1990 Will Look Like," *Medical
    Economics,* September 29, 1980
———. "Non-Surgical Practice: What's The Key to Higher Earnings,"
    Medical Economics, February 16, 1981

Kramon, Glenn. "Employees Paying Ever-Bigger Share of Medical Costs," *The New York Times*, November 22, 1988

Kravitz, Richard L., *et al*. "Malpractice Claims Data as a Quality Improvement Tool," *Journal of the American Medical Association* 266:15, October 16, 1991

Lurie, Nicole *et al*. "How Do House Officers Spend Their Nights?" *New England Journal of Medicine* 320:25, June 22, 1989

"Malpractice Research Points Towards Reform," *Advances/The Robert Wood Johnson Foundation*, Winter 1990

McCall, T.B. "No Turning Back: A Blueprint for Residency Reform," *Journal of the American Medical Association* 261, 1989

Mitka, Mike. "Pay for Primary Care Doctors in Groups Barely Beats Inflation," *American Medical News*, November 18, 1991

Pagliuso, James J., J.D. "Situations to Avoid If You Don't Want to Be Sued," *Contemporary Ob/Gyn*, March 1982

Patterson, Jane, M.D. Interview, February 1984

"Professional Liability and its Effects: Report of 1990 Survey of ACOG's Membership," *American College of Obstetricians and Gynecologists*, 1990

"The Psychological Trauma of a Medical Malpractice Suit: A Practical Guide," *American College of Surgeons Bulletin*, November 1991

Relman, Arnold S. "The Health Care Industry: Where is it Taking Us?" *New England Journal of Medicine* 325:12, September 19, 1991

Rhundle, Rhonda L. "Insurers Step up Efforts to Reduce Use of Free-Choice Health Plans," *The Wall Street Journal*, May 11, 1988

Ruddon, Kate, ACOG spokeswoman. Phone interview, November 1991

Savage, Wendy D., and Pat Tate. "Medical Students' Attitudes Towards Women: A Sex-Linked Variable?" *Medical Education* 17:15, 1983

Segal, Jack, American Medical Association spokesman. Phone interview, December 1991

Wenokur, D.O., and Linn Campbell. "Malpractice Suit Emotional Trauma," *Journal of the American Medical Association* 266:20, November 27, 1991

"Why More Doctors Won't Mean Lower Bills," *Business Week*, May 11, 1981

Wolff, Sidney. "If You Can't Find the Patients, You Can Always Find the Doctors: Hospitals Are Filling Beds by Buying Physicians," *The Washington Post*, October 26, 1987

5   Finding Dr. Right

Annas, George J. *The Rights of Patients*, Carbondale, IL: Southern Illinois University Press, 1989

Bakketeig, L.S., *et al*. "Randomised Controlled Trial of Ultrasonographic Screening in Pregnancy," *Lancet* 2, July 28, 1984

Bernaschek, G., et al. "Vaginal Sonography Versus Serum Human Chorionic Gonadotropin in Early Detection of Pregnancy," American Journal of Obstetrics and Gynecology 158:1, March 1988

Bloom, Stephen G. "As for Male Gynecologists...," Chicago Tribune, November 5, 1987

Brien, Monica, et al. "How Lamaze-Prepared Expectant Parents Select Obstetricians," Research in Nursing and Health 6, 1983

Challacombe, Christine B. "Do Women Patients Need Women Doctors?" The Practitioner 227, May 1983

Check, William A. "Question of Risk Still Hovers Over Routine Prenatal Use of Ultrasound," Journal of the American Medical Association 247:16, April 23–30, 1982

Chitkara, U., et al. "Twin Pregnancy: Routine Use of Ultrasound Examinations in the Prenatal Diagnosis of Intrauterine Growth Retardation and Discordant Growth," American Journal of Perinatology 2:1, January 1985

Cogan, Donna R. "Women in Medicine: Australia, New Zealand, Canada, and United States," Women and Health 7:1, Spring 1982

Cole, Helene M., M.D. "Legal Interventions During Pregnancy," Journal of the American Medical Association 264:20, November 28, 1990

Curran, William J., J.D. "Court-Ordered Cesarean Sections Receive Judicial Defeat," New England Journal of Medicine 323:7, August 16, 1990

De Muylder, X., et al. "Obstetrical Profile of Twin Pregnancies: A Retrospective Review of Eleven Years (1969–1979) at Hospital Notre-Dame, Montreal Canada," Acta Geneticae Medicae et Gemellologiae (Roma) 31:3–4, 1982

Feletti, G., et al. "Patient Satisfaction with Primary-Care Consultations," Journal of Behavioral Medicine 9:4, August 1986

Field, Tiffany, et al. "Effects of Ultrasound Feedback on Pregnancy Anxiety, Fetal Activity, and Neonate Outcome," Obstetrics and Gynecology 66:4, October 1985

Greenberg, Allen. Medical Records: Getting Yours, Washington, DC: Public Citizen Health Research Group, 1986

Haire, Doris. "Fetal Effects of Ultrasound: A Growing Controversy," Journal of Nurse-Midwifery 29:4, July/August 1984

Hillman, Bruce J., et al. "Frequency and Costs of Diagnostic Imaging in Office Practice—A Comparison of Self-Referring and Radiologist-Referring Physicians," New England Journal of Medicine 323:23, December 6, 1990

Holzer, James F. "The Process of Informed Consent," American College of Surgeons Bulletin 74:9, September 1989

Hunt, Morton. "Patients' Rights," The New York Times, March 5, 1989

Irwin, Susan, and Brigitte Jordan. "Knowledge, Practice and Power: Court-Ordered Cesarean Sections," Medical Anthropology Quarterly 1:3, September 1987

Johnson, C.G., et al. "Does Physician Uncertainty Affect Patient Satis-
    faction?" Journal of General Internal Medicine 3:2, March/April 1988
Jordon, Brigitte, and Susan Irwin. "The Ultimate Failure: Court-Ordered
    Cesarean Sections," New Approaches to Human Reproduction: Social
    and Ethical Decisions, Linda Whiteford and Marilyn Poland, eds.,
    Boulder, CO: Westview Press, 1988
Jurow, Ronna, and Richard H. Paul. "Cesarean Delivery for Fetal Distress
    without Maternal Consent," Obstetrics and Gynecology 63:4, April
    1984
Kletke, Phillip R., et al. "The Growing Proportion of Female Physicians:
    Implications for US Physician Supply," American Journal of Public
    Health 80:3, March 1990
Kolder, Veronika E.B., et al. "Court-Ordered Obstetrical Interventions,"
    New England Journal of Medicine 316:19, May 7, 1987
Lazare, Aaron. "Shame and Humiliation in the Medical Encounter,"
    Archives of Internal Medicine 147, September 1987
Lebrow, Morton. "Court Ordered Treatment Rarely Justified for Obstetrical
    Care," American College of Obstetricians and Gynecologists News
    Release, August 11, 1987
Li, T.C., et al. "Data Assessing the Usefulness of Screening Obstetrical
    Ultrasonography for Detecting Fetal and Placental Abnormalities
    in Uncomplicated Pregnancy: Effects of Screening a Low-Risk
    Population," Medical Decision Making 8:1, January/March 1988
Liebeskind, Doreen, et al. "Morphological Changes in the Surface
    Characteristics of Cultured Cells after Exposure to Diagnostic
    Ultrasound," Radiology 138:2, February 1981
Nelson, Alan R. "Humanism and the Art of Medicine," Journal of the
    American Medical Association 262, July 14, 1989
Nelson, Lawrence J., and Nancy Milliken. "Compelled Medical Treatment
    of Pregnant Women," Journal of the American Medical Association
    259:7, February 19, 1988
Orleans, Miriam, and Albert D. Haverkamp. "Appropriate Technology in
    Perinatal Medicine," WHO: Health for All 2000, March 1, 1987
"An Overview of Ultrasound: Theory, Measurement, Medical
    Applications, and Biological Effects," U.S. Department of Health
    and Human Services, July 1982
Page, Leigh. "Will Women Become the New Ob-gyn Majority?" American
    Medical News, December 9, 1991
"Patient Choice: Maternal-Fetal Conflict," American College of Obstetricians
    and Gynecologists, March 3, 1987
Peterson, I. "Ultrasound Safety and Collapsing Bubbles," Science News 130,
    December 13, 1986
"The Pregnant Patient's Bill of Rights," Journal of Nurse-Midwifery 20:4,
    Winter 1975
Ruddom, Kate, ACOG spokeswoman. Phone interview, July 1991

Shapiro, M.C., *et al.* "Information Control and the Exercise of Power in the Obstetrical Encounter," *Social Science and Medicine* 17:3, 1983

Shepard, Mary Jo, *et al.* "An Evaluation of Two Equations for Predicting Fetal Weight by Ultrasound," *American Journal of Obstetrics and Gynecology* 142, January 1, 1982

"Squatting May Cut Labor Time in Delivery," *Medical Tribune*, July 11, 1991

Stark, C., *et al.* "Short and Long-Term Risks After Exposure of Diagnostic Ultrasound in Utero," *Obstetrics and Gynecology* 63:2, February 1984

Stewart, H.F., and M.E. Stratmeyer. "An Overview of Ultrasound: Theory, Measurement, Medical Applications, and Biological Effects," *Bureau of Radiological Health, Food and Drug Administration*, July 1982

Stewart, Nancy. "Women's Views of Ultrasonography in Obstetrics," *Birth* 13, December 1986

Thacker, Stephen B. "Quality of Controlled Clinical Trials. The Case of Imaging Ultrasound in Obstetrics: A Review," *British Journal of Obstetrics and Gynaecology* 92, May 1985

Webster, M.A., *et al.* "Obstetric High Risk Screening and Prediction of Neonatal Morbidity," *Australian Journal of Obstetrics and Gynaecology* 28:1, February 1988

Ziskin, M.C., and Diana Petitti. "Epidemiology of Human Exposure to Ultrasound: A Critical Review," *Ultrasound in Medicine and Biology* 14:2, 1988

Zweig, S., *et al.* "Patient Satisfaction with Obstetric Care," *Journal of Family Practice* 23:2, August 1986

6   Obstetricians' Beliefs About a "Safe Birth"

Ashford, Janet Isaacs. "Unjustified Empires, Marjorie Tew's Campaign for the Truth about Birth Safety," *Childbirth Alternatives Quarterly* 8(3), Summer 1987

Aubry, Richard, M.D. "The American College of Obstetricians and Gynecologists (ACOG): Standards for Safe Childbearing," *21st Century Obstetrics Now!* Vol. 1, Lee Stewart, C.C.E., and David Stewart, Ph.D., eds., Chapel Hill, NC: NAPSAC, 1977

Brackbill, Yvonne, Ph.D., June Rice, J.D., and Diony Young. *Birth Trap*, New York: Warner Books, 1984

Campbell, Rona, and Alison Macfarlane. "Place of Delivery: A Review," *British Journal of Obstetrics and Gynaecology* 93, July 1986

Cardwell, Jewell. "Doctor Decries Trend Toward At-Home Delivery of Babies," Boulder *Daily Camera*, August 26, 1982

Chalmers, Iain, and Martin Richards. "Intervention and Causal Interference in Obstetric Practice," *Benefits and Hazards of the New*

Obstetrics, Tim Chard and Martin Richards, eds., Philadelphia: J.B. Lippincott, 1977

Chalmers, Iain, M.B., B.S., M.Sc., D.C.H. "Minimizing Harm and Maximizing Benefit during Innovation in Health Care: Controlled or Uncontrolled Experimentation?" *Birth* 13(3), September 1986

Chard, Tim, and Martin Richards, eds. *Benefits and Hazards of the New Obstetrics,* Philadelphia: J.B. Lippincott, 1977

Clark, Laura J.B. "How Fast Are Patients Abandoning Doctors for Midwives?" *Medical Economics,* November 26, 1990

Enkin, Murray, Marc J.N.C. Keirse, and Iain Chalmers. *Effective Care in Pregnancy and Childbirth,* Oxford, England: Oxford University Press, 1989

Erickson, J. David, Ph.D., and Tor Bjerkedal, M.D. "Fetal and Infant Mortality in Norway and the United States," *Journal of the American Medical Association* 247(7), February 19, 1982

Flamm, Bruce L., M.D. *Birth after Cesarean: The Medical Facts,* New York: Prentice Hall, 1990, reviewed in *Birth Gazette* 7(2), Spring 1991

Goer, Henci, A.C.C.E. "Guide Provides Information on Obstetric Management," *Genesis,* May–June 1991

Haire, Doris, D.M.S. "Maternity Practices Around the World: How Do We Measure Up?" *Safe Alternatives in Childbirth,* David Stewart, Ph.D., and Lee Stewart, C.C.E., eds., Chapel Hill, NC: NAPSAC, 1976

Kochanek, Ken, National Center for Health Statistics, Division of Vital Statistics. Phone interview, November 25, 1991 and July 1, 1992

Lake, Alice. "Childbirth in America," *McCall's,* January 1976

McCormick, Marie C., M.D., Sc.D. "The Contribution of Low Birth Weight to Infant Mortality and Childhood Morbidity," *New England Journal of Medicine* 312(2), January 10, 1985

McCoy, Jan. "County Officials Troubled by CU Hospital Limitations," Boulder *Daily Camera,* August 12, 1982

"Mexican-American Low Infant Deaths Puzzle Researchers," *Denver Post,* August 21, 1990

Mold, James W., M.D., and Howard F. Stein, Ph.D. "The Cascade Effect in the Clinical Care of Patients," *New England Journal of Medicine* 314(8), February 20, 1986

"More Women Using New Birth-Site Options," *Hospitals,* October 20, 1991

"'Natural' Childbirth Decried; High Mortality Rates Cited," *Convention Reporter* 11 (30), November 1981, reprinted in *NAPSAC News,* 7(1), Spring 1982

Odent, Michel. *Water and Sexuality,* London: Penguin, 1990

Paneth, Nigel, M.D., M.P.H., *et al.* "Newborn Intensive Care and Neonatal Mortality in Low-Birth-Weight Infants," *New England Journal of Medicine* 307(3), July 15, 1982

Placek, Paul J., Ph.D., National Center for Health Statistics. Phone interview, November 25, 1991

Poppema, Suzanne, M.D. Personal interview, January 1980

Price, Richard H. "Several Ounces of Prevention," *Psychology Today*, January 1988

Ratner, Herbert, M.D. "History of the Dehumanization of American Obstetrical Practice," *21st Century Obstetrics Now!* Vol. 1, David Stewart, Ph.D., and Lee Stewart, C.C.E., eds., Chapel Hill, NC: NAPSAC, 1977

Shearer, Madeleine H. "The Effects of Regionalization of Perinatal Care on Hospital Services for Normal Childbirth," *Birth* 4(4), Winter 1977

———. "Editor's Reply," *Birth* 6(3), Fall 1979

Stewart, Lee. Phone interview, November 15, 1991

Tew, Marjorie. "Obstetricians Over-Ruled: The Myth of Hospital Safety," *Association for Improvements in Maternity Services (AIMS) Quarterly Journal*, Spring 1984

———. "Place of Birth and Perinatal Mortality," *Journal of the Royal College of General Practitioners* 35, August 1985

———. "Do Obstetric Intranatal Interventions Make Birth Safer?" *British Journal of Obstetrics and Gynaecology* 93, July 1986

Wagner, Marsden. "The Epidemiology of Ourselves: A Light in a Dark Tunnel," *Birth Gazette* 4(3), Spring 1988

———. "Testimony before the U.S. Commission to Prevent Infant Mortality," *Birth Gazette* 4(3), Spring 1988

World Health Organization. "Appropriate Technology for Birth," *Lancet*, August 24, 1985

Young, Diony. "Effective Care in Pregnancy and Childbirth" and "Guide to Effective Care in Pregnancy and Childbirth," book reviews in *Birth* 17(1), March 1990

7   The Obstetrician's Black Bag of Interventions

Alzrich, Emily. Phone interview, January 29, 1991

Banta, H. David, M.D., M.P.H., and Stephen B. Thacker, M.D. *Costs and Benefits of Electronic Fetal Monitoring: A Review of the Literature*, National Center for Health Services Research (NCHSR), Research Report Series, DHEW Publication No. (PHS) 79-3245, April 1979

———, and Stephen B. Thacker, M.D. "The Risks and Benefits of Episiotomy," *Birth* 9(1), Spring 1982

Berman, Salee, C.N.M., and Victor Berman, M.D. *The Birth Center*, New York: Prentice Hall, 1986

Billingsley, Johanna. "Fasting in Labor," *AIMS Quarterly Journal* 1(1), 1989

Boylan, Peter, M.A.O., MRCPI, MRCOG, and Dermot MacDonald, M.A.O., FRCPI, FRCOG. "Commentary: Oxytocin: The Need to Distinguish Between Induction and Augmentation and Between Multiparas and Primiparas," *Birth* 15(4), December 1988

Brackbill, Yvonne, Ph.D. "Lasting Behavioral Effects of Obstetric Medication on Children," testimony before the U.S. Senate Subcommittee on Health and Scientific Research, April 17, 1978, reprinted in *Compulsory Hospitalization or Freedom of Choice in Childbirth?* Vol. 1, David Stewart, Ph.D., and Lee Stewart, C.C.E., eds., Marble Hill, MO: NAPSAC Reproductions, 1979

_____ , June Rice, J.D., and Diony Young. *Birth Trap,* New York: Warner Books, 1984

Caldeyro-Barcia, Roberto, M.D. "Some Consequences of Obstetrical Interference," *Birth* 2(2), Spring 1975

_____ . "The Influence of Maternal Position on Time of Spontaneous Rupture of the Membranes, Progress of Labor and Fetal Head Compression," *Birth* 6(1), Spring 1979

Carr, Katherine Camacho, C.N.M., M.S. "Obstetric Practices Which Protect Against Neonatal Morbidity: Focus on Maternal Position in Labor and Birth," *Birth* 7(4), Winter 1980

Chalmers, Iain, M.B., M.Sc., D.C.H., FRCOG. "The Perinatal Research Agenda: Whose Priorities?" *Birth* 18(3), September 1991

_____ , and Martin Richards. "Intervention and Causal Interference in Obstetric Practice," *Benefits and Hazards of the New Obstetrics,* Tim Chard and Martin Richards, eds., London: Wm. Heinemann Medical Books; Philadelphia: J.B. Lippincott, 1977

Conway, Esther, and Yvonne Brackbill. "Delivery Medication and Infant Outcome: An Empirical Study," *The Effects of Obstetrical Medication on Fetus and Infant,* Watson A. Bowes, Jr., et al., Monographs of the Society for Research in Child Development, Vol. 35, No. 4, June 1970

Curtis, Peter, M.D., and Norma Safransky. "Rethinking Oxytocin Protocols in the Augmentation of Labor," *Birth* 15(4), December 1988

Donovan, Debbi. "Exposing Epidurals: The 'Cadillac' of Anesthesia," *Clarion,* November 1989

Elsberry, Charlotte, C.N.M., M.S.N., director, Midwifery Services, North Central Bronx Hospital. Phone interviews, September 22 and 26, 1989

Enkin, Murray, Marc J.N.C. Keirse, and Iain Chalmers. *Effective Care in Pregnancy and Childbirth,* Oxford, England: Oxford University Press, 1989

Ettner, Frederic M., M.D. "Comparative Study of Obstetrics," *Safe Alternatives in Childbirth,* David Stewart, Ph.D., and Lee Stewart, C.C.E., eds., Chapel Hill, NC: NAPSAC, 1977

_____ . "Hospital Obstetrics: Do the Benefits Outweigh the Risks?" *21st Century Obstetrics Now!* Vol. 1, David Stewart, Ph.D., and Lee Stewart, C.C.E., eds., Chapel Hill, NC: NAPSAC, 1977

Floyd, Cathy, R.N., M.S., A.C.C.E. "Epidural Anesthesia: Use or Abuse?" *Genesis,* August/September 1984

Fraser, W.D., et al. "A Randomized Controlled Trial of Early Amniotomy,"

British Journal of Obstetrics and Gynaecology, abstracted in *Birth* 18(3), September 1991

Friedman, Emanuel, M.D., Sc.D. "The Obstetrician's Dilemma: How Much Fetal Monitoring and Cesarean Section is Enough?" *New England Journal of Medicine*, 315(10), September 4, 1986

Glassman, Judith. "The Changing World of Childbirth," *Cosmopolitan*, April 1981

Gordon, H., and M. Logue. "Perineal Muscle Function after Childbirth," *Lancet* 2(8447), July 20, 1985

Gray, Ann. "FDA Reviews Brackbill-Broman Research on OB Drugs," *NAPSAC News*, 1979

Haire, Doris, D.M.S. *The Cultural Warping of Childbirth*, International Childbirth Education Association, 1972

———. "Maternity Practices around the World: How Do We Measure Up?" *Safe Alternatives in Childbirth*, David Stewart, Ph.D., and Lee Stewart, C.C.E., eds., Chapel Hill, NC: NAPSAC, 1976

———. "Safety of Drugs—How Safe is 'Safe'?" American Foundation for Maternal and Child Health, 30 Beekman Pl., N.Y.C., undated

———. Testimony before Senate Health Subcommittee, April 17, 1978

———. "American Warning," *AIMS Quarterly Journal* 2(1), 1990

———. "Patient Education in Childbirth: A Long Way in Forty Years," *International Journal of Childbirth Education*, August 1991

Havercamp, Albert, M.D., *et al.* "A Controlled Trial of the Differential Effects of Intrapartum Fetal Monitoring," *American Journal of Obstetrics and Gynecology* 134(4), June 15, 1979

———. "The Evaluation of Continuous Fetal Heart Rate Monitoring in High-Risk Pregnancy," *American Journal of Obstetrics and Gynecology* 125(3), June 1, 1976

"ICEA Position Paper: Epidural Anesthesia for Labor," International Childbirth Education Association, November 1987

Kaminski, H.M., *et al.* "The Effect of Epidural Anesthesia on the Frequency of Instrumental Obstetric Delivery," *Obstetrics and Gynecology* 69, abstracted in *Birth* 14(4), December 1987

Kitzinger, Sheila. "Episiotomy," *ICEA Review* 9(2), August 1985

———. "Episiotomy," *Mothering*, Spring 1990

Kozak, Lola Jean, R.N. "Surgical and Nonsurgical Procedures Associated with Hospital Delivery in the United States: 1980–1987," *Birth* 16(4), December 1989

Lake, Alice. "Childbirth in America," *McCall's*, January 1976

Leveno, Kenneth, M.D., *et al.* "A Prospective Comparison of Selective and Universal Electronic Fetal Monitoring in 34,995 Pregnancies," *New England Journal of Medicine* 315(10), September 4, 1986

Levy, H., *et al.* "Umbilical Cord Prolapse," *Obstetrics and Gynecology* 64(4), October 1984, abstracted in *Birth* 12(1), Spring 1985

Lumley, Judith, Ph.D. "The Irresistible Rise of Electronic Fetal Monitoring," *Birth* 9(3), Fall 1982

MacArthur, C., et al. "Epidural Anesthesia and Long Term Backache after Childbirth," British Medical Journal 301, 1990, abstracted in Birth 17(4), December 1990

MacDonald, D., et al. "The Dublin Randomized Controlled Trial of Intrapartum Fetal Heart Rate Monitoring," American Journal of Obstetrics and Gynecology 152(5), 1985

McKay, Susan, R.N., Ph.D., A.C.C.E., and Charles Mahan, M.D., FACOG. "How Can Aspiration of Vomitus in Obstetrics Best Be Prevented?" Birth 15(4), December 1988

Maresh, M., et al. "Delayed Pushing with Lumbar Epidural Analgesia in Labour," British Journal of Obstetrics and Gynaecology 90(7), July 1983, abstracted in Birth 10(4), Winter 1983

Marmet, Chele. Phone interview, November 14, 1991

Minkoff, Howard L., M.D., and Richard H. Schwarz, M.D. "The Rising Cesarean Section Rate: Can It Safely Be Reversed?" Obstetrics and Gynecology 56(2), August 1980

Newcombe, R.G. "Reversal of Changes in Distribution of Gestational Age and Birth Weight among Firstborn Infants of Cardiff Residents," British Medical Journal 287(6399), October 15, 1983, abstracted in Birth 11(1), Spring 1984

Newton, Niles, Ph.D. "Oxytocin, the Hormone of Love," presentation at La Leche League International conference, Miami, July 25, 1991

Phillipson, E.H., et al. "Maternal, Fetal, and Neonatal Lidocaine Levels Following Local Perineal Infiltration," American Journal of Obstetrics and Gynecology 149(403), June 15, 1984, abstracted in Birth 11(4), Winter 1984

Prentice, A., and T. Lind. "Fetal Heart Rate Monitoring during Labor—Too Frequent Intervention, Too Little Benefit?" Lancet, December 12, 1987

Raymond, Janice. "Healthy Women in a High Tech Era," International Journal of Childbirth Education 3(4), November 1988

Read, John A., Lt. Col., M.C., U.S.A., et al. "Randomized Trial of Ambulation Versus Oxytocin for Labor Enhancement: A Preliminary Report," American Journal of Obstetrics and Gynecology 139(6), March 15, 1981

Roberts, Joyce E., R.N., C.N.M., Ph.D., Carlos Mendez-Bauer, M.D., and Deborah A. Woodell, R.N., C.N.M., M.S. "The Effects of Maternal Position on Uterine Contractility and Efficiency," Birth 10(4), Winter 1983

Scott, D.B., and B.M. Hibbard. "Serious Non-Fatal Complications Associated with Extradural Block in Obstetric Practice," British Journal of Anesthesiology 64, 1990, abstracted in Birth 17(3), September 1990

Shearer, Madeleine H., R.P.T. "Auscultation is Acceptable in Low Risk Women," editorial, Birth 6(1), Spring 1979

—————. "Fetal Monitoring: For Better or Worse?" Compulsory Hospitalization or Freedom of Choice in Childbirth? Vol. 1, David Stewart, Ph.D., and Lee Stewart, C.C.E., eds., Marble Hill, MO: NAPSAC Reproductions, 1979

Shy, Kirkwood K., et al. "Effects of Electronic Fetal-Heart-Rate Monitoring, as Compared with Periodic Auscultation, on the Neurologic Development of Premature Infants," New England Journal of Medicine 322(9), March 1, 1990

Simchak, Margery. "Has Epidural Anesthesia Made Childbirth Education Obsolete?" Childbirth Instructor, Summer 1991

"Statement of Fetal Heart Rate Monitoring," ACOG Newsletter, November 1988

"Study: Labor Pain Killers Associated with Drug Addiction," Clarion-Ledger/Jackson Daily News, July 12, 1987, reprinted in NAPSAC News 12(3), Fall 1987

Taffel, Selma, B.B.A., National Center for Health Statistics. Phone interview, December 2, 1991

———, et al. "1989 U.S. Cesarean Rate Steadies—VBAC Rate Rises to Nearly One in Five," Birth 18(2), June 1991

———, Stephanie J. Ventura, A.M., and George Gay, M.S.P.H. "Revised U.S. Certificate of Birth —New Opportunities for Research on Birth Outcome," Birth 16(4), December 1989

Thacker, Stephen, and David Banta. "Benefits and Risks of Episiotomy: An Interpretative Review of the English Language Literature 1860–1980," Obstetrics and Gynecology Survey 38(6), 1983

Thompson, Trisha. "Does Labor Have to Hurt?" Childbirth, 1990

Thorp, James A., M.D., FACOG. "Effects of Epidural on the Incidence of Cesarean Section for Dystocia in First Labors," Birth conference, San Francisco, March 16, 1989

———, Jay D. McNitt, M.D., and Phyllis C. Leppert, M.D., Ph.D., C.N.M. "Effects of Epidural Analgesia: Some Questions and Answers," Birth 17(3), September 1990

Thorp, James M., Jr., M.D., and Watson A. Bowes, Jr., M.D. "Episiotomy: Can Its Routine Use Be Defended?" American Journal of Obstetrics and Gynecology, 160(5), May 1989, abstracted in Birth Gazette 5(4), Fall 1989

Wood, C., et al. "A Controlled Trial of Fetal Heart Rate Monitoring in a Low Risk Obstetric Population," American Journal of Obstetrics and Gynecology 141(5), November 1, 1981, abstract from Birth 9(3), Fall 1982

8   The Cesarean Epidemic

Alvarez, Piera Maghella. "Birth Is Not an Illness: Fifteen Recommendations from the World Health Organization," Association for Improvements in the Maternity Services (AIMS), 40 Kingswood Avenue, London NW6, undated reprint

Banta, H. David, M.D., M.P.H., and Stephen Thacker, M.D. *Costs and Benefits of Electronic Fetal Monitoring: A Review of the Literature,* Washington, DC: DHEW Publications No. (PHS) 70-3245, April 1979

Berkowitz, Gertrud S., Ph.D., *et al.* "Delayed Childbearing and the Outcome of Pregnancy," *New England Journal of Medicine* 322(10), March 8, 1990

Boylan, Peter, M.B., D.C.I.I., M.A.O., MRCOG, MRCPI. "Failure in Active Management of Labor: Accounting for Different Cesarean Rates in Dublin, Dallas, and London Trials," Eighth Birth Conference, San Francisco, March 1989

Bruce, Gene. "So You Want to be a Mid-Life Mom?" *East West,* January 1987

Burkhart, Nancy. "Group Advocates Birth at Home," *Denver Post,* January 19, 1979

Cesarean Childbirth, Consensus Development Conference, Bethesda, MD: NIH Publication No. 82–2067, October 1981

"Cesareans Increasing but Few Study Related Maternal Deaths," *Ob/Gyn News,* July 1, 1980

Cohen, Wayne R., M.D. "Influence of the Duration of Second Stage Labor on Perinatal Outcome and Puerperal Morbidity," *Obstetrics and Gynecology* 49(3), March 1977

Coleman, Cheryl H. "Fetal Stress Response in Labor," *International Journal of Childbirth Education,* August 1986

Collea, Joseph V., M.D., *et al.* "The Randomized Management of Term Frank Breech Presentations: A Study of 208 Cases," *American Journal of Obstetrics and Gynecology* 137(2), May 15, 1980

COMA (Committee on Maternal Alternatives), *How Women Want to Have Their Babies,* Baltimore, MD: self-published, 1980

"Consensus Conference Report: Indications for Cesarean Section: Final Statement of the Panel of the National Consensus Conference on Aspects of Cesarean Birth," *Canadian Medical Association Journal* 134, June 15, 1986

Conway, D.I., *et al.* "Management of Spontaneous Rupture of the Membranes in the Absence of Labor in Primagravid Women at Term," *American Journal of Obstetrics and Gynecology* 150(8), December 1984, abstracted in *Childbirth Alternatives Quarterly* 6(4), Summer 1985

Cook, William A., M.D. *Natural Childbirth: Fact and Fallacy,* Chicago: Nelson Hall, 1982

Corea, Gena. "The Cesarean Epidemic; Who's Having This Baby, Anyway—You or the Doctor?" *Mother Jones,* July 1980

Corey, Lawrence, M.D. "The Diagnosis and Treatment of Genital Herpes," *Journal of the American Medical Association* 248(9), September 3, 1982

"Correcting a Breech Presentation," *Informed Homebirth Newsletter,* January–February 1978

Correspondence regarding Leveno, *et al.* and Haynes de Reght, *et al. New England Journal of Medicine* 316(8), February 19, 1987

Cox, Janice P. "Delivery Alternatives in the Term Breech Pregnancy," *International Journal of Childbirth Education* 12(4), November 1988

Danforth, David N., M.D. "Cesarean Section," *Journal of the American Medical Association* 253(6), February 8, 1985

Daniels, Kari. *Water Baby: Experiences of Water Birth*, video distributed by Point of View Productins, 2477 Folsom St., San Francisco, CA 94110

Davis, M. Edward, M.D. "The Expectant Mother. What Does 'Due Date' Really Mean?" *Redbook*, August 1965

Doering, Susan G., Ph.D. "Unnecessary Cesareans: Doctor's Choice, Parent's Dilemma," *Compulsory Hospitalization or Freedom of Choice in Childbirth?* Vol. 1, David Stewart, Ph.D., and Lee Stewart, C.C.E., eds., Marble Hill, MO: NAPSAC Reproductions, 1979

Enkin, Murray, Marc J.N.C. Keirse, and Iain Chalmers. *Effective Care in Pregnancy and Childbirth*, Oxford, England: Oxford University Press, 1989

Evrard, John R., M.D., M.P.H., FACOG, and Edwin M. Gold, M.D., FACOG. "Cesarean Section and Maternal Mortality in Rhode Island, Incidence and Risk Factors, 1965–1975," *Obstetrics and Gynecology* 50(5), November 1977

Feldman, Silvia, Ph.D. "Cesarean Deliveries/When and Why Are They Justified," *Self*, May 1979

––––––– . *Choices in Childbirth*, New York: Bantam, 1980

Flamm, Bruce L., M.D., *et al.* "Vaginal Birth after Cesarean Delivery: Results of a 5-Year Multicenter Collaborative Study," *Obstetrics and Gynecology* 76(5), November 1990

Frechette, Alfred L., M.D., M.P.H., and Pearl K. Russo. "A Comparison of the Quality of Maternity Care between a Health Maintenance Organization and Fee-For-Service Practices," *New England Journal of Medicine* 304(13), March 26, 1981

Friedman, Emanuel, M.D., Sc.D. "The Obstetrician's Dilemma: How Much Fetal Monitoring and Cesarean Section is Enough?" *New England Journal of Medicine* 315(10), September 4, 1986

Frye, Anne. "How Do You Handle Risks When Your Water Breaks?" *Special Delivery*, Summer 1986

Gaskin, Ina May. "Prostaglandins," *Birth Gazette* 7(2), Spring 1991

Gleicher, Norbert, M.D. "Cesarean Section Rates in the United States: The Short-Term Failure of the National Consensus Development Conference in 1980," *Journal of the American Medical Association* 252(23), December 21, 1984

Gluck, Lewis, M.D. Quoted from "current issue" of *Hospital Practice* in *Tallahassee Democrat*, April 7, 1977

Goer, Henci, A.C.C.E. "Are Cesareans Saving Babies? A Review of the

Medical Literature," *Childbirth Alternatives Quarterly* 7(4), Summer 1986

Goyert, Gregory L., M.D., *et al.* "The Physician Factor in Cesarean Birth Rates," *New England Journal of Medicine* 320(11), March 16, 1989

Grant, A., *et al.* "Routine Formal Fetal Movement Counting and Risk of Antepartum Death in Normally Formed Singletons," *Lancet* 2, 1989, abstracted in *Birth* 17(1), March 1990

"Guidelines for Vaginal Delivery after a Previous Cesarean Birth," ACOG Committee Opinion, October 1988

Halperin, Mary E., M.D., and Murray Enkin, M.D. "Induction of Labor in Postterm Pregnancy," *ICEA Review* 12(1), February 1988

Hart, S. "Cesareans Don't Help Lowest-Weight Babies," *Science News*, September 6, 1990

Havercamp, Albert D., M.D. "How to Keep Cesarean Rates Below 10% in a High Risk Population," Third Birth Conference, San Francisco, October 1984

Haynes de Reght, Roberta, M.D., *et al.* "Relation of Private or Clinic Care to the Cesarean Birth Rate," *New England Journal of Medicine* 315(10), September 4, 1986

Heilman, Jean Rattner. "Breaking the Cesarean Cycle," *New York Times Magazine,* September 7, 1980

Hellman, Louis M., and Jack A. Pritchard. *Williams Obstetrics,* 14th ed., New York: Appleton-Century-Crofts, 1971

Hemminki, Elina, M.D. "Pregnancy and Birth after Cesarean Section: A Survey Based on the Swedish Birth Register," *Birth* 14(1), March 1987

"Hospital Disclosures to Maternity Patients Now Required in Massachusetts," *Childbirth Alternatives Quarterly* 7(2), Winter 1986

Jones, M. Douglas Jr., *et al.* "Failure of Association of Premature Rupture of Membranes with Respiratory-Distress Syndrome," *New England Journal of Medicine* 292(24), June 12, 1975

Kappy, Kenneth A., M.D., *et al.* "Premature Rupture of the Membranes: A Conservative Approach," *American Journal of Obstetrics and Gynecology* 134(6), July 15, 1979

Kaye, Edward M., M.D., and Elizabeth C. Dooling, M.D. "Neonatal Herpes Simplex Meningoencephalitis Associated with Fetal Monitor Scalp Electrodes," *Neurology* 31, August 1981

Keirse, J.N.C., M.D., D. Phil. "In the Final Analysis," *Birth* 18(2), June 1991

Kitzinger, Sheila. "Sheila Kitzinger's Letter from England," *Birth* 18(3), September 1991

Klaus, Marshall H., M.D. "The Houston Randomized Controlled Trial of Effects of a Continuous Supportive Companion in Labor: A Significant Aspect of the Management of Labor," Eighth Birth Conference, San Francisco, March 1989

Kozak, Lola Jean, R.N. "Surgical and Nonsurgical Procedures Associated with Hospital Delivery in the United States: 1980–1987," *Birth* 16(4)

Lagercrantz, Hugo, and Theodore A. Slotkin. "The 'Stress' of Being Born," *Scientific American* 254(4), April 1986, abstracted in *Childbirth Alternatives Quarterly* 7(3), Spring 1986

Lenihan, J.P. "Relationship of Antepartum Pelvic Examination to Premature Rupture of the Membranes," *Obstetrics and Gynecology* 83(1), January 1984, abstracted in *Birth* 11(2), Summer 1984

Leveno, Kenneth J., *et al.* "A Prospective Comparison of Selective and Universal Electronic Fetal Monitoring in 34,995 Pregnancies," *New England Journal of Medicine* 315(10), September 4, 1986

Maloney, Basil W. "Discussion," *American Journal of Obstetrics and Gynecology* 137(2), May 15, 1980

Marieskind, Helen A., Dr. P.H. *An Evaluation of Cesarean Section in the United States*, Washington, DC: Department of Health, Education and Welfare, June 1979

———. "Cesarean Section in the United States: Has It Changed Since 1979?" *Birth* 16(4), December, 1989

"Mom's Symptomless Herpes Threatens Baby," *Science News*, May 4, 1991

Myers, Stephen A., and Norbert Gleicher. "A Successful Program to Lower Cesarean-Section Rates," *New England Journal of Medicine* 319(23), December 8, 1988

Nouhan, Joseph, M.D. Personal interview, March 17, 1989

Odent, Michel. "Birth under Water," *Lancet*, December 24/31, 1983

O'Driscoll, Kieran, M.D., and Michael Foley, M.D. "Correlation of Decrease in Perinatal Mortality and Increase in Cesarean Section Rates," *Obstetrics and Gynecology* 61(1), January 1983

"Older Mothers and Birth Defects," *Alternatives* 3(22), April 1991

Perez, Polly, R.N., A.C.C.E. "Nurturing Laboring Women in a High-Tech Town," *Childbirth Alternatives Quarterly* 6(3), Spring 1985

Placek, Paul J., *et al.* "The Cesarean Future," *American Demographics*, September 1987

———, and Selma M. Taffel, B.B.A. "Recent Patterns in Cesarean Delivery in the United States," *Obstetrics and Gynecology Clinics of North America* 15(4), December 1988

———, National Center for Health Statistics. Phone interview, November 25, 1991

Porreco, Richard, M.D., FACOG. "How Well Can Education Contain the Cesarean Birth Rate? Outcome of a Program," Eighth Birth Conference, San Francisco, March 1989

———, *et al.* "Roundtable: The U.S. Cesarean Birth Rate is 25% and Rising. How Can We Reverse the Rise?" Eighth Birth Conference, San Francisco, March 1989

———. "Decreasing Unnecessary Interventions," ICEA conference, Denver, August 17, 1991

Prober, Charles G., M.D., *et al.* "Low Risk of Herpes Simplex Virus Infections in Neonates Exposed to the Virus at the Time of Vaginal

Delivery to Mothers with Recurrent Genital Herpes Simplex Virus Infections," *New England Journal of Medicine* 316(5), January 27, 1987

Rosen, M.G., *et al.* "The Effect of Delivery Route on Outcome in Breech Presentation," *American Journal of Obstetrics and Gynecology* 148, April 1984, abstracted in *Childbirth Alternatives Quarterly* 6(2), Winter 1985

Rubin, George, M.D., *et al.* "The Risk of Childbearing Re-Evaluated," *American Journal of Public Health* 71(7), July 1981

Saunders, M.C., *et al.* "The Effects of Hospital Admission for Bed Rest on the Duration of Twin Pregnancy: A Randomized Trial," *Lancet* 2, 1985, abstracted in *Birth* 13(2), June 1986

Savage, Beverly, and Diana Simkin. *Preparation for Birth: The Complete Guide to the Lamaze Method*, New York: Ballantine Books, 1987

Shearer, Madeleine H., R.P.T. "Complications of Cesarean to Infant," *Birth* 4(3), Fall 1977

———. "Complications of Cesarean to Mothers," *Birth* 4(3), Fall 1977

———, and Milton Estes, M.D., FABFP. A Critical Review of the Recent Literature on Postterm Pregnancy and a Look at Women's Experiences," *Birth* 12(2), Summer 1985

Showstack, Jonathon A., M.P.H., *et al.* "The Role of Changing Practices in the Rising Costs of Hospital Care," *New England Journal of Medicine* 313(19), November 1, 1985

Shy, Kirkwood K., M.D., M.P.H., FACOG. "Antenatal Testing and Candid Reassurance," *Birth* 18(2), June 1991

Silberner, Joanne. "What Nationality Means to the Fine Art of Healing," *U.S. News and World Report*, December 26, 1988/January 2, 1989

Silver, Lynn, M.D., M.P.H., and Sidney Wolfe, M.D. *Unnecessary Cesarean Sections: How to Cure a National Epidemic*, Public Citizen Health Research Group, Dept. PR, 2000 P St., NW, Room 700, Washington, DC 20036

Staff members, University Medical Center, Lafayette, Louisiana. Phone interviews, July 1992

Stolzenburg, W. "Expectant Moms Take Longer than Expected," *Science News*, June 16, 1990

"Summary Report," Joint Interregional Conference on Appropriate Technology for Birth, Fortaleza, Brazil, April 22–26, 1985, English version, June 10, 1985

Sumner, Philip E., M.D., and Celeste R. Phillips, R.N., M.S. *Birthing Rooms*, London: C.V. Mosby, 1981

Szczepaniak, Jane C. "Issues in Breech Births," *International Journal of Childbirth Education*, November 1986

Taffel, Selma M., B.B.A., *et al.* "1989 U.S. Cesarean Rate Steadies—VBAC Rate Rises to Nearly One in Five," *Birth* 18(2), June 1991

———, National Center for Health Statistics. Phone interviews, April 18, 1991; December 2, 1991

Taffel, Selma M., Paul J. Placek, and Carol L. Kosary. "U.S. Cesarean Section Rates: An Update," *Birth* 19(1), March 1992

Thorp, James, M.D., FACOG. "Effects of Epidural on the Incidence of Cesarean Section for Dystocia in First Labors," Eighth Birth Conference, San Francisco, March 1989

————. Personal interview regarding use of cesarean section for women with herpes simplex virus, March 16, 1989

"Touring the Hospital by Phone," *Consumer Reports*, February 1991

Trathen, William T., M.D. "Management of Labor Following Rupture of Membranes," *ICEA Review* 8(3), December 1984

Van Tuinen, Ingrid, and Sidney Wolfe, M.D. *Unnecessary Cesarean Sections: Halting a National Epidemic*, Washington: Public Citizen's Health Research Group

Walker, T. "Most Birth Defects Don't Rise with Age," *Science News*, March 9, 1991

White, E., *et al.* "An Investigation of the Relationship between Cesarean Section Birth and Respiratory Distress Syndrome of the Newborn," *American Journal of Epidemiology* 121 (5), May 1985, abstracted in *Birth* 12(4), Winter 1985

Wolfe, Sidney M., M.D., and the Public Citizen Health Research Group with Rhoda Donkin Jones. *Women's Health Alert*, Reading, MA: Addison-Wesley, 1991

"Women Are the Recipients of Most Major Surgery," *East West*, August 1988

Young, Diony. "Cesareans in the United States: A Sobering Situation," *ICEA News* 18(41), 1979

————, and Charles Mahan, M.D. *Unnecessary Cesareans*, Minneapolis: ICEA, 1980

————. "Crisis in Obstetrics—The Management of Labor," *International Journal of Childbirth Education*, August 1987

————. "Maternity Information Act Passes in New York," *Birth* 16(4), December 1989

————. Phone interview, December 11, 1991

9 Having a Cesarean Is Having a Baby

Botlos, Kate. "Birth Dis-Illusions," *Mothering*, Summer 1979

Cohen, Nancy. Interview, September 18, 1982

Decker, C. "Cesarean Predisposes to Long Labor Later," *Science News*, March 10, 1990

"Guidelines for Vaginal Delivery after a Previous Cesarean Birth," ACOG Committee Opinion Paper, October 1988

Hansell, Richard S., M.D., Kathleen B. McMurray, M.D., and Gordon R. Huey, M.D. "Vaginal Birth After Two or More Cesarean Sections: A Five-Year Experience," *Birth* 17(3), September, 1990

Klaus, Marshall H., and John H. Kennell. *Parent-Infant Bonding*, Saint Louis, MO: C.V. Mosby, 1982

Meier, Paul R., M.D., and Richard P. Porreco, M.D. "Trial of Labor Following Cesarean Section: A Two-Year Experience," *American Journal of Obstetrics and Gynecology* 144(6), November 15, 1982

"Multiple C-sections Not a Labor Waiver," *Science News*, August 27, 1988

Myers, Stephen A., and Norbert Gleicher. "A Successful Program to Lower Cesarean Section Rates," *New England Journal of Medicine* 319(23), December 8, 1988

Once a Cesarean: Vaginal Birth after Cesarean, video distributor: Nicolas J. Kaufman Productions, 14 Clyde St., Newton, MA 02160

Perez, Polly. "VBAC: The Possible Dream," *Childbirth Alternatives Quarterly* 9(1), Fall 1987

Placek, Paul J., Ph.D., National Center for Health Statistics. Phone interview, November 25, 1991

_____ , and Selma Taffel, B.B.A. "Vaginal Birth after Cesarean (VBAC) in the 1980s," *American Journal of Public Health* 78(5), May 1988

Porreco, Richard P., M.D. Phone interview, October 1983; personal communication, February 15, 1989

Pruett, Kathleen M., *et al.* "Is Vaginal Birth after Two or More Cesareans Safe?" *Obstetrics and Gynecology* 72(2), August 1988

Shearer, Elizabeth Conner, M.Ed., M.P.H. "Education for Vaginal Birth after Cesarean," *Birth* 9(1), Spring 1982

_____ . "To the Editor," *Birth* 18(3), September 1991

Sufin-Disler, Caroline. "Vaginal Birth after Cesarean," *ICEA Review* 14(3), August 1990

Syed, Christiana. "Working for a Positive Birth," *New Beginnings*, November-December 1988

Taffel, Selma M., B.B.A., *et al.* "1989 U.S. Cesarean Rate Steadies—VBAC Rate Rises to Nearly One in Five," *Birth* 18(2), June 1991

Weston, Marianne Brorup, *et al.* "Vaginal Birth after Cesarean," reprint, Seattle: Pennypress, Inc., 1987

Zorn, Esther, president, Cesarean Prevention Movement. "Cesarean and VBAC Rates? Responses," *C/Sec Newsletter* 13(3), third quarter, 1987

_____ . Interview, November 9, 1988

10 Appreciating Your Feelings

Affonso, Dyanne D., R.N., M.S. "Missing Pieces, A Study of Postpartum Feelings," *Birth* 4:4, Winter 1977

Buesching, Don P., *et al.* "Progression and Depression in the Prenatal and Postpartum Periods," *Women and Health* 11:2, Summer 1986

Cooper, Peter J. "Non-Psychotic Psychiatric Disorder after Childbirth: A Prospective Study of Prevalence, Incidence, Course and Nature," *Journal of the American Medical Association* 260:22, December 9, 1988

Dimitroyvsky, L., *et al.* "Depression During and Following Pregnancy: Quality of Family Relationships," *Journal of Psychology* 121:3, 1987

Gottlieb, S.E., and D.E. Barrett. "Effects of Unanticipated Cesarean Section on Mothers, Infants, and Their Interaction in the First Month of Life," *Journal of Developmental and Behavioral Pediatrics* 7:3, June 1986

Halas, Celia, Ph.D., and Roberta Matteson, Ph.D. *I've Done So Well—Why Do I Feel So Bad?* New York: Macmillan, 1978: London: Collier Macmillan, 1978

Hart, Georgiana. "Maternal Attitudes in Prepared and Unprepared Cesarean Deliveries," *American Journal of Nursing*, March 1980

Hobfoll, Stevan E., *et al.* "Satisfaction with Social Support during Crisis: Intimacy and Self-Esteem as Critical Determinants," *Journal of Personality and Social Psychology* 51:2, August 1986

Jermain, Donna M. "Psycho-pharmacologic Approach to Postpartum Depression," *Journal of Women's Health* 1:1, 1992

Kendell, R.E., *et al.* "Day-to-Day Mood Changes after Childbirth: Further Data," *British Journal of Psychiatry* 145, December 1984

———. "Epidemiology of Puerperal Psychoses," *British Journal of Psychiatry* 150, May 1987

Kitzinger, Sheila. "Brief Encounters: Effects of Induction on the Mother-Baby Relationship," *Practitioner*, 1976

Knight, R.G., *et al.* "The Relationship Between Expectations of Pregnancy and Birth, and Transient Depression in the Immediate Post-Partum Period," *Journal of Psychosomatic Research* 31:3, 1987

Kumar, R., *et al.* "A Prospective Study of Emotional Disorders in Child-bearing Women," *British Journal of Psychiatry* 144, January 1984

Lang, Raven. "Delivery in the Home," *Maternal Attachment and Mothering Disorders: A Round Table*, Marshall H. Klaus, M.D., Treville Leger, and Mary Ann Trause, Ph.D., eds., Johnson and Johnson, 1975

Lipson, Juliene G. "Cesarean Support Groups: Mutual Help and Education," *Women and Health* 6:3/4, Fall-Winter 1987

———, *et al.* "Psychological Integration of the Cesarean Birth Experience," *American Journal of Orthopsychiatry* 50:4, October 1980

Loftus, Elizabeth. *Memory—Surprising New Insights into How We Remember and Why We Forget*, Reading, MA: Addison-Wesley, 1980

Lozoff, Betsy, M.D. "Birth in Non-Industrial Societies," *Birth, Interaction and Attachment: Exploring the Foundations for Modern Perinatal Care*, Marshall Klaus, M.D., and Martha Oschrin Robertson, eds., Johnson and Johnson, 1982

Morgan, B.M., *et al.* "Analgesia and Satisfaction in Childbirth (The Queen Charlotte's 1000 Mother Survey)," *Lancet* 2, October 9, 1982

Morrison, C.E., *et al.* "Pethidine Compared with Meptazinol during Labour. A Prospective Randomized Double-Blind Study in 1100 Patients," *Anaesthesia* 42:1, January 1987

Moss, Peter, *et al.* "The Hospital Inpatient Stay: The Experience of First-

Time Parents," *Child: Care, Health and Development* 13, 1987

Newton, Niles, Ph.D. Address reported in *News from H.O.M.E. (Home Oriented Maternity Experience)*, 1977

———. *Maternal Emotions*, New York: Paul B. Hoeber, 1955

O'Hara, Michael W., *et al.* "Prospective Study of Postpartum Blues: Biologic and Psychosocial Factors," *Archives of General Psychiatry* 48, 1991

Peterson, Gayle. *Birthing Normally: A Personal Growth Approach to Childbirth*, Berkeley, CA: Mindbody Press, 1981

Quadagno, D.M., *et al.* "Postpartum Moods in Men and Women," *American Journal of Obstetrics and Gynecology* 154:5, May 1986

Sandelowski, Margarete. "Expectations for Childbirth versus Actual Experiences: The Gap Widens," *Maternal Child Nursing* 9, July/August 1984

Scarf, Maggie. *Unfinished Business: Pressure Points in the Lives of Women*, Garden City, NY: Doubleday, 1980

Stern, G., and L. Kruckman. "Multi-Disciplinary Perspectives on Post-Partum Depression: An Anthropological Critique," *Social Science Medicine* 17:15, 1983

Stolte, Karen. "A Comparison of Women's Expectations of Labor with the Actual Event," *Birth* 14(2), June 1987

———. "Postpartum 'Missing Pieces': Sequel of a Passing Obstetrical Era?" *Birth* 13(2), June 1986

Tilden, V., and J. Lipson. "Cesarean Childbirth: Variables Affecting Psychological Impact," *Western Journal of Nursing Research* 3, 1981

Yarrow, Leah. "When My Baby Was Born," *Parents*, August 1982

11   Your Childbirth Support Group

Bradley, Robert, M.D. *Husband-Coached Childbirth*, New York: Harper & Row, 1981

Copstick, S.M., *et al.* "Partner Support and the Use of Coping Techniques in Labour," *Journal of Psychosomatic Research* 30:4, 1986

Dick-Read, Grantly, M.D. *Childbirth without Fear: The Principles and Practices of Natural Childbirth*, New York: Harper & Row, 1974

Gunn, T.R. "Antenatal Education: Does It Improve the Quality of Labour and Delivery?" *New Zealand Medical Journal* 96:724, January 26, 1983

Hodnett, Ellen D., Ph.D., and Richard W. Osborn, Ph.D. "A Randomized Trial of the Effects of Monitrice Support during Labor: Mothers' Views Two to Four Weeks Postpartum," *Birth* 16(4), December 1989

Hotelling, Barbara A. "The Childbirth Educator as Doula," *ICEA*, February 1988

Karmel, Marjorie. *Thank You, Dr. Lamaze: A Mother's Experience in Painless Childbirth*, New York: Doubleday, 1965

Kennell, John H., M.D. "Are We in the Midst of a Revolution?" *American Journal of Diseases of Children* 134, March 1980

——— . "The Physiologic Effects of a Supportive Companion (Doula) during Labor," *Birth, Interaction and Attachment: Exploring the Foundations for Modern Perinatal Care*, Marshall Klaus, M.D., and Martha Oschrin Robertson, eds., Johnson and Johnson, 1982

——— . Phone interview, November 1991

——— , "Continuous Emotional Support during Labor in a US Hospital," *Journal of the American Medical Association* 265:17, May 1, 1991

Kennell, John H., M.D., *et al.* "Continuous Emotional Support during Labor," *Journal of the American Medical Association* 266:11, September 18, 1991

Klaus, Marshall, M.D. Phone interview, November 1991

——— , and John H. Kennell, M.D. *Parent-Infant Bonding*, Saint Louis, MO: C.V. Mosby, 1982

Lozoff, Betsy, M.D. "Birth in Non-Industrial Societies," *Birth, Interaction and Attachment: Exploring the Foundations for Modern Perinatal Care*, Marshall Klaus, M.D., and Martha Oschrin Robertson, eds., Johnson and Johnson, 1982

Maloney, R. "Childbirth Education Classes: Expectant Parents' Expectations," *Journal of Obstetrics, Gynecology and Neonatal Nursing* 14:3, May/June 1985

McNatt, Nona L., R.N., C.N.M. "A Lesson in Empathy," *Obstetrics and Gynecology* 56:1, July 1980

Nevin, C., and K. Gijsbers. "A Study of Labour Pain Using the McGill Pain Questionnaire," *Social Science and Medicine* 19:12, 1984

Pascoe, John M. "The Cesearean Section Rate," *Journal of the American Medical Association* 264:8, August 22–29, 1990

Patton, L.L., *et al.* "Childbirth Preparation and Outcomes of Labor and Delivery in Primiparous Women," *Journal of Family Practice* 20:4, April 1985

Perez, Paulina. "Let Your Couples Know about the Role of the Professional Labor Assistant," *International Journal of Childbirth Education*, May 1989

——— , and Cheryl Snedecker. *Special Women. The Role of the Professional Labor Assistant*, Seattle: Pennypress, Inc., 1990

Raphael, Dana, Ph.D. *The Tender Gift*, Englewood Cliffs, NJ: Prentice Hall, 1973

Rosen, Mortimer G., M.D. "*Doula* at the Bedside of the Patient in Labor," *Journal of the American Medical Association* 265:17, May 1, 1991

Shearer, Madeleine H. "Commentary: When a Monitrice Is an Outsider," *Birth* 16(4), December 1989

——— , and Nenelle Bunnin. "Childbirth Educators in the 1980's: A Survey of Twenty-five Veterans," *Birth* 10(4), Winter 1983

Simkin, Penny, R.P.T. Phone interview, December 1982

Sosa, Roberto, M.D., *et al.* "The Effect of a Supportive Woman on Mother-

ing Behavior and the Duration and Complications of Labor.
Abstracted," *Pediatric Research* 13:338, 1979
_____ , et al. "The Effect of a Supportive Companion on Perinatal
Problems, Length of Labor, and Mother-Infant Interaction." *New
England Journal of Medicine* 303:11, September 11, 1980
Sumner, Philip E., M.D., and Celeste R. Phillips, R.N. *Birthing Rooms:
Concept and Reality*, Saint Louis, MO: C.V. Mosby, 1981
Tanzer, Deborah, Ph.D. "Natural Childbirth: Pain or Peak Experience?"
Psychology Today, October 1968
van der Meer, Antonia. "Doulas in Service of...," *Childbirth Educator*,
Summer 1991
Waletzky, Lucy R., M.D. "Husbands' Problems with Breastfeeding,"
American Journal of Orthopsychiatry 49(2), April 1979
Yarrow, Leah. "Fathers Who Deliver," *Parents*, June 1981

12 How to Have a Normal Vaginal Birth

Balaskas, Janet. *Active Birth*, Boston, MA: Harvard Common Press, 1992
Berman, Salee, C.N.M., and Victor Berman, M.D. "Preparation of the
Perineum," *The Birth Center*, New York: Prentice Hall, 1986
Biancuzzo, Marie, R.N. "The Patient Observer: Does the Hands-and-Knees
Posture During Labor Help to Rotate the Occiput Posterior
Fetus?" *Birth* 18(1), March 1991
Bower, B. "Alcohol Abuse Grows among Pregnant Poor," *Science News*,
October 7, 1989
Brewer, Gail Sforza, with Tom Brewer, M.D. *What Every Pregnant Woman
Should Know*, London: Penguin Books, 1985
Butler, Hilary. "Delayed Cord Clamping," *Mothering*, Fall 1986
Carr, Daniel B., M.D., et al. "Physical Conditioning Facilitates the Exercise-
Induced Secretion of Beta-Endorphins and Beta-Lipotropin in
Women," *New England Journal of Medicine* 305(10), September 3,
1981
Cox, Janice. "Effect of Warm Tub Baths during Labor," *International Journal
of Childbirth Education*, November 1988
Enkin, Murray, Marc J.N.C. Keirse, and Iain Chalmers. *Effective Care in
Pregnancy and Childbirth*, Oxford, England: Oxford University
Press, 1989
Ewy, Donna, and Rodger Ewy. *Guide to Family Centered Childbirth*, New
York: E.P. Dutton, 1981
_____ . *Preparation for Childbirth: A Lamaze Guide*, Boulder, CO: Pruett, 1970
Floyd, R. Louise, D.S.N., R.N., et al. "Smoking during Pregnancy: Preva-
lence, Effects, and Intervention Strategies," *Birth* 18(1), March
1991
"FDA Urges Label Forbidding Aspirin Use Late in Pregnancy," *Denver
Post*, November 18, 1988

Gamper, Margaret, R.N. *Preparations for the Heir Minded*, Chicago, self-published, 1971

Gillett, Jane. "Childbirth in Pithiviers, France," *Lancet* 2(8148), October 27, 1979

Gunn, Gordon C., M.D. "Premature Rupture of the Fetal Membranes," *American Journal of Obstetrics and Gynecology* 106(3), 1970

Haire, Doris, D.M.S. Comments at La Leche League International conference, Chicago, July 1981

Hartman, Rhonda Evans, R.N. *Exercises for True Natural Childbirth*, New York: Harper & Row, 1975

Kaigh, Jodi, M.D. "HIV in Pregnancy," ASPO/Lamaze conference, St. Louis, MO: October 1991

Keppel, Kenneth G., and Selma M. Taffel. "Maternal Smoking and Weight Gain in Relation to Birth Weight and the Risk of Fetal and Infant Death," *Smoking and Reproductive Health*, Littleton, MA: PSG Publishing Company, undated reprint from author

Klaus, Marshall, M.D., and Martha Oschrin Robertson, eds. *Birth, Interaction and Attachment*, Johnson and Johnson, 1982

KuroKawa, Jude, R.N., B.S.N., and Mark Zilkoski, M.D. "Adapting Hospital Obstetrics to Birth in the Squatting Position," *Birth* 12(2), Summer 1985

Lappe, Frances Moore. *Diet for a Small Planet*, New York: Ballantine Books, 1975

McCutcheon-Rosegg, Susan, with Peter Rosegg. *Natural Childbirth the Bradley Way*, New York: E.P. Dutton, 1984

Melzak, R., *et al.* "Severity of Labour Pain: Influence of Physical as Well as Psychological Variables," *Canadian Medical Association Journal* 130(5), March 1, 1984, abstracted in *Birth* 11(2), Summer 1984

Newton, Niles, Ph.D. "The Fetus Ejection Reflex Revisited," *Birth* 14(2), June 1987

Noble, Elizabeth, R.P.T. *Essential Exercises for the Childbearing Year*, Boston: Houghton Mifflin, 1982

Odent, Michel, M.D. Personal interview at Pithiviers, August 1983

——— . *Birth Reborn*, New York: Pantheon, 1984

——— . "The Evolution of Obstetrics at Pithiviers," *Birth* 8(1), Spring 1981

——— . "The Fetus Ejection Reflex," *Birth* 14(2), June 1987

——— . "The Milieu and Obstetrical Positions during Labor: A New Approach from France," reprint from Marshall Klaus, M.D., undated

Paciornik, Moyses, M.D. "Commentary: Arguments Against Episiotomy and in Favor of Squatting for Birth," *Birth* 17(2), June 1990

"Perineal Massage," Denver Birth Center reprint, undated

Phibbs, Ciaran S., Ph.D., David A. Bateman, M.D., and Rachel M. Schwartz, M.P.H. "The Neonatal Costs of Maternal Cocaine Use," *Journal of the American Medical Association* 266(11), September 18, 1991

Pietz, Carol. "Weight Gain, Nutrition and High Risk Pregnancy," *International Journal of Childbirth Education*, August 1986

Roberts, Joyce, R.N., C.N.M., Ph.D., *et al.* "The Effects of Maternal Position on Uterine Contractility and Efficiency," *Birth* 10(4), Winter 1983

Roberts, Joyce, and Donna van Lier. "Debate: Which Position for the Second Stage?" *Childbirth Educator*, Spring 1984

Scott, Rebecca Lovell, ed. "Alcohol and Pregnancy," *ICEA Review* 8(2), August 1984, reprint

Shearer, Madeleine H., R.P.T. "Malnutrition in Middle Class Pregnant Women," *Birth* 7(1), Spring 1980

"Smoking and Childbearing," *ICEA Review* 10(2), August 1986, reprint

"Study Shows Smoking Increases Fetal and Maternal Risks," *Genesis*, December/January 1981

Taffel, Selma M., B.B.A. "Association between Maternal Weight Gain and Outcome of Pregnancy," *Journal of Nurse-Midwifery* 31(2), March/April 1986

———, and Kenneth G. Keppel, Ph.D. "Advice about Weight Gain during Pregnancy and Actual Weight Gain," *American Journal of Public Health* 76(12), December 1986

———. "Implications of Mother's Weight Gain on the Outcome of Pregnancy," paper presented at the American Statistical Association Philadelphia meeting, August 1984

"Unclamped Cord Seen as Mother's Helper," *Medical World News*, March 14, 1969

Vincent, Peggy, R.N. Review of *Spiritual Midwifery*, in *Birth* 4(2), Summer 1977

White, Gregory, M.D. *Emergency Childbirth*, Franklin Park, IL: Police Training Foundation, 1958

13 The Nurse

Collins, B.A. "The Role of the Nurse in Labor and Delivery as Perceived by Nurses and Patients," *Journal of Obstetrical, Gynecological, and Neonatal Nursing* 15:5, September/October 1986

Fowler, Elizabeth M. "A Program to Recruit More Nurses," *The New York Times*, April 11, 1989

———. "Opportunities Still Abound in Nursing," *The New York Times*, October 8, 1991

Friedman, Emily. "Nursing: New Power, Old Problems," *Journal of the American Medical Association* 264:23, December 19, 1990

———. "Troubled Past of 'Invisible' Profession," *Journal of the American Medical Association* 264:22, December 12, 1990

Gartner, Lawrence M., M.D. "Facts and Fantasies About Neonatal Jaundice," address, 10th Annual Seminar for Physicians on Breastfeeding, La Leche League International, Las Vegas, July 15 and 16, 1982

Hillard, Paula J. Adams, M.D. "When an Obstetrician Has a Baby," *The Female Patient* 6:8, August 1981

"Hospitals Struck in Los Angeles," *The New York Times,* October 20, 1991

Klass, Kay, B.S.N., and Kay Capps, R.N. "Nine Years' Experience With Family-Centered Maternity Care in a Community Hospital," *Birth* 7:3, Fall 1980

Meara, Hanna, Ph.D. "A Key to Successful Breastfeeding in a Non-Supportive Culture," *Journal of Nurse Midwifery,* XXI:1 Spring 1976

Moss, P., *et al.* "The Hospital Inpatient Stay: The Experience of First-Time Parents," *Child Care and Health Development* 13:3, May/June 1987

Myers, Sheila Taylor. "Nurses' Responses to Changes in Maternity Care, Part II: Technologic Revolution, Legal Climate, and Economic Changes," *Birth* 14:2, June 1987

Stolte, Karen. "Nurses' Responses to Changes in Maternity Care, Part I. Family-Centered Changes and Short Hospitalization," *Birth* 14:2, June 1987

14   Your Baby Doctor

Auerbach, K., and L. M. Gartner. "Breastfeeding and Human Milk: Their Association with Jaundice in the Neonate," *Clinics in Perinatology* 14, 1987

Bedell, Richard, M.D. Interview, October 1982

Bell, Edward F., M.D., *et al.* "Combined Effect of Radiant Warmer and Phototherapy on Insensible Water Loss in Low-Birth-Weight Infants," *Journal of Pediatrics* 94:5, May 1979

Bell, Thomas A., M.D., *et al.* "Comparison of Ophthalmic Silver Nitrate Solution and Erythromycin Ointment for Prevention of Natally Acquired Chlamydia Trachomatis," *Sexually Transmitted Diseases* 14:4, October/December 1987

Bell, Thomas A., M.D., *et al.* "Chronic *Chlamydia trachomatis* Infections in Infants," 267:3, January 15, 1992

Bergevin, Y., M. Kramer, and C. Dougherty. "Do Infant Formula Samples Affect the Duration of Breastfeeding?" abstract presented at Annual Meeting of Ambulatory Pediatric Association, May 1981

Boylan, P., M.B. "Oxytocin and Neonatal Jaundice," *British Medical Journal,* September 4, 1976

Brown, Stephen W., Ph.D. "Survey Results: How Physicians See Themselves—and Their Image," *Medical Marketing Media* 17:2, February 1982

Buchan, Peter C. "Pathogenesis of Neonatal Hyperbilirubinaemia after Induction of Labour with Oxytocin," *British Medical Journal*

2(6200), November 17, 1979

Butterfield, Perry M., et al. "Effects of Silver Nitrate on Initial Visual Behavior," American Journal of Diseases of Children 132:426, April 1978

———. Phone interview, October 1983

Campbell, Neil, M.B., et al. "Increased Frequency of Neonatal Jaundice in a Maternity Hospital," British Medical Journal, June 7, 1975

"Canadian LLL," News, La Leche League, January–February 1981

Carmody, F., et al. "Follow Up of Babies Delivered in a Randomized Controlled Comparison of Vacuum Extraction and Forceps Delivery," Acta Obstetricia et Gynecologica Scandanavica 65:7, 1986

———. "Vacuum Extraction: A Randomized Controlled Comparison of the New Generation Cup with the Original Bird Cup," Journal of Perinatal Medicine 14:2, 1986

Carvalho, M.D., et al. "Effects of Water Supplementation on Physiological Jaundice in Breastfed Infants." Archives of Diseases in Childhood 56, 1981

———, et al. "Frequency of Breastfeeding and Serum Bilirubin Concentration," American Journal of Diseases of Children 136, 1982

Chew, W.C., and I.L. Swann. "Influence of Simultaneous Low Amniotomy and Oxytocin Infusion and Other Maternal Factors on Neonatal Jaundice: A Prospective Study," British Medical Journal, January 8, 1977

Committee on Drugs, Committee on Fetus and Newborn, Committee on Infectious Diseases. "Prophylaxis and Treatment of Neonatal Gonococcal Infections," Pediatrics 65:5, May 1980

Committee on Nutrition. "Encouraging Breastfeeding," Pediatrics 65:3, March 1980

Costich, Timothy, M.D. Correspondence, 1981

Dharamraj, Claude, M.D., et al. "Observations on Maternal Preference for Rooming-in Facilities," Pediatrics 67:5, May 1981

Drew, J.H., et al. "Short and Long-Term Complications," Archives of Disease in Childhood 51:454, 1976

D'Souza, S.W., et al. "Oxytocin Induction of Labour: Hyponatraemia and Neonatal Jaundice," European Journal of Obstetrics, Gynecology, and Reproductive Biology 22:5, September 1986

Ellis, Judith. "Home Phototherapy for Newborn Jaundice," Birth 12:3, Fall 1985

Gartner, Lawrence, and Kathleen G. Auerbach. "Jaundice and Breastfeeding," Mothering, Fall 1986

Gordon, Jay, M.D. Phone interview, 1983

Hammerschlag, Margaret R. "Efficacy of Neonatal Ocular Prophylaxis for the Prevention of Chlamydial and Gonococcal Conjunctivitis," New England Journal of Medicine 320:12, March 23, 1989

James, Frank E. "Pediatric Centers Spring Up to Provide Off-Hour Care," The Wall Street Journal, February 13, 1989

Jouppila, R., et al. "Effect of Segmental Epidural Analgesia on Neonatal

Serum Bilirubin Concentration and Incidence of Neonatal Hyper-bilirubinemia," *Acta Obstetricia et Gynecologica Scandinavica* 62:2, 1983

Khoury, Muin J., *et al.* "Recurrence Risk of Neonatal Hyperbilirubinemia in Siblings," *American Journal of Diseases of Children* 142, 1988

Laga, M., *et al.* "Prophylaxis of Gonococcal and Chlamydial Ophthalmia Neonatorum. A Comparison of Silver Nitrate and Tetracycline," *New England Journal of Medicine* 318:11, March 17, 1988

Lemons, James A. "What's New in the Newborn ICU?" *Perinatal Day* (Denver, CO), October 1984

Lewis, David D. "Circumcision and Urinary Tract Infection," *Journal of the American Medical Association* 268:1, July 1, 1992

Little, George A., *et al.* "Home Phototherapy," *Pediatrics* 76:1, July 1985

Meyer, L., *et al.* "Maternal and Neonatal Morbidity in Instrumental Deliveries with the Kobayashi Vacuum Extractor and Low Forceps," *Acta Obstetricia et Gynecologica Scandinavica* 66:7, 1987

Newman, Thomas B., M.D., *et al.* "Direct Bilirubin Measurements in Jaundiced Newborns," *American Journal of Diseases of Children* 145, November 1991

Paludetto, R., *et al.* "Moderate Hyperbilirubinemia Does Not Influence the Behavior of Jaundiced Infants," *Biology of the Neonate* 50:1, 1986

Phelps, Dale L., M.D. "Retinopathy of Prematurity," *New England Journal of Medicine* 326:16, April 16, 1992

Pryor, Karen, and Gale Pryor. *Nursing Your Baby*, New York: Pocket Books, 1991

Ramer, Cyril, M.D. Phone interview, October 1982

Rodriguez, E.M., and M.R. Hammerschlag. "Diagnostic Methods for Chlamydia Trachomatis Disease in Neonates," *Journal of Perinatology* 7:3, Summer 1987

Rogers, Mark C., M.D. "Do the Right Thing: Pain Relief in Infants and Children," *New England Journal of Medicine* 326:1, January 2, 1992

Rosta, J., *et al.* "Delayed Meconium Passage and Hyperbilirubinemia," *Lancet* 2:1138, November 23, 1968

Rubin, Rosalyn A., *et al.* "Neonatal Serum Bilirubin Levels Related to Cognitive Development at Ages Four Through Seven Years," *Pediatrics* 94:4, April 1979

Scheidt, P.C., *et al.* "Toxicity to Bilirubin in Neonates: Infant Development during First Year in Relation to Maximum Neonatal Serum Bilirubin Concentration," *Journal of Pediatrics* 91:2, August 1977

————, *et al.* "Intelligence at Six Years in Relation to Neonatal Bilirubin Level: Follow-Up of the National Institute of Child Health and Human Development Clinical Trial of Phototherapy," *Pediatrics* 87:6, June 1991

Schoen, Edgar J., M.D. "The Relationship between Circumcision and Cancer of the Penis," *CA-A Cancer Journal for Clinicians* 41:5, September/October 1991

Silverman, William A., M.D. *Retrolental Fibroplasia: A Modern Parable*, New York: Grune and Stratton, 1980

Simkin, Penny, *et al.* "Neonatal Jaundice," *Birth* 6(1), Spring 1979

Spach, David H., M.D., *et al.* "Lack of Circumcision Increases the Risk of Urinary Tract Infection in Young Men," *Journal of the American Medical Association* 267:5, February 5, 1992

Speck, W.T., C.C. Chen, and H.S. Rosenkranz. "In Vitro Studies of Effects of Light and Riboflavin on DNA and HeLa Cells," *Pediatric Research* 9:150, 1975

Stewart, David, Ph.D., ed. *The Five Standards for Safe Childbearing*, Marble Hill, MO: NAPSAC Reproductions, 1981

Taylor, Charles, M.D. Interview, January 1980

Thomas, Howard P. "Considering Newborn Circumcision," *Intensive Caring Unlimited*, July/August 1988

Van Enk, A., and R. de Leeuw. "Phototherapy: The Hospital as Risk Factor," *British Medical Journal* 294:6574, March 21, 1987

Vecchi, C., *et al.* "Green Light in Phototherapy," *Pediatric Research* 17:6, June 1983

_____ , *et al.* "Phototherapy for Neonatal Jaundice: Clinical Equivalence of Fluorescent Green and 'Special' Blue Lamps," *Journal of Pediatrics* 108:3, March 1986

Winfield, C.R., and R. MacFaul. "Clinical Study of Prolonged Jaundice in Breast- and Bottle-fed Babies," *Archives of Disease in Childhood* 53, 1978

Index

Feldman, Silvia, 53–54, 133
Fetal alcohol syndrome, 209
"Fetal distress," 37, 38, 113, 149–50, 178
Fetal monitoring. *See* Electronic fetal monitoring (EFM)
Fetal movement counting (FMC) test, 158
Fetal scalp sampling, 111–12
Fetoscope, 1, 46, 76, 84, 112, 205
First baby (primipara), 44, 140–41, 182
  cesareans for, 140, 143
  labor for, 141, 147, 218
Flamm, Bruce, 95
Florida, cesarean rates in, 136, 137
Food and Drug Administration (FDA), 83, 116, 123, 124
Forceps (instrument delivery), 20, 42, 129, 146
Formula (synthetic milk), 14, 15, 241–42, 244–45
Franklin, John, 91
Friedman, Emanuel, 112, 134, 144
"Friedman curves," 144–45
Friends, presence of, 36, 189, 202. *See also* Doulas; Women
Frye, Anne, 159

Gartner, Lawrence, 233–34, 259, 260, 262–63
Gaskin, Ina May, 51–52, 159, 183
Genital herpes, active, 153, 155–56, 254
Gleicher, Norbert, 140
Goer, Henci, 103, 138–39
Goodlin, Robert C., 37–38, 39
Gordon, Jay, 264
Great Britain, 149, 163
  mortality rates in, 50, 163
Guatemala, doulas in, 20
Gunn, Gordon C., 215

Haire, Doris, 58, 89, 114, 116, 120, 124, 126, 130, 216
Halperin, Mary, 157
Hathaway, Marjie and Jay, 17, 45
Health insurance. *See* Insurance
Health maintenance organizations (HMOs), 47, 65, 135

Heart rate, fetal, 110–13, 149, 150
Heel sticks, 259
Hemorrhage
  maternal, 37, 43, 116, 128, 142
  newborn, 129
Herpes. *See* Genital herpes
High blood pressure
  as "high-risk" factor, 82, 89, 114
  in labor, 37
  in newborn, 12
"High-risk" women, 62, 82, 88–91, 112, 141
High-tech trends in childbirth, 1–2, 61, 65–66, 130. *See also* Electronic fetal monitoring; Interventions; Testing, prenatal; Ultrasound
Hillard, Paula J. Adams, 234
Hispanic-Americans, mortality rates and, 100
HIV-positive pregnant women, 209–10
Hodnett, Ellen, 19
Home, remaining at, in early labor, 44, 146, 147, 215–17
Home birth, 1, 11, 33, 37, 48–52, 183, 299–300
  costs of, 34, 48
  doctor's opposition to, 45, 68
  and mortality rates, 57
  safety considerations, 37, 49
  satisfaction with, 35
Hon, Edward H., 144, 150
Hormones, and postpartum emotions, 183
Hospital(s), 1, 3–4, 34, 76–77, 186, 193, 253
  birth centers in, 94–95
  cesarean rates of, 136–39
  choosing a, 36, 74, 76 77
  costs of delivery in, 34, 39–40, 77
  negotiating with, 175 76, 197, 253
  safety considerations, 37–39, 49, 95 96, 197
  single-room maternity care in, 34, 39–43
  staff of, 8, 18–19
  traditonal maternity care in, 34, 36–39
Humenick, Sharron, 23–24